GASTRIC CARCINOMA-
NEW INSIGHTS INTO
CURRENT MANAGEMENT

Edited by **Daniela Lazăr**

Gastric Carcinoma- New Insights into Current Management
http://dx.doi.org/10.5772/45896
Edited by Daniela Lazăr

Contributors

Ekambaram Ganapathy, Devaraja Rajasekaran, Asokan Devarajan, Muhammad Farooq Shukkur, Muhammed Farooq Abdul Shukkur, Sakthisekaran Dhanapal, Murugan Sivalingam, Eriko Maeda, Kuo-Wang Tsai, Chung-Man Leung, Hung-Wei Pan, Takehiro Okabayashi, Yasuo Shima, Okan Akturk, Jolanta Czyzewska, Daniela Lazar, Elvira Garza Gonzalez, Guillermo Perez Perez, Shinya Shimada, Masafumi Kuramoto, Jae Y. Ro, Sun - Mi Lee, Kyoung-Mee Kim

Published by InTech

Janeza Trdine 9, 51000 Rijeka, Croatia

Publishing Process Manager Danijela Duric

Technical Editor InTech DTP team

Cover InTech Design team

Additional hard copies can be obtained from orders@intechopen.com

Gastric Carcinoma- New Insights into Current Management, Edited by Daniela Lazăr

p. cm.

ISBN 978-953-51-0914-3

For EU product safety concerns:
IN TECH d.o.o., Prolaz Marije Krucifikse Kozulić 3, 51000 Rijeka, Croatia,
info@intechopen.com or visit our website at intechopen.com.

Meet the editor

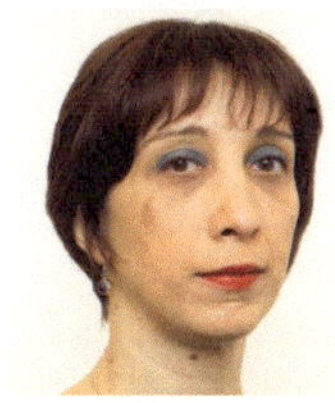

Dr. Daniela Lazar began her career in a center of excellence in Romania. It is the Department of Gastroenterology and Hepatology, University of Medicine and Pharmacy Timisoara, where she has acquired clinical skills in gastroenterology, learned the techniques of endoscopy and abdominal ultrasonography and began her research activity. She is specialized in Gastroenterology and Medical Oncology and underwent her PhD thesis in the field of gastric cancer. The research interests of Dr. Daniela Lazar are concerned mainly with the neoplasms of the gastrointestinal tract, especially gastric cancer. Dr. Lazar has participated at many national and international congresses with research studies in the field of gastroenterology and digestive oncology. She published many studies regarding angiogenesis, premalignant lesions and prognostic factors in gastric cancer. She is interested also in aspects regarding the epidemiology, phenotypes and treatment of inflammatory bowel diseases, being part of the national and international working groups in this domain. Dr. Lazar is a reviewer in many international journals.

Contents

Preface

Although gastric cancer was in the past the second most common cancer in the world, its incidence has dropped to fourth place, after cancers of the lung, breast, and colon and rectum. In most developed countries, rates of stomach cancer have shown a dramatically decline over the past half century. Nevertheless, gastric cancer is still the second most common cause of cancer-related death in the world, causing about 800,000 deaths worldwide per year.

Gastric neoplasm is often either asymptomatic or it may cause only nonspecific symptoms in its early stages; by the time symptoms occur, the tumor has often reached a locally advanced stage or may have also metastasized, which is one of the main reasons for the delayed diagnosis and relatively poor prognosis of this cancer.

Gastric cancer may often be multifactorial, involving both genetic predisposition (e.g hereditary non-polyposis colorectal cancer, familial adenomatous polyposis, hereditary diffuse gastric cancer and Peutz–Jeghers syndrome) and environmental factors, such as Helicobacter pylori infection.

Multidisciplinary treatment approach is compulsory for stomach cancer, including surgeons, gastroenterologists, medical and radiation oncologists, radiologists and pathologists. Surgical resection represents the only modality that is potentially curative. In the last years, in the case of early gastric cancer, endoscopic resection may replace the surgical procedure.

Literature data have shown that the 5-year survival rate for curative surgical resection ranges from 30-50% for patients with stage II disease and from 10-25% for patients with stage III disease. Because these patients have a high likelihood of local and systemic relapse, the treatment is completed by adjuvant chemotherapy.

Many trials have demonstrated a survival benefit for adjuvant chemotherapy or chemoradiotherapy in patients with stage II/III gastric cancer. Patients with inoperable, locally advanced gastric cancer should be treated with palliative chemotherapy; afterwards, they may be reassessed for surgery if a good response is achieved. Patients with metastatic disease should be considered for palliative chemotherapy, which improves survival. Recent data have shown the benefit of adding targeted therapy to the chemotherapy schemes on the survival of selected gastric cancer patients (e.g the addition of trastuzumab to chemotherapy in patients with HER2-positive gastric cancer).

This book contains a comprehensive overview of most recent data concerning a multitude of facets of the gastric cancer. The book highlights various aspects of gastric neoplasm, from the epidemiology, preneoplastic lesions, the complex process of carcinogenesis, the risk and protective factors, morphological and molecular changes, up to the modern diagnostic tools and current management of early and advanced gastric cancer, revealing the valuable contribution of the multidisciplinary treatment approach.

This publication is appropriate for students, clinicians and researchers in the field of gastroenterology, oncology, pathology, immunology, genetics, molecular biology, radiology, and many other specialties. They will find interesting data and hot topics in this book, from fundamental research knowledge to clinical issues that may be helpful in daily practice.

This book, written in an easy-to-read style, makes an insight into the diagnosis and assessment of premalignant gastric lesions and into the current management of gastric cancer in its early stages. The authors focus on novel risk factors in gastric carcinogenesis, such as fetal-type glycogen phosphorylase expression in intestinal metaplasia and also new discovered protective factors such as naringenin that inhibits oxidative stress induced macromolecular damage in a model of gastric carcinogenesis in rats. Also, one of the topics refers to the importance of the host factors in gastric neoplasm associated with H. pylori infection. Furthermore, this publication is presenting the role of endoscopic and histological assessment in order to obtain a proper diagnostic of the premalignant gastric lesions.

"Gastric cancer-new insights into current management" provides a detailed description of the morphologic classification and of the molecular changes encountered in the case of this tumor. Moreover, it depicts some rare histological types of gastric cancers that may help young scientists recognize them. An important topic refers to the epigenetic gene regulation mechanisms and the biological behavior of the tumors, focusing on DNA methylation aspects in aggressive gastric neoplasm. The identification of the molecular mechanisms of gastric carcinogenesis and its progression using recent advances in genomic science allows finding markers for early detection of stomach cancer, and can provide better information on tumor aggressiveness, prognosis and prediction of response to cancer therapy.

The publication reveals some distinct and particular imaging findings that may accompany different histological types of gastric tumors and also, the most important factors contributing to the prognosis of gastric cancer.

There are no screening tests available for diagnosis of gastric cancer, therefore patients usually presents in late stages. The preoperative evaluation stratifies patients in those with loco-regional, potentially resectable disease, and those with systemic involvement. The book describes the role of different diagnostic tools in the preoperative assessment of patients with gastric carcinoma. Currently, early gastric cancer is treated with endoscopic resection, gastrectomy, antibiotic therapy for H.pylori infection and adjuvant treatment. Surgical resection remains the curative treatment for local and locoregional cancer. The authors highlights the fact that adjuvant chemoradiotherapy is an essential part of the treatment schedule as 80% of the cases develop local recurrence.

"Gastric cancer-new insights into current management" represents an important tool for clinicians in the process of continuing medical education by updating with novel information offered by a valuable team of well-known scientist who belong to different specialties. Moreover, it may open new and interesting gates for further research concerning carcinogenesis, genetic and epigenetic alterations, signaling pathways, H. pylori infection, the discovery of protective factors against gastric cancer and of revolutionary therapies of this tumor.

I wish to express my gratitude to all the scientists-authors and co-authors- who have contributed to the elaboration of this comprehensive book, and also to the publisher with his entire team, especially to Ms. Danijela Duric, for the support.

Finally, I wish to dedicate this book to my beloved parents who are my models in life and profession.

Daniela Lazar
Assistant Professor of Gastroenterology,
Gastroenterology and Hepatology Department
University of Medicine and Pharmacy "Victor Babes"
Timisoara, Romania

Section 1

Preneoplastic Lesions and Early Gastric Cancer

The Role of Endoscopy and Biopsy in Evaluating Preneoplastic and Particular Gastric Lesions

Daniela Lazăr, Sorina Tăban and Sorin Ursoniu

Additional information is available at the end of the chapter

http://dx.doi.org/10.5772/52676

1. Introduction

Although incidence has declined in recent years, gastric cancer still represents the second most frequent cause of cancer-related mortality in the world [1]. The prognosis of stomach cancer is related to the stage of disease at the time of diagnosis, with a good prognosis associated with early gastric cancer [2]. Therefore, it is essential an early diagnosis of gastric carcinoma, at present only about 10-20% of cancers being diagnosed in an early phase [3]. A great interest has arisen in recent years in the detection and management of premalignant conditions and early gastric cancer because of the high cure rate achieved treating these lesions, compared with advanced gastric cancer. The well known multistep cascade of carcinogenesis developed by Correa [4] is represented by superficial gastritis followed by atrophic gastritis, intestinal metaplasia and increasing grades of dysplasia, leading to gastric adenocarcinoma. Surveillance of the premalignant lesions could determine an early detection of patients with disease progression, with the possibility of early therapeutic intervention and improved survival of these patients [5].

Diagnosis and localization of premalignant lesions and early gastric cancer is difficult because of the possible lack of evident gross endoscopic signs, even with the performance of multiple random biopsies [6]. Another problem with conventional white light endoscopic diagnosis of these lesions consists in finding the exact location of previously sampled sites for endoscopic or surgical treatment [7]. Recently developed new endoscopic techniques have surpassed some of these drawbacks and have an improved accuracy of diagnosing early cancers and precancerous lesions.

2. Material and methods

In order to evaluate the role of endoscopy and biopsy in assessing preneoplastic gastric lesions, we prospectively included in our study 96 consecutive patients with dyspeptic symptoms, admitted at the Department of Gastroenterology of the County Emergency Hospital Timisoara, Romania, between April 2010 and March 2011. The patients with various conditions which prevented satisfactory endoscopic examination were excluded from the study. Previously, the patients were informed and given their written consent regarding the protocol and the maneuvers of intervention included in the study.

All the endoscopic investigations were performed by senior endoscopists, with a conventional endoscope of the type Olympus Exera 140 (Japan). According to the criteria of the Sydney system of endoscopic evaluation of the gastritis [8,9,10], we designed a protocol (completed for each case) including: location of lesions, endoscopic aspect at the antral and body level (normal, focal or diffuse erythematous gastritis, erosive gastritis, erosive-hemorrhagic gastritis, atrophic gastritis, petechial gastritis), maintaining of certain particular elements (hypertrophy of the folds, nodularity, etc.), the severity of gastritis on endoscopy (mild, moderate, and severe).

For each case 5 biopsies were taken and processed: two biopsies from the antral level (A1 = the small curvature; A2 = the large curvature), two biopsies from the gastric body (C1 = the small curvature; C2 = the large curvature) and a biopsy from the gastric angle (U). Moreover, all macroscopically visible lesions have been biopsied with specification of their location and clinical diagnosis.

Tissue fragments were processed in the same manner, with fixation in 4% formaldehyde, paraffin inclusion and stained with hematoxylin-eosin. For histological identification of H. pylori we utilized the Giemsa modified stain. Histochemical reactions AA-PAS pH 2.5 and HID-AA allowed to appreciate the profile of mucins on sections examined. Morphological investigation was performed by a pathologist with experience in digestive pathology.

Statistical analysis of data was performed in a computerized manner, on the folder created, with specialized programs: Epi Info 6.04, SPSS 10 and Open Epi. This analysis consisted of:

- calculating the arithmetic means and standard deviations, for the quantitative variables;
- calculating the frequencies and percentages for the qualitative variables;
- statistical comparison of percentages with the χ^2 (square Chi) test;
- statistical estimation of results was performed using the criteria of decision of statistical tests:
- $p<0.05$- significant differences
- $p<0.01$- very significant differences
- $p<0.001$- extremely significant differences.

3. Results

A total of 96 patients (58 females and 38 males) aged between 24 and 86 years (mean age 60.1±15.1 years) were included in the study. Age groups and gender distribution are shown in Table 1 and Graphic 1.

Age groups	Males (no. of cases; %)	Females (no. of cases; %)
21-30 years	0 (0%)	6 (10.35%)
31-40 years	4 (10.53%)	0 (0%)
41-50 years	6 (15.79%)	12 (20.69%)
51-60 years	6 (15.79%)	8 (13.79%)
61-70 years	8 (21.05%)	20 (34.48%)
≥ 71 years	14 (36.84%)	12 (20.69%)
Total patients	38 (100%)	58 (100%)

Table 1. Age groups and gender distribution of cases

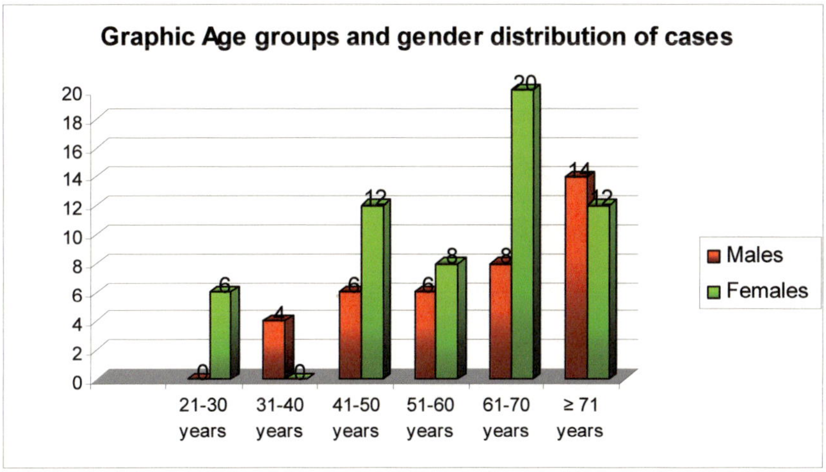

Graphic 1. Distribution of cases according to age groups and gender

Gastric biopsies (480 samples) were taken and processed from these patients (two antral biopsies, two biopsies from the body, and one biopsy from the gastric angle for each case).

Atrophic gastritis, defined endoscopically by the appearance of submucosal vessels, giving rise to a mucosal vascular pattern similar to that found in the colon, sometimes associated with other features, e.g, mucosal discoloration, smoothness, or flattened rugal folds, constituted a rarely encountered entity in our study. In the cases studied we did not observe any case of antral atrophic gastritis. In the gastric body, atrophic gastritis, was noted in 6 elderly patients (Tab 2).

Endoscopic aspect	Antrum No. of cases (%)	Body No. of cases (%)
Focal erythematous gastritis	12 (12.5 %)	0 (0%)
Diffuse erythematous gastritis	54 (56.1 %)	22 (23%)
Erosive gastritis	4 (4.2 %)	0 (0%)
Erosive-hemorrhagic gastritis	2 (2.1 %)	0 (0%)
Petechial gastritis	22 (23 %)	10 (10.4%)
Atrophic gastritis	0 (0 %)	6 (6.3%)
Normal aspect	2 (2.1 %)	58 (60.3%)

Table 2. Frequency of gastritis diagnosed endoscopically

For this lesion we noted a poor correlation between the conventional endoscopic investigation and histopathological examination (Tab. 3).

In accordance with the Sydney system, the morphological criteria of quantification applied to cases with gastric atrophy are the following:

- 0 = absent;
- 1 = mild (disappearance of less than 25% of glands);
- 2 = moderate (disappearance of 25 - 50% of glands);
- 3 = severe (disappearance of over 50% of glands);
- 4 = biopsy inappropriate for histopathological interpretation.

Age groups	Antral atrophy score (no. of cases; %)				Gastric body atrophy score (no. of cases; %)			
	0	1	2	3	0	1	2	3
21-30 years	6	-	-	-	6	-	-	-
31-40 years	2	-	2	-	2	-	2	-
41-50 years	10	2	6	-	8	4	6	-
51-60 years	8	-	6	-	8	2	4	-
61-70 years	20	4	4	-	18	2	8	-
≥ 71 years	4	4	16	2	2	6	14	4
Total patients	50 (52.1%)	10 (10.4%)	34 (35.4%)	2 (2.1%)	44 (45.8%)	14 (14.6%)	34 (35.4%)	4 (4.2%)

Table 3. Distribution of the histological score of atrophy identified histopathologically

http://dx.doi.org/10.5772/52676

Atrophic chronic gastritis is characterized histopathologically by the numeric decrease in glandular structures of the gastric mucosa and development of new metaplastic glands lined by intestinal and/or pseudo-pyloric epithelium. We did not consider as real atrophy certain modifications of the gastric mucosa that produce a false reduction in gastric glands, such as the massive inflammatory infiltrate or the edema of the lamina propria.

From the total number of cases included in the study, we observed lesions of atrophic type in 46 antral biopsies (48%) and 52 gastric body biopsies (54.2%).

For antral location (Graphic 2) 10 cases with mild atrophy were noted (21.7%), 34 cases with moderate atrophy (74%) and 2 cases with severe atrophy (4.3% - Fig. 2). Glandular atrophy of gastric mucosa was observed much more frequently in patients with older ages (over 61 years). Biopsies noted with score 3 for atrophy pertain only to patients with ages ≥ 71 years.

Glandular atrophy was more frequently encountered in gastric body biopsies (but without significant differences compared with the antrum, p=0.386), being predominant in patients with average or old ages. Especially moderate and mild forms of atrophy were noted (14 cases with mild atrophy – 27%; 34 cases with moderate atrophy – 65.4% - Fig. 3; 4 cases with severe atrophy – 7.6%). All patients with severe glandular atrophy pertain to the age group ≥ 71 years.

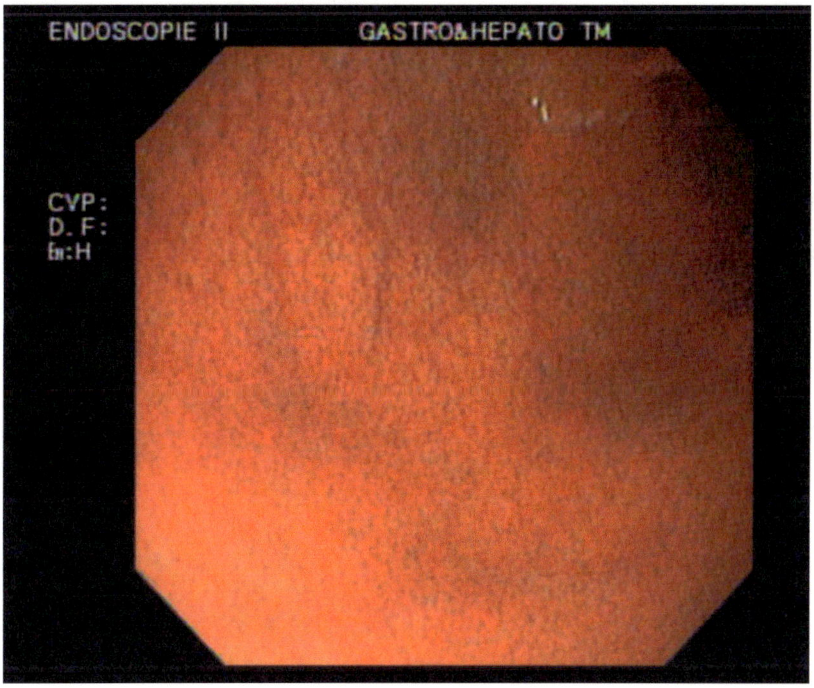

Figure 1. Congestive gastritis of gastric body, with mild atrophy of the mucosa

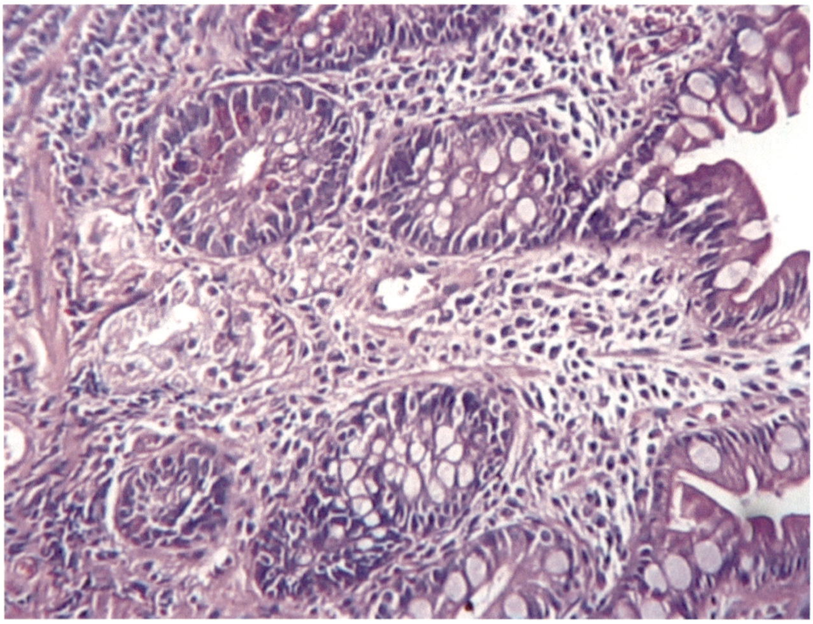

Figure 2. Antral chronic gastritis with severe atrophy and intestinal metaplasia. HE x 200.

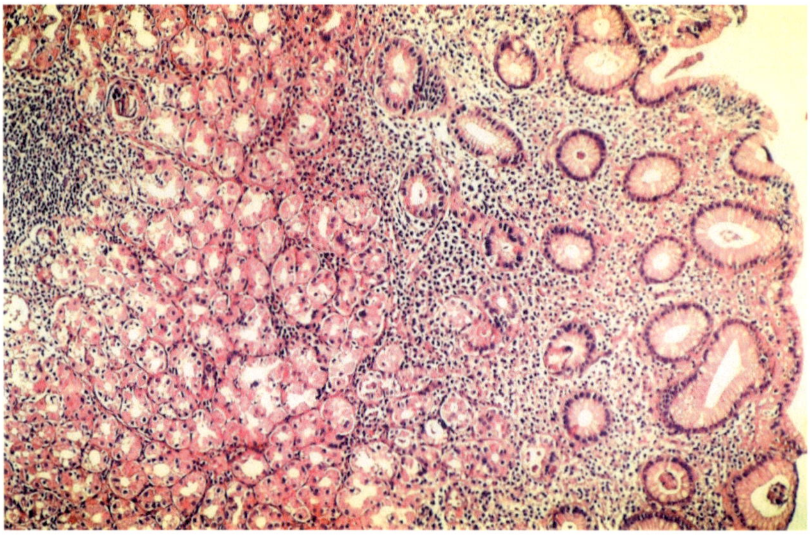

Figure 3. Chronic gastritis of the gastric body with moderate atrophy. HE x 100.

http://dx.doi.org/10.5772/52676

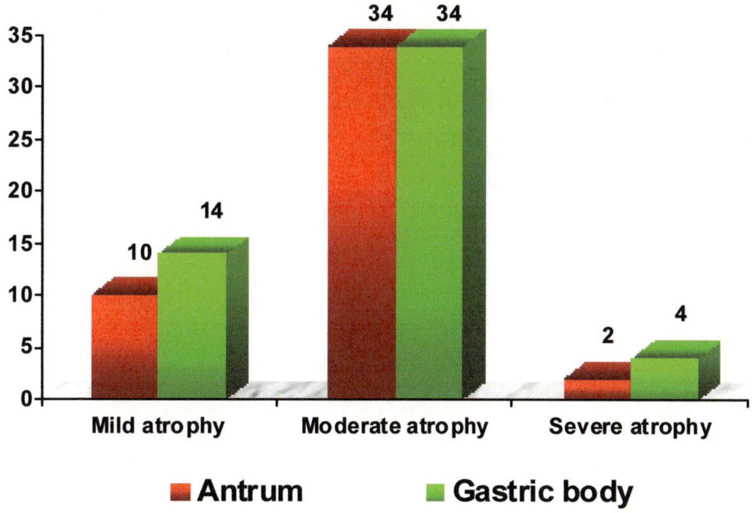

Graphic 2. Histological evaluation of gastric atrophy

Intestinal metaplasia (IM) represents the replacement of the surface and glandular gastric epithelium by one composed of cells of the intestinal type (small or large intestine).

In conventional endoscopy, modifications such as nodules of yellow and white-nacreous color, aspect like fish scales or diffuse granular are suggestive for intestinal metaplasia of gastric mucosa. Such lesions were evident in 7 patients (4 males and 3 females) with ages between 54 and 76 years, with location in the gastric body.

In histopathological examination, preparations stained through usual morphological methods do not allow for the certainty diagnosis, nor do they allow for classification of intestinal metaplasia. For these reasons we used histochemical stain methods which give exact information on the composition of the mucus synthesized by the modified glands, respectively the neutral mucins, sialo- and sulfomucins.

Among histochemical methods recommended by the specialty literature, we used staining methods PAS-AA at pH 2.5 and reaction with colloidal iron diamine-AA (HID-AA).

Type I intestinal metaplasia (complete) is characterized by relatively normal glandular architecture, with straight crypts and glands lined by absorbing cells which do not secrete mucus and goblet cells with flattened nuclei and with widened apical pole, these two cellular types being encountered in approximately equal proportions. Occasionally, at the base of the glands one can observe Paneth cells. We identified this form of intestinal metaplasia with the PAS-AA stain, due to the presence of blue sialomucins in goblet cells (Fig. 4). Reaction with paraphenyldiamine is negative.

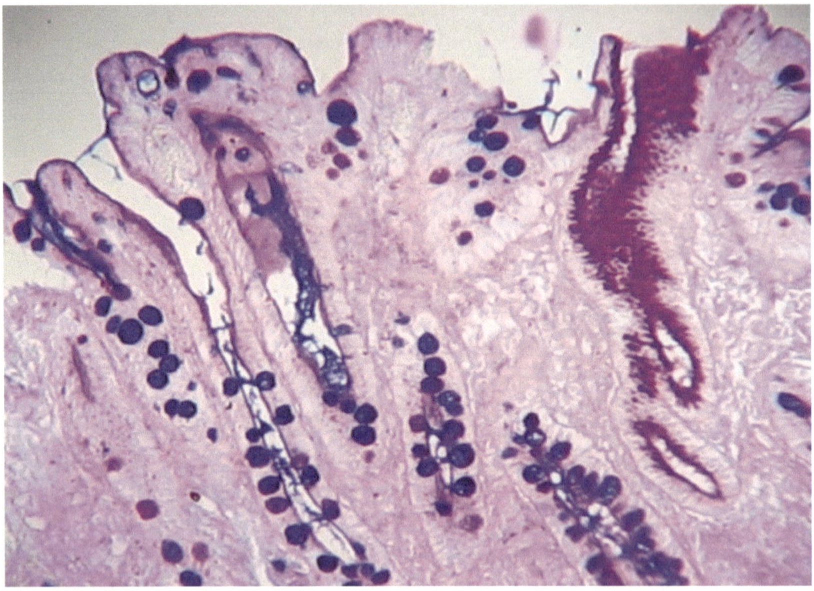

Figure 4. Type I intestinal metaplasia. AA-PAS x 200.

Type II intestinal metaplasia presents slight architectural modifications, with elongated and tortuous crypts, with focal areas of foveolar hyperplasia and columnar cells in variable number, which contain a mixture of neutral mucines and sialomucins, but not sulfomucins. The proportion of the goblet cells is greater than in type I. PAS-AA positive reaction is translated by mixed areas, PAS-positive and alcyanophil, representing neutral and acid mucines. The positive material is located in the apical portion of epithelial cells, in the lumen of some glands and in goblet cells (Fig. 5).

Type III of intestinal metaplasia is characterized morphologically by important glandular distortions, with ramified glands, lined with columnar cells which secrete sulfomucins and goblet cells secreting sialomucins. PAS reaction is negative, but the HID-AA reaction appears intensely positive, through both dyeing solutions. The positive substrate appears in goblet cells (blue), in the apical portion of columnar cells and in the lumen of metaplastic glands (dark brown) (Fig. 6 and Fig. 7).

The prevalence of intestinal metaplasia identified histopathologically at the antral level was of 20.8% (20 cases), and at the level of the gastric body of 25% (24 cases – Tab. 3) (p=0.492). At the antral level we noted 18 cases with focal distribution (score given 1 and 2) and only two cases with diffuse distribution (score 3) interesting almost entirely the gastric glandular epithelium. Following the extension of intestinal metaplasia according to patients' age, we observed the great frequency of types II and III in patients over 61 years old. For gastric body biopsies we did not encountered intestinal metaplasias with score 3, but 18 cases of metaplasias with score 1 and 6 cases with score 2 were identified. These metaplastic transformations occur more frequently in older patients, but also in patients from the age groups 31-40 years and 41-50 years (Tab 4).

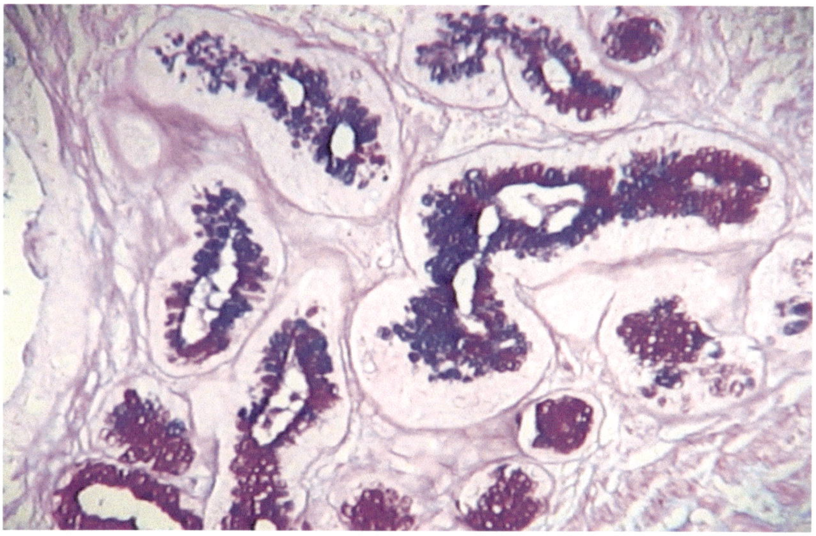

Figure 5. Type II intestinal metaplasia. AA-PAS x 200.

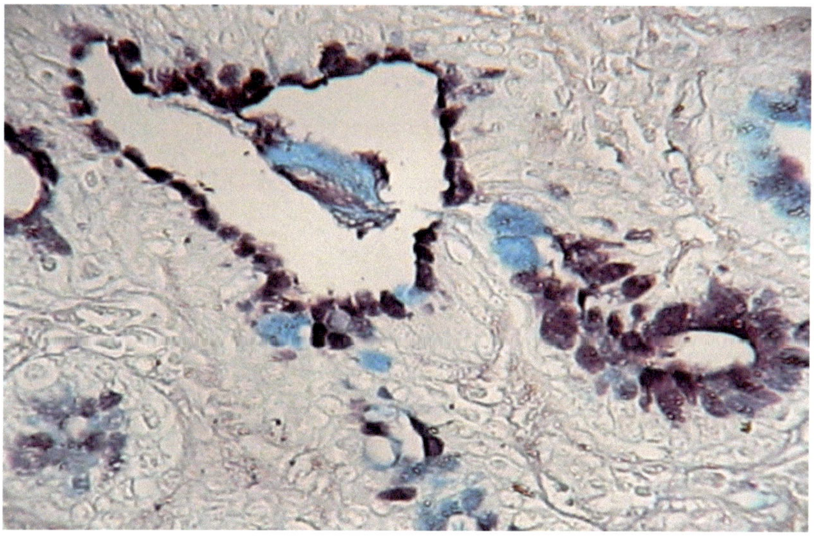

Figure 6. Type III intestinal metaplasia. HID-AA x 400.

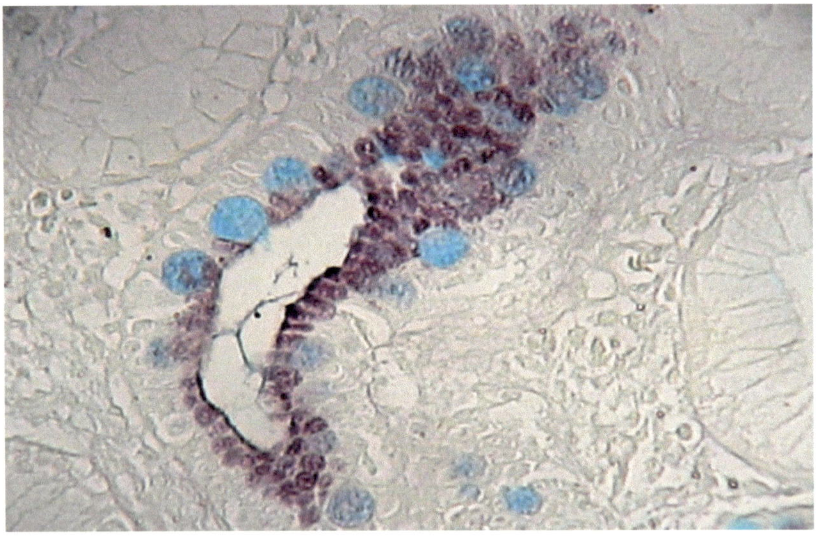

Figure 7. Secretion of sulfomucins (brown) and sialomucins (blue) from intestinal metaplasia type III. HID-AA x 400.

In accordance with the Sydney system, the morphological criteria of quantification applied to cases with intestinal metaplasia are the following:

- 0 = absent;
- 1 = mild (intestinal metaplasia in a focus of 1-4 glands);
- 2 =moderate (intestinal metaplasia in separate foci, but limited as extension);
- 3 = severe (intestinal metaplasia in over 50% from the gastric epithelium);
- 4 = biopsy inappropriate for histopathological interpretation.

Age groups	**IM – antral biopsies (no. cases; %)**				**IM – gastric body biopsies (no. cases; %)**			
	0	**1**	**2**	**3**	**0**	**1**	**2**	**3**
21-30 years	6	-		-	6	-	-	-
31-40 years	4	-	-	-	2	-	2	-
41-50 years	18	-	-	-	16	2	-	-
51-60 years	10	4	-	-	12	2	-	-
61-70 years	24	2	-	2	24	2	2	-
≥ 71 years	14	10	2	-	12	12	2	-
Total patients	76 (79.2%)	16 (16.6%)	2 (2.1%)	2 (2.1%)	72 (75%)	18 (18.7%)	6 (6.3%)	0 (0%)

IM –intestinal metaplasia

Table 4. Distribution of the histological score given to intestinal metaplasia

http://dx.doi.org/10.5772/52676

For both locations, type I intestinal metaplasia was the most frequent encountered type (11.4% for antral biopsies and 15.6% for gastric body biopsies). The distribution of the three types of intestinal metaplasia at the antrum and gastric body level, respectively, did not differ significantly (p=0.560). Type II of intestinal metaplasia presented a relatively uniform distribution in all age groups (Tab. 5).

Age groups	IM – antral biopsies			IM – gastric body biopsies		
	I	II	III	I	II	III
21-30 years	-	-	-	-	-	-
31-40 years	-	-	-	-	1	1
41-50 years	-		-	1	1	-
51-60 years	3	1	-	1	1	-
61-70 years	-	3	1	3	-	1
≥ 71 years	8	2	2	10	1	3
Total patients	11 (11.4%)	6 (6.25%)	3 (3.1%)	15 (15.6%)	4 (4.2%)	5 (5.2%)

Table 5. Types of intestinal metaplasia

In our study we evaluated the incidence and types of **epithelial dysplasia** encountered in patients with dyspeptic symptoms. In accordance with the Vienna classification, dysplastic modifications were divided in low-grade dysplasia and high-grade dysplasia.

Histopathological examination of the 96 cases showed dysplastic lesions in 10 patients, prevalence being of 10.4%.

Low-grade dysplasia, observed in 8 patients (Tab. 6, Graphic 3), is characterized by glandular architecture mostly preserved, sometimes with the presence of pseudovilli, cystic dilated glands or slightly irregular glands, with discrete intraluminal papillary projections or serrated aspect. Glandular structures are lined with high, crowded cells, with or without mucous vacuoles at the apical pole. The nuclei appear elongated and pseudostratified, discretely pleomorphic, being situated in the lower half of the cytoplasm (Fig. 8 and Fig. 9). Mitotic activity is discrete.

Age groups	Gastric epithelial dysplasia	
	Low-grade dysplasia	High-grade dysplasia
21-30 years	-	-
31-40 years	1	-
41-50 years	-	-
51-60 years	1	-
61-70 years	2	1
≥ 71 years	4	1
Total patients	8 (8.33%)	2 (2.1%)

Table 6. Epithelial dysplasia in the cases studied

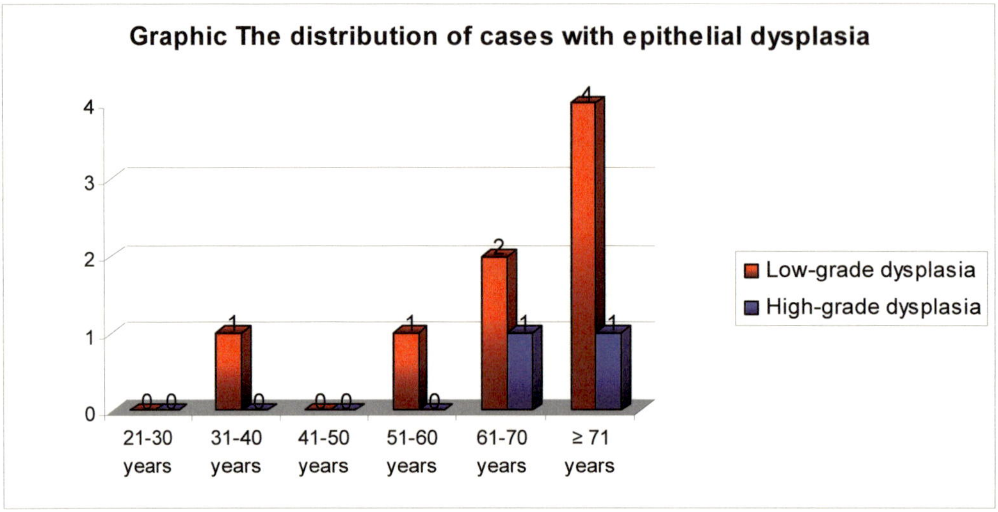

Graphic 3. The distribution of cases with epithelial dysplasia

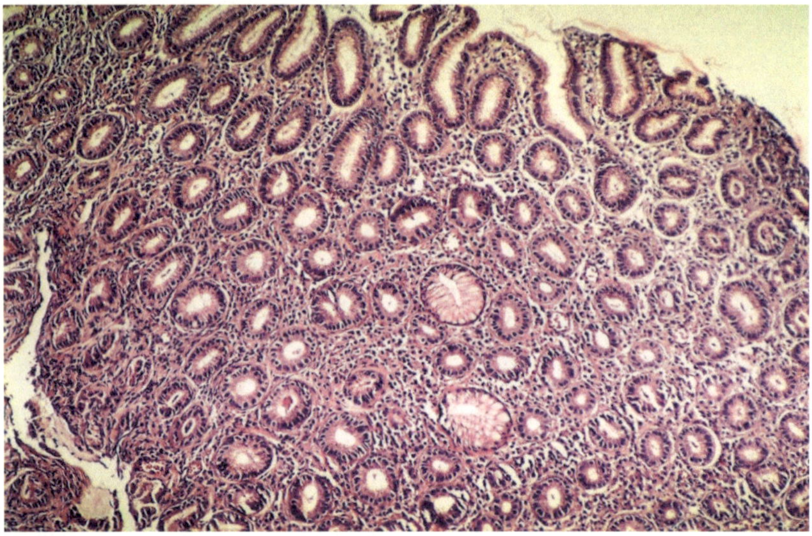

Figure 8. Low-grade epithelial dysplasia. HE x 100.

In all cases, dysplastic lesions were diagnosed histopathologically in the biopsies taken from the antrum. From an endoscopic point of view, patients presented more frequently aspects of antral diffuse erythematous gastritis (in 7 cases). In the case of a 66 year-old patient, the antral mucosa did not show macroscopic modifications which were visible with conventional gastroscopy. Epithelial dysplasia is observed mostly in patients in age groups 51-60 years, 61-70 years, and ≥71 years. In the cases studied we noted low-grade dysplastic lesions in a young patient, of age 36.

http://dx.doi.org/10.5772/52676

Only in 2 patients we noted high-grade dysplastic modifications. High-grade epithelial dysplasia is characterized histopathologically by highly distorted glandular architecture, with crowded, irregular and ramified glands, with frequent papillary intraluminal projections, lined with stratified epithelium, with crowded, pleomorphic nuclei overlapping, with intense mitotic activity, losing of normal polarity, nuclei that touch the apical pole of the cell. In the neoplastic epithelium, goblet cells and Paneth cells are absent (Fig. 10).

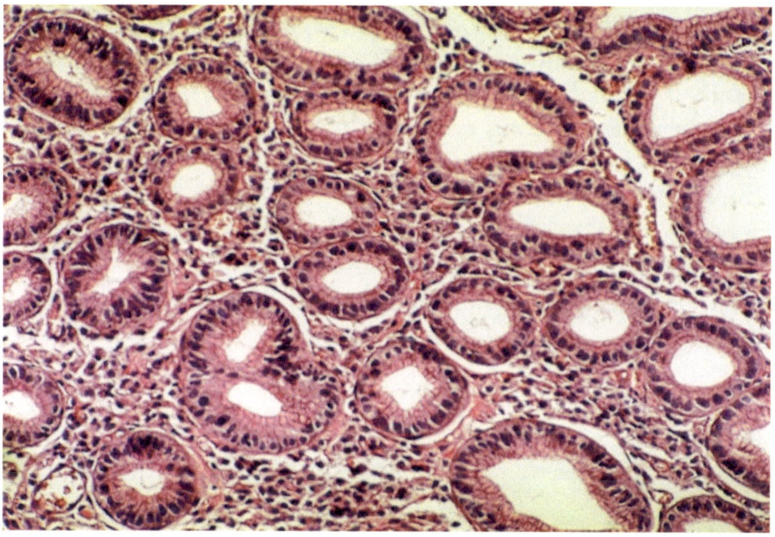

Figure 9. Low-grade epithelial dysplasia (detail). HE x 200.

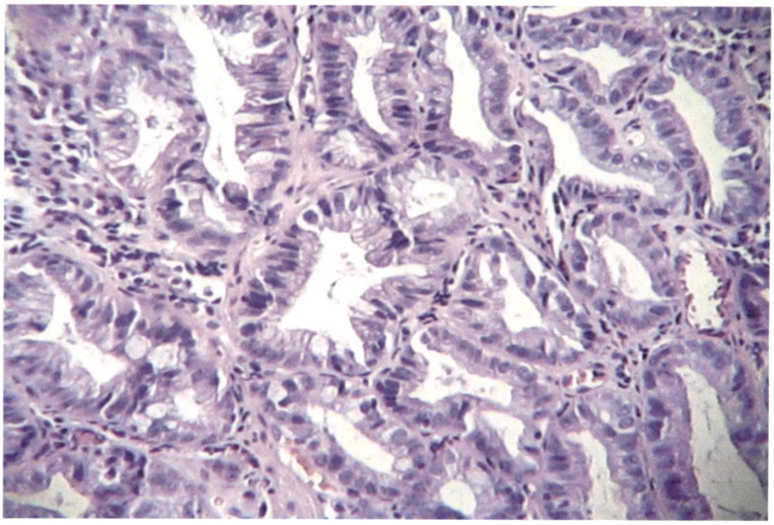

Figure 10. High-grade epithelial dysplasia. HE x 200.

These 2 patients were males of 64 and 75 years, respectively. In the case of the 75-year old patient, pangastritis obvious endoscopically was characterized through aspects of focal erythematous gastritis of the antrum with mild intensity and petechial gastritis of the gastric body, of severe intensity. For the second patient, gastroscopy showed only aspects of erythematous diffuse antral gastritis with moderate intensity. In both patients, infection with H. pylori proved to be negative histopathologically.

From **the particular lesions** observed, we mention the case of a 79-year old patient who presented in endoscopic investigation a nodular aspect of the mucosa of the antrum and gastric body, on the background of a petechial antral gastritis with mild intensity (Fig. 11). Histopathologically a particular form of pangastritis was diagnosed, granulomatous gastritis with non-necrotizing granulomas consisting of epitheloid cells and multinuclear cells, surrounded by lymphocytes, accompanied by a rich inflammatory lymphoplasmocytic infiltrate and atrophic modifications of the mucosa (Fig. 12 and Fig. 13). Lesions were more intense on the large curvature, for antral biopsy as well as for the biopsy taken from the gastric body. Anamnestic data and other investigations performed excluded a possible sarcoidosis or an idiopathic granulomatous gastritis, diagnostic conclusion being that of gastric Crohn's disease.

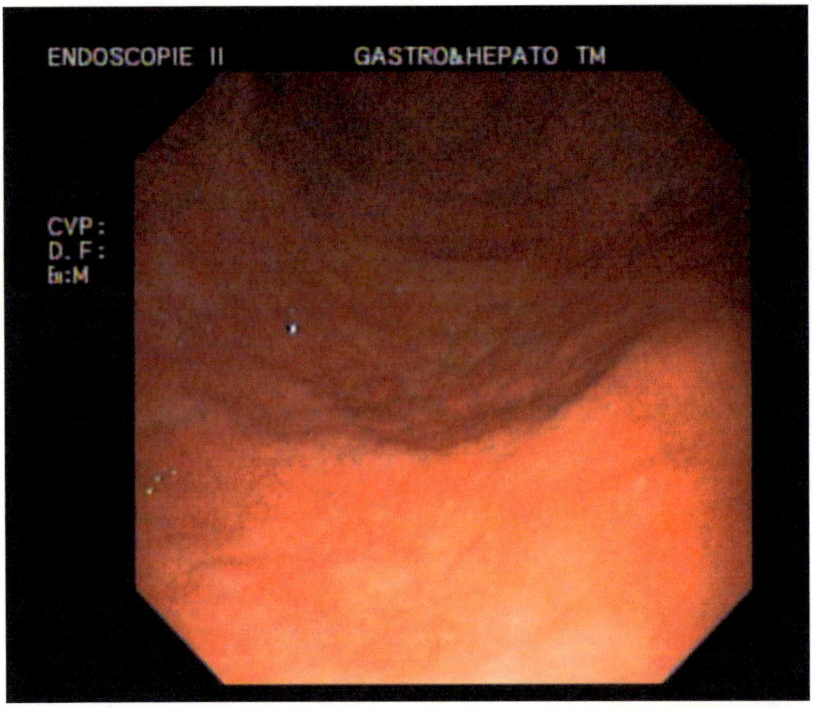

Figure 11. Congestive gastritis of the gastric body, at the large curvature, with nodular aspect.

http://dx.doi.org/10.5772/52676

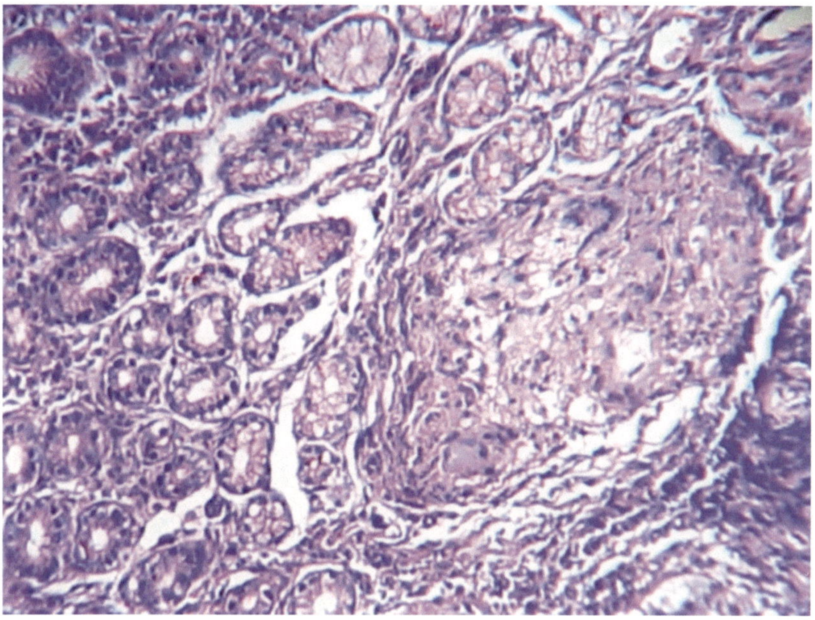

Figure 12. Gastric Crohn's disease. HE x 200.

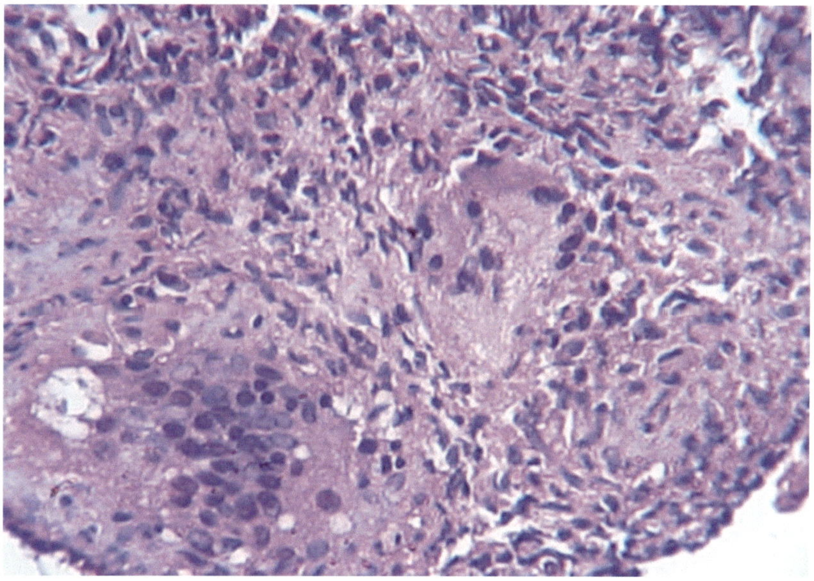

Figure 13. Non-necrotizing granulomas in the deep mucosa. HE x 400.

Another particular case is that of a patient aged 77, with gastroscopic modifications of diffuse erythematous gastritis of the antrum, of mild intensity. Although the gastric body did not appear modified, histopathological exam showed a rich lymphoplasmocytic infiltrate in the lamina propria, very frequent intraepithelial lymphocytes (at the level of the surface epithelium and in superficial glands), vacuolizations of epithelial cells, a slight glandular atrophy, discrete activity and absence of bacterial colonization (Fig. 14 and 15). Histopathological image was characteristic for lymphocytic gastritis, a rarely encountered form.

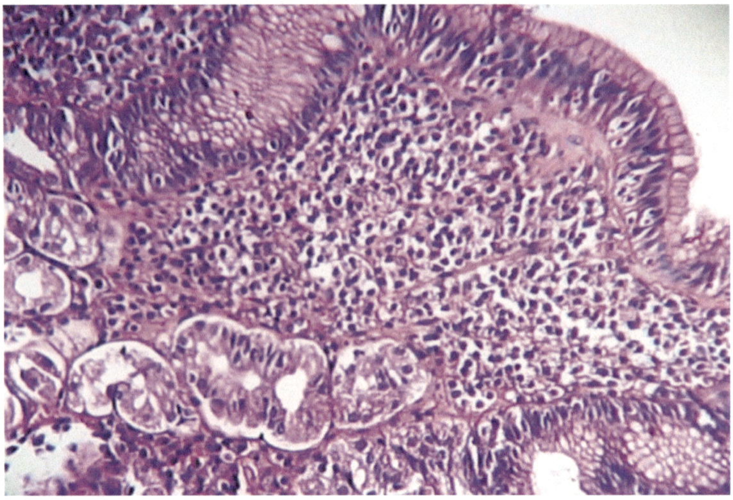

Figure 14. Lymphocytic gastritis. HE x 200.

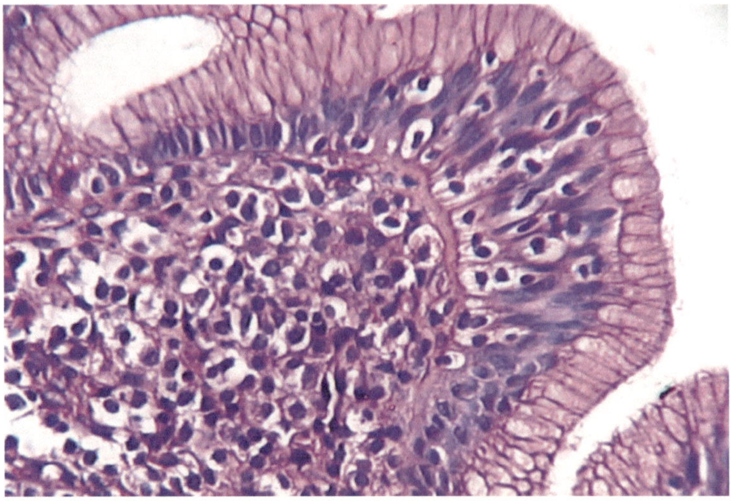

Figure 15. Lymphocytic gastritis. Numerous intraepithelial lymphocytes. HE x 400.

http://dx.doi.org/10.5772/52676

4. Discussions

For the endoscopists, evaluation the presence or absence of gastritis based on the endoscopic aspect of the gastric mucosa represents a common practice. Throughout the years, the concept of "endoscopic gastritis" has gained credibility, its existence being recognized by the Sydney System of classifying gastritis [8,9,10]. Numerous studies followed the concordance between endoscopy and histopathological exam regarding the diagnosis of gastritis. The results of these works are contradictory, most of them supporting a low degree of concordance. However, the significant correlation between the gastroscopic and histopathological aspects in severe forms of gastritis are mentioned, and exclusion of active gastritis in case of a normal endoscopic aspect [11].

Epidemiological and clinicopathological studies have proved that the extent, the intensity and the distribution of gastric atrophy and inflammation are closely correlated with the incidence of gastric cancer [12,13]. Presently, the idea is accepted that only histopathological examination of gastric mucosa can correctly assess the risk of neoplastic progression of a gastric lesion, through identifying the modifications called preneoplastic: atrophy, intestinal or pyloric metaplasia, epithelial dysplasia [14].

Following the studies performed by Siurala M. in Finland and Estonia [15], Correa P. in Columbia and numerous Japanese authors [4], initially separate entities such as superficial chronic gastritis, atrophy, metaplasia, dysplasia and carcinoma were integrated in a hypothetical sequence, called "the cascade of Correa" [16]. This hypothesis of gastric carcinogenesis, presented in 1984, was lacking the triggering etiologic element. The discovery in the same year of H. pylori [17] placed the infection of gastric mucosa with this bacterium on the first step of the carcinogenesis cascade [18].

Histopathological lesions regarded as preneoplastic are represented by chronic atrophic gastritis, intestinal metaplasia and dysplasia. In their evolution, these entities can be regarded as a pyramid with a very wide base, composed of the population infected with H. pylori. A segment of this population (greater in the developing countries, compared with industrialized countries) will present the evolution of lesions towards atrophic gastritis, with or without intestinal metaplasia. Only a small part of the population will develop lesions of dysplasia and possibly gastric adenocarcinoma. In the cascade of carcinogenesis, the closer a lesion is of neoplasia, the greater is its risk to progress towards gastric carcinoma [14]. Thus, chronic gastritis is a remote and uncertain precursor of gastric cancer, which constitutes rather a predisposing condition. High-grade dysplasia is a true neoplastic lesion [19,20].

Gastric atrophy is defined as a numeric reduction of the self glandular structures of the gastric mucosa [21,22]. This definition, purely morphological, implies a disappearance of glands characteristic for an area of the gastric mucosa, for instance specialized glands from the gastric body, and their replacement either with extracellular matrix, fibroblasts or collagen, or by intestinal type or pseudopyloric glands. These modifications imply the alteration of physiological mechanisms, for instance, anomalies of the secretion of mucins and acid.

Atrophic lesion is defined by the presence of atrophy areas in the gastric mucosa. The most frequent causes are the long-term infection with H. pylori and autoimmune gastritis. In the actualized Sydney system, the term of "atrophic gastritis" is used to differentiate this entity by the "non-atrophic gastritis" or simply "gastritis", a lesion with severity expressed in the antrum and identified in most patients infected with H. pylori.

Atrophic gastritis is characterized by the numeric decrease or disappearance of typical gastric glands, the expansion of antral type mucosa in the gastric body (antralization or pseudopyloric metaplasia) and areas of intestinal metaplasia. This entity presents a significant epidemiologic risk for the gastric adenocarcinoma, the prognostic implications being determined by the extent and distribution of atrophic areas [14,16,23,24].

Studies from literature have shown that the presence of atrophic gastritis has an annual incidence of progression to gastric cancer of approximately 0.5-1%, and that the extent of atrophic gastritis within the stomach correlates with the risk of progression to carcinoma [25-28].

The two forms of atrophic gastritis are represented by corporal autoimmune and by multifocal atrophic gastritis, the later being more common, associated with H. pylori infection, and with lesions of metaplasia. The presence of infection has been associated with an approximately 10-fold increased risk of atrophic gastritis development. There has been demonstrated an important regional variation in the prevalence of atrophic gastritis in H. pylori-infected individuals, with an increase of about 3-fold in Asia, in comparison with Western countries [29,30].

The pathophysiology associated with the increased risk of gastric cancer in patients with gastric atrophy may be related to achlorhydria, which predisposes to gastric bacterial overgrowth, accumulation of N-nitroso compounds, and diminished ascorbate secretion into the gastric lumen. Moreover, low acid output determines increased serum gastrin levels that may contribute to abnormal cell growth and increased risk of neoplastic progression [31].

In our study, the endoscopic aspect of atrophic gastritis was rarely encountered. Some authors signal the reduced percentage of atrophic gastritis cases diagnosed endoscopically, the lesions being obvious only for the severe forms as intensity [32]. In the cases studied we did not observe any case of antral atrophic gastritis. In the gastric body, atrophic gastritis, was noted in 6 elderly patients

For this lesion we noted a poor correlation between the conventional endoscopic investigation and histopathological examination. Out of the total number of biopsies included in the study, we observed lesions of atrophic type in 46 antral biopsies (48%) and 52 biopsies of the gastric body (54.2%); location of the atrophy was encountered more frequently at the level of the gastric body, but without statistical significance ($p=0.386$). Location of the chronic atrophic gastritis predominantly at the level of the gastric body is mentioned in specialty literature. This lesion presents a multifocal disposition with individual foci, initially developed at the level of the gastric angle. The foci extend and merge along the small curvature and on the anterior and posterior walls of the stomach [27]. In a recent study it is shown that most gastric carcinomas of intestinal type develop on the background of a wide terrain of atrophic gastritis, with small dispersed areas of intestinal metaplasia, which progresses proximally towards the large gastric curvature [33].

For the antral location we noted 10 cases with mild atrophy (21.7%), 34 cases with moderate atrophy (74%) and 2 cases with severe atrophy (4.3%). The glandular atrophy of the gastric mucosa was encountered much more frequently in patients with older ages (over 61 years old). The biopsies graded with score 3 for atrophy pertain only to patients with ages ≥ 71 year.

Glandular atrophy was encountered more frequently in biopsies of the gastric body, being predominant in patients with average and old ages. Especially moderate and mild forms of atrophy were noted (14 cases with mild atrophy – 27%; 34 cases with moderate atrophy – 65.4%; 4 cases with severe atrophy – 7.6%). All patients with severe glandular atrophy pertain to the age group of ≥ 71 years. In concordance with other studies [27,34] we noted an association between atrophic gastritis, and gastritis in general, predominant in the gastric body and old age of patients.

Intestinal metaplasia represents the replacement of the gastric lining and glandular epithelium by one composed of cells of the intestinal type (small or large intestine). Multiple attempts to classify the various forms of intestinal metaplasia led to a complex terminology, difficult to apply in the medical practice (complete or incomplete, type 1, 2a and 2b, etc.). The most used classification is the one proposed by Jass and Filipe, which includes 3 types of intestinal metaplasias:

- type I intestinal metaplasia (the complete type or of small intestine type) is characterized by relatively normal glandular architecture, with straight crypts and glands lined with absorbent cells non-secreting mucus, with striated plate and goblet cells with flattened nuclei and with widened apical pole, these two cellular types being encountered in approximately equal proportions. Occasionally, at the base of the glands Paneth cells can be observed. Goblet cells secrete AA-positive sialomucins. Reaction with paraphenyldiamine is negative;

- type II intestinal metaplasia (the incomplete type or enterocolic type) presents slight architectural modifications, with prolonged and tortuous crypts, with focal areas of foveolar hyperplasia and columnar cells in variable number, which contain a mixture of neutral mucines and sialomucins, but not sulfated material. The proportion of goblet cells is greater than in type I. PAS-AA positive reaction translates through mixed PAS-positive and alcyanophil areas, representing neutral and acid mucines. The positive material is located in the apical portion of epithelial cells, in the lumen of certain glands and in goblet cells;

- type III of intestinal metaplasia (the incomplete type or colonic type) is characterized morphologically through important glandular distortions, with ramified glands, lined with columnar cells which secrete sulfomucins and goblet cells secreting sialomucins and sulfomucins. PAS reaction is negative, but the HID-AA reaction appears intensely positive, through both coloring solutions. The positive substrate appears in goblet cells (blue), in the apical portion of columnar cells and in the lumen of some metaplastic glands (dark-brown) [14,27,35].

Currently use classifications take into consideration the presence of Paneth cells (complete metaplasia) or crescent architecture changings, dedifferentiation, and degree of absence of Paneth cells (incomplete metaplasia), and also the pattern and type of mucin expression. Type I metaplasia displays decreased expression of gastric mucins (MUC1, MUC5AC, and MUC6), and expression of the intestinal mucin MUC2. In type II and III metaplasia gastric mucins (MUC1, MUC5AC, and MUC6) are coexpressed with MUC2 [36]. However, the use of immunohistochemistry or other special techniques in order to subtype intestinal metaplasia is not widespread in routine practice.

Another pattern of metaplasia- spasmolytic polypeptide expressing metaplasia (SPEM), has been described in recent years. This type is characterized by the expression of the TFF2 spasmolytic polypeptide that is associated with oxyntic atrophy and usually develops in the gastric body and fundus. SPEM appears to share some characteristics with pseudopyloric metaplasia, and has a strong association with chronic infection with Helicobacter pylori and with gastric cancer. Studies suggests that it may represent another pathway to gastric neoplasia [37].

The presence of type I intestinal metaplasia confers a very low risk of malignant transformation. However, type III is considered a true dysplastic lesion

Type I metaplasia does not seems to raise the risk of gastric carcinoma. Numerous studies have shown that the presence of type II or III intestinal metaplasia is associated with a 20-fold increased risk of gastric cancer [38-40]. Intestinal metaplasia represents a preneoplastic lesion for the intestinal type of gastric cancer, 42% of patients with type III intestinal metaplasia developing early gastric cancer within five years of follow-up [41].

It remains unclear whether gastric carcinoma arises from areas of intestinal metaplasia or whether this lesion represents only a marker for higher cancer risk. The prevalence of intestinal metaplasia (similar to atrophic gastritis) in H. pylori-infected individuals is higher in Asia (about 40%) in comparison with Western countries [29,30].

Atrophic gastritis and intestinal metaplasia are often unevenly distributed throughout the stomach. The updated Sydney System is the most widely accepted for classification of gastritis and recommends five biopsies, two from the antrum (3 cm from the pylorus, greater and lesser curvatures), one from the incisura and two from the corpus (one from the lesser curvature, 4 cm proximal to the incisura, and one from the middle of the greater curvature) [10]. Although this biopsy protocol generally establishes with accuracy H. pylori status and chronic gastritis, the number of biopsies is controversial with regard to staging of precancerous gastric lesions, mainly because of their multifocal disposition [42-44].

For an accurate staging and grading of gastric precancerous conditions, the Guideline of the European Gastrointestinal Endoscopy recommends at least four non-targeted biopsies of two topographic sites (at the lesser and greater curvature, from both the antrum and the corpus) and additional target biopsies of lesions [45].

http://dx.doi.org/10.5772/52676

Although the updated Sydney system have contributed to a uniform description of preneoplastic lesions, in order to predict gastric cancer risk it has been established OLGA staging system (operative link for gastritis assessment). This system offers a standardized report of histopathological data with information about the topography and the extent of the atrophic changes and subgrouping of patients by gastric cancer risk [46,47]. Gastritis stages (0 to IV) express increasing extents of atrophy, proved on antral and corpus biopsies. Studies have allocated a small minority of gastritis patients to stages III and IV, associating this subgroup of population with a significantly higher cancer risk and thus with endoscopic follow-up programs [48,49]. Because the OLGA system is based on the severity and extent of atrophy, which held a low interobserver agreement, it was introduced a modified system-based on intestinal metaplasia, OLGIM (operative link for gastric intestinal metaplasia), with a high level of interobserver concordance [50]. Implementation of OLGIM system was associated with an easier histological assessment and the advantage of including of fewer patients into the high risk stages, therefore a smaller population for whom endoscopic surveillance would be needed [51].

The surveillance of premalignant gastric lesions may be important for early detection of gastric cancer and improved survival. Globally, gastric cancer risk is too low to justify endoscopic follow-up in all patients with atrophic gastritis and intestinal metaplasia. Studies have shown that cancer risk increases in patients with extensive intragastric lesions [26,28,52]. The two forms of extensive intestinal metaplasia, the so-called "magenstrasse" or "transitional zones" distribution (intestinal metaplasia found over the lesser curvature from cardia to pylorus) and the "diffuse distribution" show an increase risk for cancer (odds ratio [OR] = 5.7 and 12.2, respectively) [53]. In order to establish the extent of atrophy and intestinal metaplasia, it can be used endoscopic assessment, histological assessment of multiple biopsies and serology. Serologic testing for pepsinogens, gastrin and H.pylori antibodies can establish the extent of atrophic gastritis and identifies patients at increased risk of developing gastric cancer [54].

The Guideline of the European Gastrointestinal Endoscopy recommends that endoscopic surveillance should be offered to patients with extensive atrophy and/or intestinal metaplasia every 3 years after diagnosis [45].

Correct classification of intestinal metaplasia requires performing some relatively sophisticate histochemical techniques, whose interpretation was not standardized up to present day. From the histochemical methods recommended by specialty literature, in our study we used coloration methods PAS-AA at a pH of 2.5 and reaction with colloidal iron diamine-AA (HID-AA).

In conventional endoscopy, modifications of the type of intestinal metaplasia of gastric mucosa were evident in 7 patients (4 males and 3 females) with ages between 54 and 76 years, with location at the level of the gastric body.

The incidence of intestinal metaplasia identified histopathologically at the level of the antrum was of 20.8% (20 cases), and at the level of the gastric body of 25% (24 cases), without any significant differences between the antral location and the location at the level of the gastric body, respectively, of the metaplasia (p=0.492). At the antral level we noted 18 cases with focal disposition (score given 1 and 2) and only 2 cases with diffuse disposition (score 3), interesting almost entirely the gastric glandular epithelium. Following the extension of the intestinal metaplasia in relation with patients` age, we observed the great frequency of types II and III in patients over 61 years old. For the biopsies of the gastric body we did not note intestinal metaplasias with score 3, but we identified 18 cases of metaplasias with score 1 and 6 cases with score 2. These metaplastic transformations appear more frequently in elderly patients, but also in patients from the age groups 31-40 years and 41-50 years.

For both locations we remarked the predominance of type I intestinal metaplasia (11.4% for antral biopsies and15.6% for biopsies of the gastric body, without statistically significant differences between the two locations, p=0.398). Type III was a lesion rarely encountered in our study, being slightly more frequent in the gastric body (5.2%), in comparison with the antrum (3.1%) and noted especially in patients over the age of 50. Type II intestinal metaplasia presented a relatively uniform distribution in all age groups. In the large study of Suriani R. and collaborators [55], which included 1750 patients, type III intestinal metaplasia was noted in 6.7% of cases, from which 5.7% identified only in the antral mucosa.

Neoplasia constitutes the final stage of phenotypic and genetic progressive changings which affect the normal cellular morphology, resulting in a new cell characterized through uncontrolled proliferation and potential of migrating and implanting. In epithelial tissues, the first noticeable modification in optical microscopy is the alteration of cell morphology. Tumoral cells present large nuclei, with prominent nucleoli and granular chromatin or in rough blocks. In comparison with the nucleus, the cytoplasm is poorly represented, the nucleus-cytoplasm ratio being much increased. Cytological alterations are associated with various degrees of architectural anomalies. Such epithelial changings can appear in two situations: in epithelial injuries, followed by processes of reparation and in neoplastic alterations. For the first situation the term of reactive atypia is used, and for the second the term of dysplasia.

Throughout several decades, the pathologists have tried to standardize the criteria of diagnosis and grading for epithelial dysplasia. Pathologists from around the world united their efforts, but their opinions have coincided only in regard to the epithelial dysplasia of the mucosa of large intestine and the dysplasia in the Barrett epithelium. The discovery of the H. pylori bacterium and its relationship with gastric cancer focused the attention of researchers upon the gastric preneoplastic lesions. It was suggested that the eradication of this infection can prevent or even reduce the regression of these lesions. Unlike metaplasia or atrophy, whose types and classifications were established without major disputes, specifying the definition and diagnosis criteria for dysplasia created significant controversies among the Western and the Japanese pathologists. Japan represents one of the countries with the greatest incidences for gastric adenocarcinoma and at the same time, with the best survival rates in gastric cancer. The reasons invoked for exceptional results are: implementing the early diagnosis programs, introducing innovating endoscopic techniques and especially including some borderline lesions in the group of carcinomas, while other pathologists include them in the category of dysplasia [14].

http://dx.doi.org/10.5772/52676

There were differences between Japanese and European/North American pathologists in categorizing intraepithelial neoplasia; for instance, lesions interpreted by the latter as high-grade intraepithelial neoplasia (dysplasia) have been frequently classified by Japanese pathologists as "noninvasive intramucosal carcinoma". In an attempt to resolve this issue, several proposals have been made regarding terminology of the morphological spectrum of lesions ranging from non-neoplastic changes to early invasive cancer.

Thus, in order to eliminate the existent dissensions, an international forum was formed, and in 1996, Schlemper RJ organized a seminar with this topic, the results being published in the Lancet magazine in 1997 [56]. Subsequently, several study groups were constituted formed by Japanese pathologists and Western pathologists who made their goal to establish a consensus on the classification of preneoplastic lesions. One of these classifications, accepted by the World Health Organization, was presented at the seminar from Padua, Italy in 1998, and represents a model of histopathological interpretation and of choosing the therapeutic conduit [57,58].

The Padua Model includes the definition of dysplasia as pre-invasive neoplasia and the classification of gastric neoplasia in 5 categories:

1. negative for dysplasia;
2. non-defined for dysplasia;
3. non-invasive neoplasia;
4. suspicion of invasive cancer;
5. gastric cancer.

These lesional categories are similar with the lesions included in the Japanese Classification of the Gastric Cancer. Each category corresponds to one or several sub-categories, in order to cover the entire spectrum of epithelial alterations [14].

In 1998, on occasion of the World Congress of Gastroenterology in Vienna, a consensus was reached in regard to the terminology for the gastrointestinal epithelial dysplasia, named **"The VIENNA Classification"** [19]. In this classification, the diagnosis of "high-grade dysplasia/adenoma", "carcinoma *in situ* (CIS)", and "suspicion of invasive carcinoma" were grouped in a single category (category 4), called "high-grade non-invasive neoplasm", due to the therapeutic recommendation which was similar for all these sub-groups.

At the beginning of the year 2000, the Vienna classification was reviewed, in category 4 including a new subcategory, namely, the intramucous carcinoma [59]. The terminology of this consensus makes a distinction between high-grade intraepithelial neoplasia, without the actual invasion of the lamina propria, and respectively with the invasion of the lamina propria, the last term being named intramucous carcinoma at the level of the esophagus and of the stomach. At the level of the colon, the risk of nodal invasion is null in this situation, for which reason in the West there is the tendency to avoid the term "carcinoma" for the lesions without invasion of the submucosa, since they are treated completely only through local excision. Beyond this stage, all neoplastic lesions with invasion of the submucosa are termed invasive carcinomas.

The Vienna Classification reviewed of gastrointestinal epithelial neoplasia:

Category 1: Negative for dysplasia/neoplasia

Category 2: Non-defined for dysplasia/neoplasia

Category 3: Low-grade epithelial neoplasia:

- low-grade adenoma/dysplasia

Category 4: High-grade epithelial neoplasia:

4.1. High-grade adenoma/dysplasia

4.2. Non-invasive carcinoma (carcinoma „in situ")

4.3. Suspect of invasive carcinoma

4.4. Intramucous carcinoma

Category 5: Carcinoma with invasion of the submucosa.

At the end of the year 2000 the work Classification of the WHO revised was published, in which category 4 in the Vienna classification was adopted under the name of "high-grade intraepithelial neoplasia" and is defined as "modification of the mucosa with cytological and architectural aspects of malignity without the invasion of the stroma; it includes the lesions of severe dysplasia and carcinoma in situ" [60].

In our study we evaluated the incidence and forms of epithelial dysplasia encountered in patients with dyspeptic symptoms. In accordance with the Vienna classification, the dysplastic modifications were classified in low-grade dysplasia and high-grade dysplasia.

Current **WHO classification** [61] considers the following conditions as precursor lesions of invasive neoplasia (intraepithelial neoplasia) of the stomach:

- gastritis-associated dysplasia:

– adenomatous (type 1)

– foveolar (type 2)

- adenoma:

– intestinal type

– pyloric-gland type

– foveolar type

- fundic gland polyp-associated dysplasia.

According to the **WHO classification of tumors of the stomach 2010**, the following categories of gastric intraepithelial neoplasia (dysplasia) should be considered:

http://dx.doi.org/10.5772/52676

1. *Negative for intraepithelial neoplasia (dysplasia).* This subgroup includes benign mucosal processes that are inflammatory, metaplastic, or reactive in nature.
2. *Indefinite for intraepithelial neoplasia (dysplasia).* This term is usually used when an ambiguous morphological pattern is encountered, but is not a final diagnosis. This category is usually used were there is doubt as to whether a lesion is neoplastic or non-neoplastic (i.e. reactive or regenerative), particularly in small biopsies exhibiting inflammation. The dilemma is usually solved by cutting deeper levels, by obtaining additional biopsies, or after treating for possible etiologies.
3. *Intraepithelial neoplasia (dysplasia).* This category includes epithelial neoplastic proliferation characterized by variable cellular and architectural atypia, but without convincing evidence of invasive growth. Intraepithelial neoplasia (gastric epithelial dysplasia) can have polypoid, flat or slightly depressed growth patterns. The flat or slightly depressed patterns may show an irregular appearance on chromoendoscopy or microvasculature anomalies on narrow-band imaging, aspects that are not apparent with conventional white-light endoscopy. In the western countries, the term "adenoma" has been applied when the neoplastic proliferation produces a protruding lesion. By contrast, in Japan, "adenomas" include all gross types (flat, elevated and depressed).

In the stomach, most cases of dysplasia have an intestinal phenotype (adenomatous; type I) resembling colonic adenomas with crowded, tubular glands lined by atypical columnar cells; the cells present overlapping, hyperchromatic and/or pleomorphic nuclei, with pseudostratification and inconspicuous nucleoli, mucin depletion, and lack of surface maturation [62].

The other variant is represented by the gastric phenotype (foveolar or pyloric phenotype; type II) in which the cells are cuboidal or low-columnar, with clear or eosinophilic cytoplasm, and round to oval nuclei [62].

These two variants may be differentiated by expression of mucin, CD10, and CDX2, as well as by background changes in the gastric mucosa. The intestinal/adenomatous type expresses MUC2, CD10, and CDX2, and the gastric/foveolar type expresses MUC5AC, the absence of CD10 and low positivity of CDX2 [63,64]. Intraepithelial neoplasia (dysplasia) is stratified into two grades, low or high.

5. Intramucosal invasive neoplasia/intramucosal carcinoma

This category defines carcinomas invading lamina propria and that are distinguished from intraepithelial neoplasia by desmoplastic changes that can be minimal or absent, and also by marked glandular crowding, excessive branching, and budding.

The diagnosis of intramucosal carcinoma indicates that there is an increased risk of lymphatic invasion and lymph-node metastasis. Novel endoscopic techniques can allow treatment of some of these patients without open surgery, particularly for lesions of < 2 cm in size and for those that are well-differentiated [65].

6. Invasive neoplasia

This category defines carcinomas that show invasion beyond lamina propria. In the stomach, this diagnosis is associated with a varying risk of nodal and distant metastasis and overall prognosis. The recommended treatment consists in surgical resection, sometimes with neoadjuvant therapy.

Histopathological examination of the 96 cases showed dysplastic lesions in 10 patients, the incidence being of only 10.4%. According to the data in the literature, the prevalence of dysplasia varies between 0.5 - 4% in Western countries and between 9-20% in areas with high risk for gastric cancer [66]. The high frequency of epithelial dysplasia, observed in our study, can also be explained through the modality of taking the biopsies for each case (the large number of biopsies/case, the different location of taking the sample), method of work that eliminates somehow the errors connected with the focal, dispersed characteristic of dysplastic lesions.

Low-grade dysplasia, encountered in 8 patients, is characterized by glandular architecture mostly preserved, sometimes with the presence of pseudovilli, cystically dilated glands or slightly irregular glands, with discrete intraluminal papillary projections or serrated aspect. Glandular structures are lined with high, crowded cells, with or without mucous vacuoles. The nuclei, discretely pleomorphic, appear elongated and pseudostratified, situated in the inferior half of the cytoplasm. The mitotic activity is discrete.

In all cases, dysplastic lesions were diagnosed histopathologically at the level of the biopsies taken from the antrum. In literature the predominantly antral location of premalignant gastric lesions is mentioned, except for the atrophic gastritis associated with pernicious anemia, which is identified especially at the level of the gastric body [27].

Epithelial dysplasia is encountered especially in patients over 51 years old. In the cases studied we encountered dysplastic lesions of low grade in a young 36-year-old patient.

Data reveal that low-grade dysplasia may regress in up to 60% of cases, and progress to high-grade dysplasia in 10-20% of cases [67,68]. High-grade dysplasia rarely regresses, being associated with an annual incidence of progression to carcinoma of 2-6%; it can be uni- or multifocal, and it is often associated with synchronous cancer. A prospective study from the Netherlands has shown that high-grade dysplasia was associated with a markedly increased risk of progression to carcinoma (adjusted hazard ratio, 40.1) [5,69].

While routine surveillance for Barrett's esophagus is recommended and guidelines for the surveillance for other gastrointestinal premalignant conditions are available [70,71], in the last years the management for gastric premalignant conditions varied from surgery to annual surveillance for dysplasia and from no treatment to surveillance every 3 to 5 years for less advanced lesions [72-75]. Data showed that endoscopic mucosal resection and routine surveillance of advanced premalignant gastric lesions may significantly decrease the mortality and morbidity associated with gastric cancer. Yeh and collaborators [76] have elaborated a simulation model of gastric cancer natural history for a cohort of U.S. men with a recent incidental diagnosis of gastric precancerous lesions, and they estimated that among 50-year old men with dysplasia, approximately one in every twenty will develop gastric cancer in their lifetime, which is similar to the risk of colorectal cancer in the like-aged general U.S population or persons with Barrett's esophagus. This study highlighted that EMR with surveillance every 1 to 5 years for dysplasia is promising for secondary cancer prevention because it can reduce gastric cancer risk by 90%, and it is considered cost-effective in the U.S. Endoscopic surveillance of less advanced lesions does not appear to be cost-effective, except possibly immigrants from high-risk countries.

The Guideline of the European Gastrointestinal Endoscopy [45] recommends that patients with low grade dysplasia, in the absence of an endoscopically defined lesion, should receive follow-up within 1 year after diagnosis. If there is an endoscopically visible lesion, endoscopic resection should be considered in order to obtain a more accurate diagnosis. For patients with high grade dysplasia, if there are no endoscopically defined lesions, endoscopic reassessment with extensive biopsy sampling and surveillance at 6-month to 1-year intervals is recommended. In the case of endoscopically defined lesions, resection needs to be considered, either through endoscopy (endoscopic mucosal resection) or surgery.

From an endoscopic point of view, the patients presented more frequently aspects of antral diffuse erythematous gastritis (in 7 cases). In the case of a 66-year old patient, the antral mucosa did not show visible macroscopic modifications on conventional endoscopy. Though the quality of the images obtained through standard endoscopy was improved substantially in the past few decades, the modifications observed during conventional endoscopy are correlated in a smaller measure with the histopathologicaldiagnosis of atrophic gastritis, intestinal metaplasia and dysplasia. These results are due to the unsatisfactory viewing of the structure of the mucosa, its color and vascularization, important elements in the differential diagnosis between premalignant lesions and incipient gastric cancer [27]. So, data show that conventional white light endoscopy cannot accurately diagnose premalignant gastric lesions. Magnification endoscopy and narrow band imaging (NBI), with or without magnification, improve the diagnosis of these conditions [45]. Some studies concluded that correlation between white light endoscopy and histology was poor [77]. Absence of rugae and presence of visible vessels in the gastric mucosa can predict severe atrophy but with a low sensitivity [78]. Intestinal metaplasia may appear endoscopically as thin, white mucosal deposits, but the value of some endoscopic signs for its diagnosis it is still unclear [79]. In addition to low accuracy, the lesions detected on conventional endoscopy were associated also with low reproducibility [80,81]. Therefore current data show that white light endoscopy cannot be relied upon to accurately diagnose patients with atrophy and intestinal metaplasia.

Recent studies have followed the performances of endoscopy by magnification in the detection of premalignant gastric lesions. The correlation between the endoscopic aspects and histopathological diagnosis proved to be exceptional [82-84]. Detailed visualization of the superficial gastric mucosa allows classifying the patterns that the gastric folds and foveoles can take in different pathological conditions. The model of superficial micro-vascularization identifies the chronic gastritis induced by H. pylori and other entities classified as preneoplastic. In H. pylori positive gastritis, collector venules lose their regular aspect, "sea star"-like, in some cases being invisible. In atrophic gastritis, the alterations in the subepithelial capillary network and of the collector venules are correlated with the degree of atrophy. The areas of intestinal metaplasia are suspected in the presence of depressions with wide and elongated epithelial rigs, separated by deep grooves [83]. Data show that high resolution magnifying endoscopy appears superior to standard endoscopy, allowing accuracy for the diagnosis of H. pylori gastritis, intestinal metaplasia and dysplasia [85,86].

The techniques of in vivo coloration represent adjuvant methods for the optimal viewing of the lesions during the conventional endoscopy, or with magnification. Methylene blue visualizes the areas of intestinal metaplasia. Architectural modifications from the neoplastic areas are emphasized by using the indigo carmine solution. Unlike conventional endoscopy, chromoendoscopy can identify limited foci of incipient gastric carcinoma [32,87]. Studies suggest that chromoendoscopy, particularly with magnification, helps to identify lesions of intestinal metaplasia and dysplasia. Dinis-Ribeiro et al. proposed a chromoendoscopy classification with methylene blue for these lesions that proved to be reproducible and highly accurate [87]. The use of other solutions, such as indigo carmine, acetic acid, or hematoxylin, has shown a high diagnostic accuracy, especially for dysplasia [88,89].

No comparative study of magnification with or without chromoendoscopy has been made, despite the fact that Tanaka et al [89] have suggested that magnification chromoendoscopy with acetic acid is superior to conventional magnification endoscopy and indigo carmine chromoendoscopy.

However, magnification chromoendoscopy lengthens the time of the endoscopic procedure and may compromise patient tolerance. For these reasons, performance of this technique should be restricted to experienced centers [45].

In the last years new endoscopic techniques were introduced, which utilize certain spectral features of the light, for instance image obtained through narrow band, autofluorescence or fluorescence capturing. The results of implementing this new methods of investigation are only preliminary and in some studies even conflicting, thus their follow-up on long periods of time is necessary [27].

The technique of narrow band imaging (NBI) has been found to have good sensitivity and specificity for the diagnosis of gastric lesions [90-95]. The principle of this new method is based on modification of the spectral characteristics of the optical filter in the light source, leading to improved visibility of mucosal components. With the use of NBI in combination with image magnification, mucosal structures are highlighted with accuracy, because of the increased contrast between surface and vascular pattern [96]. The study of Capelle et al [97] provides evidence that NBI yields more accurate results in the surveillance of patients with intestinal metaplasia and dysplasia than conventional endoscopy. They have shown that considerably more lesions of intestinal metaplasia were detected by NBI compared to white light endoscopy and that the sensitivity for the detection of advanced premalignant gastric lesions increased by 20-71% for NBI.

http://dx.doi.org/10.5772/52676

Both NBI and chromoendoscopy can reveal the mucosal pattern and microvascular structure of the mucosa that have been considered as distinctive characteristics of early gastric cancer and premalignant gastric lesions. The study of Zhang et al [98] showed that the image quality of magnifying NBI is superior to magnifying conventional endoscopy in respect of morphology, pit pattern and blood capillary form of abnormal gastric zones, but also to magnifying chromoendoscopy concerning blood capillary form.

Angiogenesis represents an important element in gastric carcinogenesis [99], the vascular pattern of gastric cancer and precancerous lesions being differ from that of normal mucosa [100]. Nakayoshi et al [101] studied 165 patients with early gastric cancer with magnifying NBI, showing that 66.1% of differentiated adenocarcinoma had fine microvascular networks, and 85.7% of undifferentiated carcinoma had corkscrew microvascular networks.

The use of auto-fluorescence endoscopy demonstrated a high correlation between Barrett's esophagus and histological diagnosis, but the correlation between gastric cancer and this method is still controversial [102,103].

Confocal endomicroscopy is an endoscopic technique that produces 1000-fold magnification cross-sectional images and can accurately diagnose the presence of early cancer in targeted areas. A recent gastric pit-pattern classification for assessment of gastritis and atrophy showed a high correlation with histological changing and needs further evaluation [104,105]. This technique is too elaborate to be used for assessment of the entire gastric mucosa.

Liu et al [106] studied the microvascular architecture of early gastric cancer with confocal microscopy, and revealed that differentiated gastric cancerous mucosa presented hypervascularity and microvessels of different caliber and shapes, and undifferentiated gastric cancer showed hypovascularity and irregular short branched vessels.

Only in 2 patients we observed high-grade dysplastic modifications. High-grade epithelial dysplasia is characterized histopathologically through intensely distorted glandular architecture, with crowded glands, irregular and ramified, with frequent intraluminal papillary projections, lined with stratified epithelium, with crowded and overlapping nuclei, pleiomorphic, with intense mitotic activity, loss of normal polarity, nuclei that touch the apical pole of the cell. In the neoplastic epithelium, goblet cells and Paneth cells are absent.

The patients diagnosed histopathologically with high-grade epithelial dysplasia were both males, with ages of 64 and 75 years, respectively. In the case of the 75-year old patient, the pangastritis evident endoscopically was characterized by aspects of focal erythematous gastritis of the antrum with mild intensity and petechial gastritis of the gastric body, of severe intensity. For the second patient, gastroscopy showed only aspects of antral diffuse erythematous gastritis with moderate intensity. In both patients, the infection with H. pylori proved negative histopathologically.

7. Conclusions

For the diagnoses of atrophy we noted a poor correlation between the conventional endoscopic investigation and histopathological examination. Type I intestinal metaplasia predominated both for antrum and gastric body. Type III intestinal metaplasia was encountered slightly more frequent at the level of gastric body, especially in patients over 50 years old. About 2% of patients presented high-grade dysplasia needing resection treatment. The use of modern endoscopic techniques may help identifying gastric precancerous lesions. Among our study group, we found some rare types of gastritis, such as gastric Crohn's disease and lymphocytic gastritis, emphasizing the importance of performing multiple biopsies for an accurate histopathological diagnosis of gastritis.

Author details

Daniela Lazăr[1], Sorina Tăban[2] and Sorin Ursoniu[3]

1 Department of Gastroenterology, University of Medicine and Pharmacy „Victor Babeş" Timişoara, Romania

2 Department of Pathology, University of Medicine and Pharmacy „Victor Babeş" Timişoara, Romania

3 Department of Public Health, University of Medicine and Pharmacy „Victor Babeş" Timişoara, Romania

References

[1] Ferlay J, Bray F, Forman D, et al. GLOBOCAN 2008. Cancer Incidence and Mortality Worldwide: IARC Cancer Base No. 10, Lyon, 2010.

[2] Onodera H, Tokunaga A, Yoshiyuki T, et al. Surgical oucome of 483 patients with early gastric cancer: prognosis, postoperative morbidity and mortality, and gastric remnant cancer. Hepatogastroenterology 2004, 51: 82-85.

[3] Tan YK, Fielding JW. Early diagnosis of early gastric cancer. Eur J GastroenterolHepatol 2006, 18: 821-829.

[4] Correa P – A human model of gastric carcinogenesis. Cancer Res, 1988; 48: 3554-3560.

[5] de Vries AC, van Grieken NC, Looman CW, et al. Gastric cancer risk in patients with premalignant gastric lesions: a nationwide cohort study in the Nederlands. Gastroenterology 2008; 134: 945-952.

[6] Taghavi SA, Membari ME, Eshraghian A, et al. Comparison of chromoendoscopy and conventional endoscopy in the detection of premalignant gastric lesions. Can J Gastroenterol 2009; 23 (2): 105-108.

[7] Ida K, Hashimoto Y, Takeda S, et al. Endoscopic diagnosis of gastric cancer with dye scattering. Am J Gastroenterol 1975; 63: 316-20.

[8] Tytgat GNJ – The Sydney System: Endoscopic Division. Endoscopic appearances in gastritis/duodenitis. J GastroenterolHepatol, 1991; 6: 223-234

[9] Price AB – The Sydney System: histological division. J GastroenterolHepatol, 1991; 6: 209-222.

[10] Dixon Mf, Genta RM, Yardley JH, Correa P – Classification and grading of gastritis. The updated Sydney System. International Workshop on the histopathology of gastritis, Houston, 1994. Am J SurgPathol, 1996; 20: 1161-1181.

[11] Kaur G, Raj M – A study of the concordance between endoscopic gastritis and histological gastritis in an area with a low background prevalence of Helicobacter pylori infection. Singapore Med J, 2002; 43(2): 90-92.

[12] Sipponen P, Kekki M, Siurala M – Atrophic chronic gastritis and intestinal metaplasia in gastric carcinoma. Comparison with a representative population sample. Cancer, 1983; 52: 1062-1068.

[13] Correa P – The biological model of gastric carcinogenesis. IARC SciPubl, 2004; 157: 301-310.

[14] Genta RM, Rugge M – Assessing risks for gastric cancer: new tools for pathologists. World J Gastroenterol, 2006; 12(35): 5622 – 5627.

[15] Thamaki T, Saukkonen M, Siurala M – The sequelae and course of chronic gastritis during 30+ to 34+zear bioptic follow-up study. Scand J Gastroenterol, 1985; 20: 485-491.

[16] Correa P – Chronic gastritis as a cancer precursor. Scand J Gastroenterolsuppl 1984; 104: 131-136.

[17] Marshall BJ, Warren JR – Unidentified curved bacilli in the stomachof patients with gastritis and peptic ulceration. Lancet, 1984; 1: 1311-1315.

[18] Correa P – Human gastric carcinogenesis: a multistep and multifactorial process – First American cancer Society Award Lecture on Cancer Epidemiology and Prevention. Cancer Res, 1992; 52: 6735-6740.

[19] Schlemper RJ, Riddel RH, Kato Y et al – The Vienna classification of gastrointestinal epithelial neoplasia. Gut, 2000; 47: 251-255.

[20] Rugge M, Correa P, Dixon MF et al – Gastric dysplasia: the Padova international classification. Am J SurgPathol, 2000; 24: 167-176.

[21] Rugge M, Correa P, Dixon MF et al – Gastric mucosal atrophy: interobserver consistency using new criteria for classification and grading. Aliment PharmacolTher, 2002: 16: 1249-1259.

[22] Ruiz B, Garay J, Johnson W, Li D et al – Morphometric assessment of gastric antral atrophy: comparison with visual evaluation. Histopathology, 2001; 39: 235-242.

[23] Thamaki T, Sipponen P, Varis K et al – Characteristics of gastric mucosa which precede occurenceof gastric malignancy: results of long-term follow-up of three family samples. Scand J Gastroenterol, 1991; 186: 16-23.

[24] Correa P – Helicobacter pylori and gastric cancer: state of the art. Cancer Epidemiol Biomarkers Prev, 1996; 5: 477-481.

[25] Abrams JA and Wang TC. Adenocarcinoma and other tumors of the stomach. In Gastrointestinal and Liver Disease, vol 1, 887-904. Saunders, Elsevier 2010.

[26] Lahner E, Bordi C, Cattaruzza MS, et al: Long-term follow-up in atrophic body gastritis patients: Atrophy and intestinal metaplasia are persistent lesions irrespective of Helicobacter pylori infection. Aliment PharmacolTher 2005; 22:471-481.

[27] deVries AC, Haringsma J, Kuipers EJ. The detection, surveillance and treatment of premalignant gastric lesions related to Helicobacter pylori infection. Helicobacter 2007; 12:1-15.

[28] Cassaro M, Rugge M, Gutierrez O, et al. Topographic patterns of intestinal metaplasia and gastric cancer. Am J Gastroenterol 2000; 95:1431-1438.

[29] Kuipers EJ, Uyterlinde AM, Pena AS, et al. Long-term sequelae of Helicobacter pylori gastritis. Lancet 1995; 345:1525-1528.

[30] Asaka M, Sugiyama T, Nobuta A, et al. Atrophic gastritis and intestinal metaplasia in Japan: Results of a large multicenter study. Helicobacter 2001; 6:294-299.

[31] Watson SA, Grabowska AM, El-Zaatari M, Takhar A. Gastrin—Active participant or bystander in gastric carcinogenesis?. Nat Rev Cancer 2006; 6:936-946.

[32] Yang JM, Chen L, Fan YL et al – Endoscopic patterns of gastric mucosa and its clinicopathological significance. World J Gastroenterol, 2003; 9(11): 2552-2556.

[33] El-Zimaity HM, Ota H, Graham DZ et al – Patterns of gastric atrophy in intestinal type gastric carcinoma. Cancer, 2002; 94: 1428-1436.

[34] Leodolter A, Ebert MP, Peitz U et al – Prevalence of H pylori associated high risk gastritis for development of gastric cancer in patients with normal endoscopic findings. World J Gastroenterol, 2006; 12(34): 5509-5512.

[35] Fenoglio-Preiser CM – Chronic Gastritis. In Gastrointestinal Pathology. An atlas and text. Second edition, Lippincott-Raven, Philadephia, 1999, chapter 6: 184-202.

[36] Reis CA, David L, Correa P, et al. Intestinal metaplasia of human stomach displays distinct patterns of mucin (MUC1, MUC2, MUC5AC and MUC6) expression. Cancer Res. 1999; 59:1003–1007.

[37] Gutiérrez-González L, Wright NA. Biology of intestinal metaplasia in 2008: more than a simple phenotypic alteration. Dig Liver Dis. 2008; 40:510–522.

[38] Jass JR, Filipe MI – The mucin profiles of normal gastric mucosa, intestinal metaplasia and its variants and gastric carcinoma. Histochem J, 1981; 13: 931-939.

[39] Tosi P, Filipe MI, Luzi P et al – Gastric intestinal metaplasia type III cases are classified as low-grade dysplasia on the basis of morphometry. J Pathol, 1993; 169: 73-78.

[40] Filipe MI, Munoz N, Matko I et al – Intestinal metaplasia types and the risk of gastric cancer: a cohort study in Slovenia. Int J Cancer, 1994; 57: 324-329.

[41] Rokkas T, Filipe MI, Sladen GE: Detection of an increased incidence of early gastric cancer in patients with intestinal metaplasia type III who are closely followed up. Gut 1991.

[42] Eriksson NK, Färkkilä MA, Voutilainen ME, et al. The clinical value of taking routine biopsies from the incisuraangularis during gastroscopy. Endoscopy. 2005; 37:532–536.

[43] Rugge M, Genta RM. Staging and grading of chronic gastritis. Hum Pathol. 2005; 36:228–233.

[44] Kashin, S.; Pavlov, A.; Gono, K.; Nadezhin, A. Endoscopic diagnosis of early gastric cancer and gastric precancerous lesions. In: Pasechnikov, VD., editor. Gastric cancer: diagnosis, early prevention, and treatment. 1: edn.. Nova Science Publishers; New York: 2010. p. 197-233.

[45] Dinis-Ribeiro M, Areia M, de Vries AC, et al. Management of precancerous conditions and lesions in the stomach (MAPS): guideline from the European Society of Gastrointestinal Endoscopy (ESGE), European Helicobacter Study Group (EHSG), European Society of Pathology (ESP), and the Sociedade Portuguesa de Endoscopia-Digestiva (SPED). Endoscopy. 2012; 44(1): 74–94.

[46] Rugge M, Correa P, Di Mario F, et al. OLGA staging for gastritis: a tutorial. Dig Liver Dis. 2008; 40:650–658.

[47] Rugge M. Genta RM OLGA groupeStaging gastritis: an international proposal. Gastroenterology. 2005; 129:1807–1808.

[48] Graham DY, Rugge M. Clinical practice: diagnosis and evaluation of dyspepsia. J ClinGastroenterol 2010; 44: 167-172.

[49] Rugge M, Meggio A, Pennelli G, et al. Gastritis staging in clinical practice: the OLGA staging system. Gut 2007; 56: 631-636.

[50] Capelle LG, de Vries AC, Haringsma J, et al. The staging of gastritis with the OLGA system by using intestinal metaplasia as an accurate alternative for atrophic gastritis. GastrointestEndosc. 2010; 71:1150–1158.

[51] Rugge M, Fassan M, Pizzi M, et al. Operative link for gastritis assessment versus operative link on intestinal metaplasia assessment. World J Gastroenterol 2011; 17 (41): 4596-4661.

[52] Vannella L, Lahner E, Osborn J, et al. Risk factors for progression to gastric neoplastic lesions in patients with atrophic gastritis. Aliment PharmacolTher. 2010; 31:1042–1050.

[53] Van Zanten SJ, Dixon MF, Lee A. The gastric transitional zones: neglected links between gastroduodenal pathology and helicobacter ecology. Gastroenterology. 1999; 116:1217–1229.

[54] Dinis-Ribeiro M, Yamaki G, Miki K, et al. Meta-analysis on the validity of pepsinogen test for gastric carcinoma, dysplasia or chronic atrophic gastritis screening. J Med Screen. 2004; 11:141–147.

[55] Suriani R, Venturini I, Taraglio S, et al. Type III intestinal metaplasia, Helicobacter pylori infection and gastric carcinoma risk index in an Italian series of 1750 patients. Hepatogastroenterology. 2005;52(61):285-8.

[56] Schlemper RJ, Itabashi M, Kato Y et al – Differences in diagnostic criteria for gastric carcinoma between Japanese and western pathologists. Lancet, 1997; 349: 1725-1729.

[57] Rugge M, Correa P, Dixon MF et al – Gastric dysplasia: the Padova international classification. Am J SurgPathol, 2000; 24: 167-176.

[58] Schlemper RJ, Kato Y, Stolte M – Diagnostic criteria for gastrointestinal carcinomas in Japan and Western countries: proposal for a new classification system of gastrointestinal epithelial neoplasia. J GastroenterolHepatol, 2000; 15: G49-G57.

[59] Dixon MF. Gastrointestinal epithelial neoplasia: Vienna revisited. Gut 2002; 51: 130-131.

[60] Hamilton SR, Aalfonen LA (eds). Pathology and genetics of tumours of the digestive system. WHO classification of tumours. DARC Press, Lyon, 2000.

[61] Lauwers GY, Carneiro F, Graham DY, et al. Gastric carcinoma. In: WHO Classification of Tumors of the Digestive System, IARC Lyon, France, 2010, 48-58.

[62] Jass JR. Aclassification of gastric dysplasia. Hystopathology 1983; 7: 181-193.

[63] Park do Y, Srivastava A, Kim GH, et al. Adenomatous and foveolar gastric dysplasia: distinct patterns of mucin expression and backgroung intestinal metaplasia. Am J Surg Pathol 2008; 32: 524-533.

[64] Park DY, Srivastava A, Kim GH, et al. CDX2 expression in the intestinal-type gastric epithelial neoplasia: frequency and significance. Mod Pathol 2010; 23: 54-61.

[65] Nakajima T. Gastric cancer treatment guidelines in Japan. Gastric Cancer 2002; 5:1-5.

[66] Lauwers GY, Riddell RH – Gastric epithelial dysplasia. Gut, 1999; 45: 784-790.

[67] Di Gregorio C, Morandi P, Fante R, De Gaetani C: Gastric dysplasia. A follow-up study. Am J Gastroenterol 1993; 88:1714-1719.

[68] Rugge M, Cassaro M, Di Mario F, et al: The long term outcome of gastric non-invasive neoplasia. Gut 2003; 52:1111-1116.

[69] Kokkola A, Haapiainen R, Laxen F, et al: Risk of gastric carcinoma in patients with mucosal dysplasia associated with atrophic gastritis: a follow up study. J Clin Pathol 1996; 49:979-984.

[70] Wang KK, Sampliner RE. Updated guidelines 2008 for the diagnosis, surveillance and therapy of Barrett's esophagus. Am J Gastroenterol. 2008; 103(3):788–97.

[71] Hirota WK, Zuckerman MJ, Adler DG, Davila RE, Egan J, Leighton JA, et al. ASGE guideline: the role of endoscopy in the surveillance of premalignant conditions of the upper GI tract. Gastrointest Endosc. 2006; 63(4):570–80.

[72] Weinstein WM, Goldstein NS. Gastric dysplasia and its management. Gastroenterology. 1994; 107(5):1543–5.

[73] Whiting JL, Sigurdsson A, Rowlands DC, Hallissey MT, Fielding JW. The long term results of endoscopic surveillance of premalignant gastric lesions. Gut. 2002; 50(3): 378–81.

[74] West AB, Fischer R, Kapadia C, Genta RM, Wang TC, Lauwers GY. What and whom to treat with metaplasia. J Clin Gastroenterol. 2003; 36(Suppl1):S61–62.

[75] Dinis-Ribeiro M, Lopes C, da Costa-Pereira A, Moreira-Dias L. We would welcome guidelines for surveillance of patients with gastric atrophic chronic and intestinal metaplasia! Helicobacter. 2008; 13(1):75–6.

[76] Yeh JM, Chin Hur MD, Kuntz KM, et al. Cost-Effectiveness of Treatment and Endoscopic Surveillance of Precancerous Lesions to Prevent Gastric Cancer. Cancer. 2010; 116(12): 2941–2953.

[77] Bah A, Saraga E, Armstrong D, et al. Endoscopic features of Helicobacter pylori-related gastritis. Endoscopy 1995; 27:593–596.

[78] Redéen S, Petersson F, Jönsson KA, et al. Relationship of gastroscopic features to histological findings in gastritis and Helicobacter pylori infection in a general population sample. Endoscopy 2003; 35:946–950.

[79] Stathopoulos G, Goldberg RD, Blackstone MO. Endoscopic diagnosis of intestinal metaplasia. Gastrointest Endosc. 1990; 36:544–545.

[80] Eshmuratov A, Nah JC, Kim N, et al. The correlation of endoscopic and histological diagnosis of gastric atrophy. Dig Dis Sci. 2010; 55:1364–1375.

[81] Laine L, Cohen H, Sloane R, et al. Interobserver agreement and predictive value of endoscopic findings for H. pylori and gastritis in normal volunteers. Gastrointest Endosc. 1995; 42:420–423.

[82] Nakagawa S, Kato M, Shimizu Y et al – Relationship between histopathologic gastritis and mucosal microvascularity: observations with magnifying endoscopy. GastrointestEndosc. 2003; 58: 71-75.

[83] Kim S, Harum K, Ito M et al – Magnifying gastroendoscopy for diagnosis of histologic gastritis in the gastric antrum. Dig Liver Dis, 2004; 36: 286-291.

[84] Yagi K, Nakamura A, Sekine A – Comparison between magnifying endoscopy and histological, culture and urease test findings from the gastric mucosa of the corpus. Endoscopy, 2002; 34: 376-381.

[85] Anagnostopoulos GK, Yao K, Kaye P, et al. High-resolution magnification endoscopy can reliably identify normal gastric mucosa, Helicobacter pylori-associated gastritis, and gastric atrophy. Endoscopy. 2007; 39:202–207.

[86] Gonen C, Simsek I, Sarioglu S, et al. Comparison of high resolution magnifying endoscopy and standard videoendoscopy for the diagnosis of Helicobacter pylori gastritis in routine clinical practice: a prospective study. Helicobacter. 2009; 14:12–21.

[87] Dinis-Ribeiro M, da Costa-Pereira A, Lopez C et al – Magnification chromoendoscopy for the diagnosis of gastric intestinal metaplasia and dysplasia. GastrointestEndosc 2003; 57: 498-504.

[88] Mouzyka S, Fedoseeva A. Chromoendoscopy with hematoxylin in the classification of gastric lesions. Gastric Cancer. 2008; 11:15–21. discussion 21–22.

[89] Tanaka K, Toyoda H, Kadowaki S, et al. Surface pattern classification by enhanced magnification endoscopy for identifying early gastric cancers. GastrointestEndosc. 2008; 67:430–437.

[90] Tahara T, Shibata T, Nakamura M, et al. Gastric mucosal pattern by using magnifying narrow-band imaging endoscopy clearly distinguishes histological and serological severity of chronic gastritis. GastrointestEndosc. 2009; 70:246–253.

[91] Kato M, Kaise M, Yonezawa J, et al. Magnifying endoscopy with narrow-band imaging achieves superior accuracy in the differential diagnosis of superficial gastric lesions identified with white-light endoscopy: a prospective study. GastrointestEndosc. 2010; 72:523–529.

[92] Ezoe Y, Muto M, Horimatsu T, et al. Magnifying narrow-band imaging versus magnifying white-light imaging for the differential diagnosis of gastric small depressive lesions: a prospective study. GastrointestEndosc. 2010; 71:477–484.

[93] Kadowaki S, Tanaka K, Toyoda H, et al. Ease of early gastric cancer demarcation recognition: a comparison of four magnifying endoscopy methods. J GastroenterolHepatol. 2009; 24:1625–1630.

[94] Okubo M, Tahara T, Shibata T, et al. Changes in gastric mucosal patterns seen by magnifying NBI during H. pylori eradication. J Gastroenterol. 2011; 46:175–182.

[95] Kaise M, Kato M, Urashima M, et al. Magnifying endoscopy combined with narrow-band imaging or differential diagnosis of superficial depressed gastric lesions. Endoscopy. 2009; 41:310–315.

[96] Uedo N, Ishihara R, Iishi H, et al. A new method of diagnosing gastric intestinal metaplasia: narrow-band imaging with magnifying endoscopy. Endoscopy. 2006; 38:819–824.

[97] Capelle LG, Haringsma J, da Vries AC, et al. Narrow band imaging for the detection of gastric intestinal metaplasia and dysplasia during surveillance endoscopy. Dig Dis Sci. 2010; 55:3442–3448.

[98] Zhang J, Guo SB, Duan ZJ. Application of magnifying narrow-band imaging endoscopy for diagnosis of early gastric cancer and precancerous lesion. BMC Gastroenterology 2011, 11: 135.

[99] Folkman J, Klagsbrun M. Angiogenic factors. Science 1987, 235: 442-447.

[100] Lambert R, Kuznetsov K, Rey JF. Narrow-band imaging in digestive endoscopy. Scientific World Journal 2007, 7: 449-465.

[101] Nakayoshi T, Tajiri H, Matsuda K, et al. Magnifying endoscopy combined with narrow band imaging system for early gastric cancer: correlation of vascular pattern with histopathology. Endoscopy 2004; 36: 1080-1084.

[102] Ortner MA, Ebert B, Hein E, et al. Time gated fluorescence spectroscopy in Barrett's esophagus. Gut 2003; 52: 28-33.

[103] Kato M, Kaise M, Yonezawa J, et al. Autofluorescence endoscopy versus conventional white light endoscopy for the detection of gastric superficial neoplasia: a prospective comparative study. Endoscopy 2007; 39: 937-941.

[104] Zhang JN, Li YQ, Zhao YA, et al. Classification of gastric pit patterns by confocal endomicroscopy. GastrointestEndosc 2008; 67: 843-853

[105] Dunbar K, Canto M. Confocal endomicroscopy. CurrOpinGastroenterol 2008; 24: 631-637.

[106] Liu H, Li YQ, Yu T, et al. Confocal endomicroscopy for in vivo detection of microvascular architecture in normal and malignant lesions of upper gastrointestinal tract. J GastroenterolHepatol 2008; 23: 56-61.

Chapter 2

Management of Early Gastric Cancer

Takehiro Okabayashi and Yasuo Shima

Additional information is available at the end of the chapter

http://dx.doi.org/10.5772/50781

1. Introduction

Gastric carcinoma is the second most common malignancy worldwide and surgical treatment remains the only curative management option. Early gastric carcinoma (EGC) is defined as a lesion of the stomach confined to the mucosa and/or submucosa, regardless of the lymph node metastatic status. The incidence of EGC has gradually increased with advances in diagnostic techniques and equipment [1-3]. In the West, EGC accounts for 4 - 16% of all gastric carcinoma cases [4.5], whereas the proportion of EGC in Japan is approximately 30 - 50% [4-6].

The presence of a lymph node metastasis is one of the most important prognostic indicators for EGC. Lymph node metastases occur during the early stage of gastric carcinoma, and regional lymphadenectomy is the recommended surgical treatment of this disease. Excellent curative outcomes for patients with EGC have been obtained with regional lymphadenectomy [4,7].

In this article, the basic concept of EGC is revisited and recent published articles on both new diagnostic and treatment modalities are reviewed.

2. Classification of EGC

2.1. Macroscopic classification

The Japanese "gastric cancer" classification groups all gastric cancers into types 1 to 4 according to their morphological appearance [8]. EGC has been added as type 0, which is subdivided according to the macroscopic appearance of the lesion: 0-I, protruded or polypoid; 0-II, superficial; 0-III, excavated lesion characterized by a deep ulcer-like excavation that can resemble benign ulceration. Type 0-II lesions are most prevalent and are further subdivided into IIa (elevated), IIb (superficial spread), and IIc (depressed).

2.2. Microscopic classification

There has been considerable controversy between Japanese and Western pathologists regarding the histological reporting of mucosal lesions. Some observers have suggested that the reported incidence of EGC in Japan could be attributed to the over-diagnosis of dysplastic lesions as invasive cancer. Japanese pathologists often use the term, gastric cancer, whereas western pathologists use the term, dysplasia. Western pathologists require evidence of cellular invasion into the lamina propria before they consider that the basement membrane has been breached and can make a diagnosis of invasive cancer. Japanese pathologists have traditionally relied on nuclear features such as enlargement, pleomorphism, prominent nucleoli, and loss of polarity along with glandular architectural cancer diagnosis.

In 1965, Lauren described two histological subtypes of gastric cancer: intestinal and diffuse [9]. Since that time the Lauren classification scheme has been used worldwide. The intestinal-type gastric cancer consists of a cohesive group of neoplastic cells that form distinct well-defined tubular structures. In contrast, cell cohesion is lost in diffuse-type gastric cancer and individual cells infiltrate the gastric wall without a glandular structure. This description closely resembles the Japanese classification of differentiated (papillary, well-differentiated adenocarcinoma or moderately-differentiated adenocarcinoma) and undifferentiated types (poorly-differentiated adenocarcinoma, signet ring cell carcinoma, mucinous carcinoma).

3. Diagnostic challenges for early gastric cancer

Double contrast barium meal studies have been employed for more than 40 years in Japan, but endoscopy shows higher sensitivity in EGC detection.

3.1. Indigo carmine chromoendoscopy

To achieve a successful outcome, it is very important to accurately determine the lateral extent of a tumor. Traditionally, this has been done with conventional endoscopy and chromoendoscopy using indigo carmine dye [3]. However, it is sometimes difficult to identify the margins of the tumors, especially those of superficial or flat-type tumors. Chromoendoscopy with indigo carmine dye added to acetic acid (AI chromoendoscopy) has been recently reported to improve the diagnostic yield by aiding the recognition of the tumor borders in patients with EGC [10].

Chromoendoscopy of a differentiated adenocarcinoma is shown in Fig. 1. A combined flat and elevated lesion with an unclear border is located at the middle of the stomach (Fig. 1a). The borders of the lesion becomes distinct with high image clarity in an endoscopic view after indigo carmine was sprinkled onto the lesion (Fig. 1b). The lesion was resected by endoscopic submucosal dissection (ESD) and was shown to be a differentiated adenocarcinoma.

http://dx.doi.org/10.5772/50781

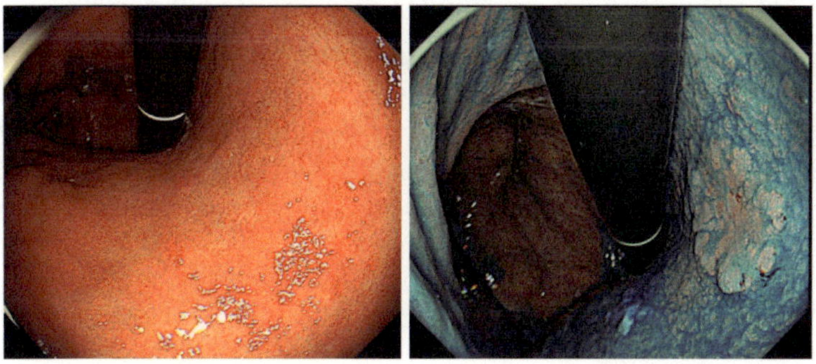

(a) (b)

Figure 1. Chromoendoscopic imaging. (a) A combined flat and elevated lesion with an unclear border at the middle of the stomach is shown. (b) Endoscopic view of the lesion after indigo carmine was sprinkled onto it. The borders of the lesion became distinct with high clarity images after chromoendoscopy with indigo carmine dye.

3.2. Magnifying narrow-band imaging endoscopy

The survival rate for patients who were treated for EGC is excellent, but the prognosis for advanced gastric cancer is very poor. Therefore, an early diagnosis of gastric cancer is very important but diagnosis is difficult because most patients with EGC do not have specific symptoms and it is difficult to distinguish EGC from a benign peptic ulcer or gastritis. Technological developments have enabled novel endoscopic imaging modalities such as magnifying narrow-band imaging (NBI) endoscopy to be used recently for the diagnosis of early gastric cancer [11,12].

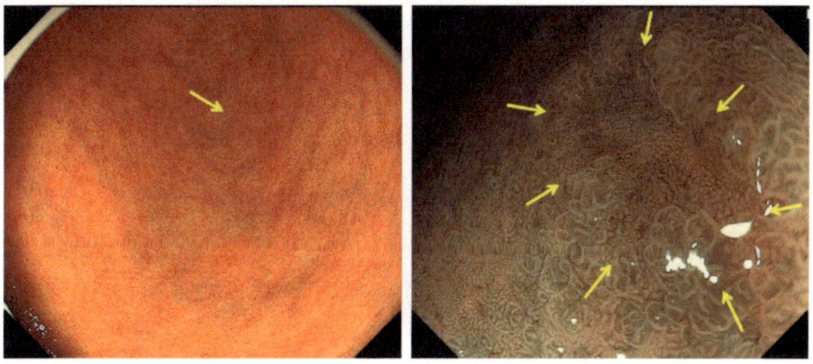

(a) (b)

Figure 2. Magnifying endoscopy with narrow-band imaging findings. (a) Conventional endoscopy with white light imaging demonstrates that this lesion (arrow) should be classified as a pale lesion rather than a red-colored lesion. (b) Magnifying endoscopy with narrow-band imaging findings (arrows) showed that this lesion should be diagnosed as cancer by the presence of an irregular microvascular pattern plus an irregular microsurface pattern using the vessel plus surface classification system.

A representative case of EGC is shown in Fig. 2. Conventional endoscopy with white light imaging demonstrated that this lesion (arrow) should be classified as a pale lesion rather than a red-colored lesion (Fig. 2a). Magnifying endoscopy with narrow-band imaging was used to diagnose the lesion as cancerous. The vessel plus surface classification system was used to identify features including the presence of an irregular microvascular pattern together with an irregular microsurface pattern (Fig. 2b). The histopathological diagnosis of the resected specimen was EGC.

4. Management of early gastric cancer

4.1. Endoscopic mucosal resection (EMR)

EMR has been used as the standard treatment of EGR because there is no risk of lymph node metastasis, and it is a minimally invasive, safe, convenient, and efficacious procedure. In order for EMR to be considered potentially curative, there are two important conditions that should be met: complete en-bloc removal with a clear margin around the primary tumor, and zero or extremely low possibility of lymph node metastasis. The Japanese Gastric Cancer Association has proposed the following indications for curative EMR: (a) invasion is clinically confined to the mucosa, (b) tumor size of 2 cm or smaller, (c) histologically differentiated type, (d) no ulcer or ulcer scar in the lesion [13]. A tumor that satisfies all of these indications can be safely removed by EMR but if the tumor depth is histologically diagnosed as mucosal, then lymph node metastasis should be absent.

Endoscopic submucosal dissection (ESD) is a newly developed technique in the field of endoscopic treatments for EGC in Japan. This technique uses specialized devices, including an insulation-tipped diathermy knife (IT knife), to dissect directly along the submucosal layer. Although the drawbacks of ESD include its technical difficulty and a higher risk of procedure-related complications, it has replaced EMR in Japan, and it has been introduced in Korea and Europe. Large numbers of ESD procedures are promising with high rates of both en-bloc resection and curative resection. The risk factors associated with the resectability and curability of ESD have been recently reported [14].

EGCs without any lymph node metastasis were treated with ESD using an IT knife (Fig. 3a). Briefly, the markings along the presumed cutting line were first defined relative to the normal mucosa that surrounded the lesion. This was performed with a standard needle knife at least 5 mm away from the tumor (Fig. 3b). An epinephrine solution (0.025 mg/mL in saline solution) was injected into the submucosa along the presumed cutting line and a standard needle-knife was used to make a pre-cut outside the indicated area. The IT knife was inserted into the incision, and an electrosurgical current was applied by a standard electrosurgical generator to complete the incision around the lesion (Fig. 3c). After the circumferential cut was completed, a solution of epinephrine was injected into the submucosa below the lesion when needed. The IT knife was then used to dissect the submucosa. If the tissue did not lift during or after injection, the IT knife or the standard needle-knife was used to carefully dissect the tissue along the plane of the submucosa (Fig. 3d).

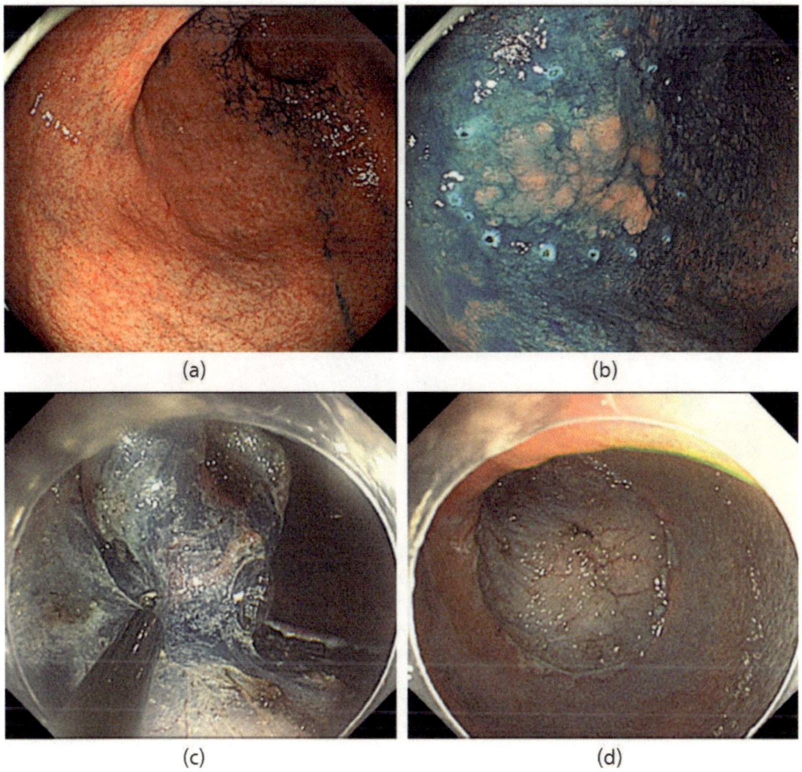

Figure 3. ESD technique. (a) EGCs that were diagnosed with no lymph node metastasis were treated with ESD with an IT knife. (b) Electrocautery marking surrounding the target lesion. (c) Submucosal injection of diluted epinephrine with indigo carmine, and circumferential cutting around the lesion. (d) Completion of resection. ESD was performed by an experienced gastrointestinal endoscopist (Dr. Hajime Yamaoka at Kochi Medical School, JAPAN).

4.2. Gastric surgery

Subtotal or total gastrectomy with regional lymphadenectomy is the standard treatment for resectable gastric cancer in Japan and Korea as well as high-volume centers in other countries. Less invasive gastrectomy with limited lymphadenectomy, such as pylorus-preserving gastrectomy and proximal gastrectomy, has been proposed for EGC that has a low possibility of nodal metastasis and a high probability of cure [15].

A typical gastrectomy with regional lymphadenectomy is shown in Fig. 4. After division of the left gastric artery, the lymphatic and connective tissue was removed from the surface of diaphragmatic crus that covers the aorta and the posterior aspect of the esophageal hiatus was exposed (Fig. 4a). Immediate inspection of the resected stomach revealed a tumor of the distal stomach, and the lymphadenectomy of supramesentric vein was performed (Fig. 4b).

Laparoscopic-assisted gastrectomy (LAG) has been used to treat EGC, which requires less extensive lymph node dissection. The use of LAG for EGC was first reported in 1994 [16] and many studies have since reported on the benefits of the technique, which include reduced blood loss, decreased pain, early recovery of bowel movements, and a short hospital stay [17]. Other studies have focused on its oncologic equivalency to open gastrectomy but the technique does involve a steep surgical learning curve [18]. Recently, the indication for LAG in some high-volume centers has been extended to include advanced gastric cancer [19].

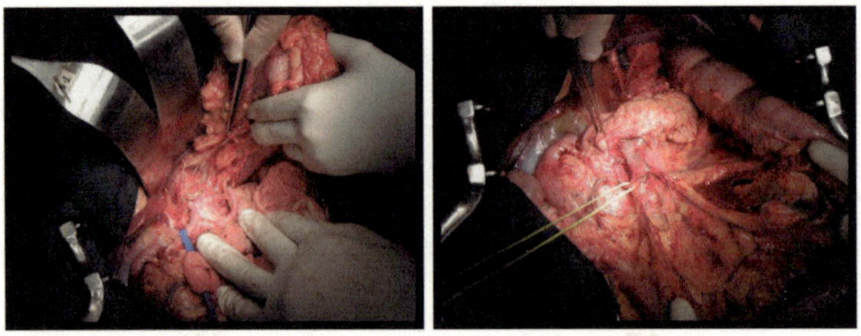

(a) (b)

Figure 4. Standard gastrectomy. (a) The lymphatic and connective tissue was removed from the surface of diaphragmatic crus that covers the aorta after division of the left gastric artery. The posterior aspect of the esophageal hiatus was exposed. (b) Immediate inspection of the resected stomach revealed a tumor of the distal stomach, and the lymphadenectomy of supramesentric vein was added. Total gastrectomy was performed by Dr. Takeshi Sano (Cancer Institute Hospital, JAPAN).

4.3. Reconstruction after gastric resection

Various reconstructive procedures have been proposed for patients undergoing distal gastrectomy for gastric cancer. In general, Billroth I (BI) reconstruction is the most common technique used clinically because it involves relatively simple reconstruction. However, bile reflux resulting in remnant gastritis and gastroesophageal reflux disease (GERD) has been noted as a problem associated with BI reconstruction after distal gastrectomy. Some studies have indicated that Roux-en-Y (RY) reconstruction following distal gastrectomy is superior to BI reconstruction in preventing remnant gastritis and reflux esophagitis because it reduces duodenogastric and gastroesophageal reflux [20]. The disadvantages of RY reconstruction include the possible development of stomal ulcers, increased probability of cholelithiasis, increased difficulty with an endoscopic approach to the papilla of Vater, and the possibility of Roux stasis syndrome. Furthermore, the RY reconstruction technique has a different route of reconstruction whereby all food passes through the jejunum and bypasses the duodenum, which causes one of the disadvantages of this procedure. An additional problem caused by RY reconstruction is the considerable difficulty with endoscopic access to the papilla of Vater for the diagnosis or treatment of pancreatobiliary disorders that may develop after the distal gastrectomy. Recently, double tract reconstruction (DT) after either total or subtotal gastrectomy have been introduced to remove the disadvantage of RY reconstruction [21]. DT reconstruction is as simple as RY reconstruction and can be performed safely after distal gastrectomy with regional lymphadenectomy. The advantages of DT reconstruction following both total and distal gastrectomy include maintaining the physiological passage of food and allowing future diagnostic and therapeutic endoscopic interventions to be safely performed. The technique chosen for surgical reconstruction of the gastrointestinal tract to perform gastrojejunostomy should take potential future endoscopic requirements into account (Fig. 5).

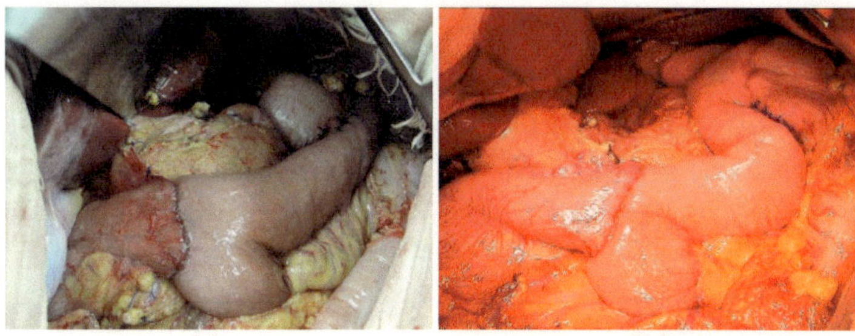

(a) (b)

Figure 5. Double tract reconstruction after gastrectomy. (a) Double tract reconstruction (DT) after subtotal gastrectomy. (b) DT after total gastrectomy. Gastrectomy was performed by Dr. Tsutomu Namikawa and Dr. Michiya Kobayashi (Kochi Medical School, JAPAN).

5. Prognosis of EGC

The incidence of lymph node metastasis has been reported to be 5.7 - 20% and it is one of the most important factors in determining the prognosis of patients with EGC [22-24]. Excellent curative treatment for patients with EGC has been obtained with regional lymphadenectomy [25]. Less invasive treatments, including EMR and ESD, have been performed recently for EGC and these options should be considered when deciding on a treatment method [26-29].

Experienced endoscopists are able to accurately evaluate the extent of lesions in gastric carcinoma and therefore, less invasive treatments such as EMR or ESD, may become possible for EGC with tumors less than 2 cm in diameter [30]. Use of the endoscopic scale for measuring the size of the EGC and endoscopic ultrasonography can be effective because the exact tumor diameter is not always easy to determine endoscopically. The use of EMR and/or ESD has become a reasonable and convenient diagnostic and treatment modality, because histological information about the whole tumor can be obtained. Furthermore, a curative treatment is achieved in the case of localized tumors without lymph node metastasis, which preserves the whole stomach. In recent years, the use of EMR and/or ESD has become safe and effective curative treatment option with feasible clinical outcomes in patients with EGC. As a result, the use of EMR and/or ESD has ensured an excellent prognosis, and should be the first choice of treatment in patients with EGC, although careful histological examination and long-term endoscopic surveillance remain important. When lymphatic permeation or vascular invasion is recognized in post-resection specimens, additional surgical resection of the stomach with lymphadenectomy is recommended [31,32]. Further prospective studies are warranted to evaluate the efficacy of this therapeutic strategy.

6. Conclusion

EGC is a curable disease in many cases, and a variety of less invasive, function-preserving treatments have been proposed. The use of EMR and/or ESD has ensured an excellent prognosis for patients who were suffering from EGC with no lymph node metastasis. Lymph node metastasis was one of the most important factors in determining the prognosis of patients with EGC. Therefore, when lymphatic permeation or vascular invasion is recognized in post-resection specimens of either EMR or ESD, additional surgical resection of the stomach with lymphadenectomy is recommended.

Author details

Takehiro Okabayashi* and Yasuo Shima

*Address all correspondence to: tokabaya@kochi-u.ac.jp

Department of Surgery, Kochi Health Sciences Center, Japan

References

[1] Huguier, M., Ferro, L., & Barrier, A. (2002). Early gastric carcinoma: spread and multicentricity. . Gastric Cancer , 5, 125-128.

[2] Seto, Y., Shimoyama, S., Kitayama, J., Mafune, K., Kaminishi, M., Aikou, T., Arai, K., Ohta, K., Nashimoto, A., Honda, I., Yamagishi, H., & Yamamura, Y. (2001). Lymph node metastasis and preoperative diagnosis of depth of invasion in early gastric cancer. *Gastric Cancer*, 4, 34-38.

[3] Okabayashi, T., Gotoda, T., Kondo, H., Ono, H., Oda, I., Fujishiro, M., & Yachida, S. (2000). Usefulness of indigo carmine chromoendoscopy and endoscopic clipping for accurate preoperative assessment of proximal gastric cancer. *Endoscopy*, 32, S62.

[4] Piso, P., Werner, U., Benten, D., Bektas, H., Meuer, U., & Klempnauer, J. (2001). Early gastric cancer- excellent prognosis after curative resection in 87 patients irrespective of submucosal infiltration, lymph-node metastases or tumor size. *Langenbecks Arch Surg.*, 386, 26-30.

[5] Borie, F., Millat, B., Fingerhut, A., Hay, J. M., Fagniez, P. L., & De Saxce, B. (2000). Lymphatic involvement in early gastric cancer. *Arch Surg.*, 135, 1218-1223.

[6] Folli, S., Morgagni, P., Roviello, F., De Manzoni, G., Marrelli, D., Saragoni, L., Di Leo, A., Gaudio, M., Nanni, O., Carli, A., Cordiano, C., Dell'Amore, D., & Vio, A. (2001). Risk factors for lymph node metastases and their prognostic significance in early gas-

tric cancer (EGC) for the Italian Research Group for Gastric Cancer (IRGGC). *Jpn J Clin Oncol.*, 31, 495-499.

[7] Popiela, T., Kulig, J., Kolodziejczyk, P., & Sierzega, M. (2002). Long-term results of surgery for early gastric cancer. *Br J Surg.*, 89, 1035-1042.

[8] Japanese classification of gastric carcinoma-2nd English edition Gastric Cancer. (1998)., 1, 10-24.

[9] Lauren, P. (1965). The two histological main types of gastric carcinoma. *Acta Pathol Microbiol Scand.*, 64, 31-49.

[10] Zhang, J., Guo, S. B., & Duan, Z. J. (2011). Application of magnifying narrow-band imaging endoscopy for diagnosis of early gastric cancer and precancerous lesion. *BMC Gastroenterol.*, 11, 135.

[11] Maki, S., Yao, K., Nagahama, T., Beppu, T., Hisabe, T., Takaki, Y., Hirai, F., Matsui, T., Tanabe, H., & Iwashita, A. (2012). Magnifying endoscopy with narrow-band imaging is useful in the differential diagnosis between low-grade adenoma and early cancer of superficial elevated gastric lesions. *Gastric Cancer (in press).*

[12] Nagahama, T., Yao, K., Maki, S., Yasaka, M., Takaki, Y., Matsui, T., Tanabe, H., Iwashita, A., & Ota, A. (2011). Usefulness of magnifying endoscopy with narrow-band imaging for determining the horizontal extent of early gastric cancer when there is an unclear margin by chromoendoscopy (with video). *Gastrointest Endosc.*, 74, 1259-1267.

[13] Nakajima, T. (2002). Gastric cancer treatment guidelines in Japan. *Gastric Cancer*, 5, 1-5.

[14] Hirasawa, K., Kokawa, A., Oka, H., Yahara, S., Sasaki, T., Nozawa, A., Morimoto, M., Numata, K., Taguri, M., Morita, S., Maeda, S., & Tanaka, K. (2011). Risk assessment chart for curability of early gastric cancer with endoscopic submucosal dissection. *Gastrointest Endosc.*, 74, 1268-1275.

[15] Sano, T., & Hollowood, A. (2006). Early gastric cancer: diagnosis and less invasive treatments. *Scand J Surg.*, 95, 249-255.

[16] Kitano, S., Iso, Y., Moriyama, M., & Sugimachi, K. (1994). Laparoscopy-assisted Billroth I gastrectomy. *Surg Laparosc Endosc.*, 4, 146-148.

[17] Lee, J. H., Han, H. S., & Lee, J. H. (2005). A prospective randomized study comparing open vs laparoscopy-assisted distal gastrectomy in early gastric cancer: early results. *Surg Endosc.*, 19, 168-173.

[18] Kunisaki, C., Makino, H., Yamamoto, N., Sato, T., Oshima, T., Nagano, Y., Fujii, S., Akiyama, H., Otsuka, Y., Ono, H. A., Kosaka, T., Takagawa, R., & Shimada, H. (2008). Learning curve for laparoscopy-assisted distal gastrectomy with regional lymph node dissection for early gastric cancer. *Surg Laparosc Endosc Percutan Tech.*, 18, 236-241.

[19] Kunisaki, C., Makino, H., Kosaka, T., Oshima, T., Fujii, S., Takagawa, R., Kimura, J., Ono, H. A., Akiyama, H., Taguri, M., Morita, S., & Endo, I. (2012). Surgical outcomes of laparoscopy-assisted gastrectomy versus open gastrectomy for gastric cancer: a case-control study. *Surg Endosc.*, 26, 804-810.

[20] Namikawa, T., Kitagawa, H., Okabayashi, T., Sugimoto, T., Kobayashi, M., & Hanazaki, K. (2010). Roux-en-Y reconstruction is superior to billroth I reconstruction in reducing reflux esophagitis after distal gastrectomy: special relationship with the angle of his. *World J Surg.*, 34, 1022-1027.

[21] Namikawa, T., Kitagawa, H., Okabayashi, T., Sugimoto, T., Kobayashi, M., & Hanazaki, K. (2011). Double tract reconstruction after distal gastrectomy for gastric cancer is effective in reducing reflux esophagitis and remnant gastritis with duodenal passage preservation. *Langenbecks Arch Surg.*, 396, 769-776.

[22] Wu, C. Y., Chen, J. T., Chen, G. H., & Yeh, H. Z. (2002). Lymph node metastasis in early gastric cancer: clinicopathological analysis. *Hepato-gastroenterology*, 49, 1465-1468.

[23] Arai, K., Iwasaki, Y., & Takahashi, T. (2002). Clinicopathological analysis of early gastric cancer with solitary lymph node metastasis. *Br J Surg.*, 89, 1435-1437.

[24] Choi, H. J., Kim, Y. H., Kim, S. S., & Hong, S. H. (2002). Occurrence and prognostic implications of micrometastases in lymph nodes from patients with submucosal gastric carcinoma. *Ann Surg Oncol.*, 9, 13-9.

[25] Okabayashi, T., Gotoda, T., Kondo, H., Inui, T., Ono, H., Saito, D., Yoshida, S., Sasako, M., & Shimoda, T. (2000). Early carcinoma of the gastric cardia in Japan: is it different from that in the West? *Cancer*, 89, 2555-2559.

[26] Tsujitani, S., Oka, S., Saito, H., Kondo, A., Ikeguchi, M., Maeta, M., et al. (1999). Less invasive surgery for early gastric cancer based on the low probability of lymph node metastasis. *Surgery*, 125, 148-154.

[27] Kunisaki, C., Shimada, H., Nomura, M., & Akiyama, H. (2001). Appropriate lymph node dissection for early gastric cancer based on lymph node metastases. *Surgery*, 129, 153-157.

[28] Noguchi, Y., Morinaga, S., Yamamoto, Y., & Yoshikawa, T. (2002). Is there a role for nontraditional resection of early gastric cancer? *Surg Oncol Clin N Am.*, 11, 387-403.

[29] Yoshikawa, T., Tsuburaya, A., Kobayashi, O., Sairenji, M., Motohashi, H., & Noguchi, Y. (2002). Is D2 lymph node dissection necessary for early gastric cancer? *Ann Surg Oncol.*, 9, 401-405.

[30] Gotoda, T., Sasako, M., Ono, H., Katai, H., Sano, T., & Shimoda, T. (2001). Evaluation of the necessity for gastrectomy with lymph node dissection for patients with submucosal invasive gastric cancer. *Br J Surg.*, 88, 444-449.

[31] Okabayashi, T., Kobayashi, M., Nishimori, I., Sugimoto, T., Namikawa, T., Onishi, S., & Hanazaki, K. (2008). Clinicopathological features and medical management of early gastric cancer. *Am J Surg.*, 195, 229-232.

[32] Okabayashi, T., Kobayashi, M., Sugimoto, T., Okamoto, K., Hokimoto, N., & Araki, K. (2007). Clinicopathological investigation of early gastric carcinoma; is less invasive surgery right for early gastric carcinoma? *Hepatogastroenterology*, 54, 609-612.

Section 2

Risk and Protective Factors

Chapter 3

Risk Factors in Gastric Cancer

Jolanta Czyzewska

Additional information is available at the end of the chapter

http://dx.doi.org/10.5772/52136

1. Introduction

Gastric cancer is one of the most commonly occurring malignant cancers in the world. During the second half of the 20th century a drastic rise has been observed in the number of cases and deaths caused by this cancer. Gastric cancer is the second, after pulmonary cancer, cause of death due to malignant cancers in the world. There is a geographic diversification in the occurrence of gastric cancer. Most cases are recorded in Japan, China, South America, and significantly less in Western Europe and in the United States [1].

The frequency of the occurrence of gastric cancer throughout the world is conditioned by various factors. The following factors increase the risk of occurrence of gastric cancer: chronic atrophic gastritis with intestinal metaplasia, peptic ulcer, dysplasia, partial gastrectomy and polyps. Environmental factors which can cause an increase in the risk of occurrence of gastric cancer include, among others, dietary factors, smoking as well as a *Helicobacter pylori* infection [2].

2. Risk factors in gastric cancer

2.1. Age

One of the risk factors for contracting gastric cancer is age (above 45 years of age). The number of cases involving this tumor increases with age, reaching a peak between the ages of 50 and 70 [3,4]. Most deaths are recorded in the 55-75 age group; and the number of fatalities decreases after 75. The frequency of gastric cancer occurrence rising with age can be explained by the accumulation of somatic mutations connected with the occurrence of malignant tumors [5,1].

2.2. Sex

Gastric cancer definitely develops more often in men. The coefficient of contracting this type of cancer is 1.8 – 2 times higher for men in comparison to women. Generally, percentages show 68% of gastric cases to be men and only 32% to be women [3, 6].

2.3. Obesity

Obesity is one of the causes facilitating spreading of the cancer in the cardia since discharging of food contents into the esophagus can occur. Research results have indicated a 2.3- fold increase of the risk of contracting gastric cancer in the cardia in obese persons in comparison to non-obese people [4]. It has been shown that obesity in men (BMI $\geq$ 30 kg/m^2) was connected not only to an increased risk of development of gastric cancer but also of colorectal cancer, cancers of the liver and the gallbladder. In turn, obesity in women (BMI $\geq$ 30 kg/m^2) was tied to an increased risk of development of tumors of the liver, pancreas and breasts in women above 50 years of age [7].

2.4. Diet

Diet, especially one rich in salt, smoked or marinated foods, grilled meat or smoked fish, preserved food, rich in red meat, deficient in vitamins and antioxidants, significantly increases the probability of cancer occurrence. Salt and consumption of salted foods causes an increase in the risk of stomach cancer occurrence even up to 50-100%. This happens because sodium chloride damages the mucous membrane of the stomach leading to infections and consequently facilitates colonization and growth of *Helicobacter pylori*. Increasing the supply of salt while at the same time decreasing the number of consumed fruit and vegetables is particularly dangerous [2, 3, 8].

This risk can be reduced by increasing the amount of vegetables and fruit consumed. Increasing the number of consumed vegetables and fruit in every day diet reduces the risk of contracting gastric cancer by as much as 30-50%. It is connected to the antioxidant effect of the substances contained in vegetables such as ascorbic acid (vitamin C), carotenoids and tacopherols. Moreover, soy products and green tea reduce the risk of contracting this type of cancer. Catechins contained in green tea inhibit polyphenol nitrosation, have an anti-inflammatory and antineoplastic effect modulating the path of signal transfer, inhibiting cell proliferation and transformation, as well as inducement of apoptosis, and in effect inhibit the development of tumors [4,8].

Reducing the amount of chemically preserved products in the foods ingested also contributes to reducing the risk of gastric cancer occurrence. Antioxidants such as vitamins C and E, beta-carotene, or microelements like selenium, zinc or magnesium [2] have a protective effect.

2.5. Stimulants

The risk of gastric cancer development correlates with the frequency and duration of smoking cigarettes. A nearly 5-fold increase occurs in the probability of contracting this disease in persons who smoke over 20 cigarettes a day and using alcohol more than 5 times in a two week period of time. Furthermore, the probability of contracting this type of cancer increased approximately 1.3 times for passive smokers in comparison to people who do not smoke and are not passive smokers. This is caused by the carcinogenic effects contained in cigarette smoke (for example tar and its polycyclic hydrocarbons) [3-5,9]. Carcinogens are able to form covalent bonds with DNA, which alters the correct function of the DNA and can lead to the development of gastric cancer [10].

Similarly, overuse of spirits, especially those with high alcohol content, significantly increases the risk of contracting gastric cancer and other tumors of the digestive tract (cancers of the mouth, throat, larynx and esophagus). Overconsumption of alcohol (4 or more drinks a day) is connected to a significant increase in the risk of contracting gastric cancer, equally for smokers as well as non-smokers (10). Alcohol stimulates the production of gastric juices and gastric motility. Intragastric supply of 70-100% ethanol causes extensive mucous membrane damage, with simultaneous reduction of blood flow in the blood vessels of the stomach, reduced generation of mucus, increase in the activity of proinflammatory cytokines (including IL-1), tumor necrosis factor alpha (TNFα), the level of leucotriene B4 and causing of oxidative stress [11].

Ethanol is not a carcinogen but the nitrosamines present in alcoholic beverages, especially in vodka, can be responsible for heightened risk of gastric cancer development. Acetic aldehyde, a metabolite of ethanol, is a known to be a carcinogen in animals. Acetic aldehyde created during ethanol metabolizing is mainly eliminated from the organism by aldehyde dehydrogenase-2 (ALDH2). ALDH2 is polymorphic and in people it has two alleles: ALDH2*1 and ALDH2*2. Reduced activity of the enzyme ALDH2*2 in homozygous individuals results in approximately 6-20 times higher level of acetic aldehyde in blood in comparison to homozygote ALDH2*1 and is connected with an elevated risk of developing gastric cancer [10].

2.6. Medicines

Aspirin is one of the medicines which increase the risk of contracting gastric cancer. For people who regularly take aspirin the risk of contracting gastric cancer increases up to 30%. Regular application of non-steroid anti-inflammatory drugs (NSAID) increased the risk of developing peptic ulcers and digestive tract bleeding, while at the same time, depending on the dosage, decreasing the growth of *H. pylori* and bacterial virulence factors. Aspirin increases the permeability of the external bacterial membrane causing an increased sensitivity of *H. pylori* to antibiotics [12]. Occurrence of damage to the gastric mucosa (bleeding and ulceration of the stomach, duodenum and small intestine) connected to aspirin intake at a dosage of 75-325 mg/day has been described. In patients taking aspirin occasionally bleeding of the digestive tract occurred 5.5 times more often and in patients regularly taking this drug approximately 7.7 times more frequently in relation to persons who did not take aspirin [13]. Furthermore, aspirin significantly decreases the amount of claudin-7, a protein produced by the MNK28 cells, connected to damage of the digestive tract and aspirin related dysfunction of the epithelium in the stomach. Aspirin related concentration decrease of the protein claudin-7 has been completely eradicated by the SB-203580 (inhibitor p38MAPK) treatment. These results demonstrate that the protein claudin-7 plays a significant role in the occurrence of aspirin related dysfunction of the stomach and that the activation of p28MAPK also takes a part in this dysfunction [14].

On the other hand it has been shown that patients who regularly take NSAIDs had a significantly reduced risk of gastric cancer occurrence in relation to persons occasionally taking these drugs or not taking them at all. However, the protective role of the NSAIDs was observed only in patients with non-cardia gastric cancer [15].

2.7. *H. pylori* infection

In many studies a close connection has been shown between a *Helicobacter pylori (H. pylori)* infection and an infection of the mucous membrane of the stomach wall, peptic ulcer and cancer [4]. The World Health Organization (WHO) classified *H. pylori* as a group 1 carcinogen, even though the exact mechanism through which this bacterium contributes to the development of gastric cancer is not completely understood [5]. It has been ascertained that in patients with an *H. pylori* infection the risk of the development of gastric cancer increases seven fold in comparison with a group of people without such an infection. It seems that an *H. pylori* infection connected with cagA genes (cytotoxin-associated gene A) and VacA (valulocating cytotoxin A) induces a more severe infection [6]. These genes are responsible for the production of cytotoxins which increase virulence. Especially the presence of *Helicobacter pylori* CagA + contributes to the rise of the risk of carcinogenesis occurrence. CagA intensifies immunological response, and through stimulation releases IL-8, a chemokine which leads to damage to the mucosa [4,16,17]. Additionally, *Helicobacter pylori* produce large amounts of urease which breaks urea into ammonia and carbon dioxide. The ammonia neutralizes the hydrochloric acid contained in stomach juices leading to it gaining a higher pH therefore making it easier for the bacteria to survive and reproduction [18]. Chronic inflammation caused by a *Helicobacter pylori* infection can result in damage to cell DNA by disrupting antioxidant processes, while at the same time raising the level of reactive forms of oxygen, as well as the amount of nitric oxide (NO), eventually elevating the risk of carcinogenesis. What is more, *Helicobacter pylori* causes the release of interleukins such as IL-1β, IL-6, IL-8, IL-18 as well as of the tumor necrosis factor α (TNF-α), through this intensifying the immunological response of the body and development of cancer[19, 16, 20].

H. pylori have a carcinogenic effect in the stomach through one of two possible mechanisms:

i. direct transformation of the stomach's mucous membrane using the metabolic products of the body or

ii. quick transformation of the mucosa cells causing infection related damage to the mucous membrane which may elevate the risk of DNA damage, predisposing the mucosa to transformation by absorption or endogenic mutagens [21] and byproducts of the infection [22] such as peroxides and hydroxyl ions which can cause oxidative damage, mutation and malignant transformation [23].

Furthermore, it has been proven that the eradication of *H. pylori* in patients below the age of 40 can reduce the risk of gastric cancer occurrence [24].

2.8. Epstein-Barr virus infection

The Epstein-Barr virus (EBV) is a herpes gamma virus, which causes opportunistic lymphomas in immunologically compromised hosts, and in individuals without immunologic suppression. Mechanisms of EBV- related tumorigenesis may include:

- DNA methylation, which regulates host gene expressions and signal pathway through viral proteins
- viral small RNAs that can target host genes
- altered expression of microRNAs (miRNA) of host cells and
- other epigenetic alterations (chromatin conformation and histone modification) [25].

It has been shown that the frequency of EBV infections in patients with gastric cancer differs in different countries and ranges from 1.3% to 20.1%, an average of approximately 10%. In association with the presence of the EBV in cancerous cells this type of gastric cancer has been called the EBV-associated gastric carcinoma (EBVaGC). EBVaGC is a non-endemic disease since it is distributed throughout the world. This carcinoma shows some distinct clinicopathologic characteristics, such as male predominance, predisposition to the proximal part of the stomach, and a high proportion in diffuse-type gastric carcinomas. Also, EBVaGC shows some characteristic of molecular abnormality, like global and nonrandom CpG-island methylation of the promoter region of many cancer-related genes (p16, p73, CDH1). EBVaGC presents a relatively favorable prognosis [26-30].

2.9. Socioeconomic status

Throughout the world in 2002 2/3 of gastric cancer cases have been recorded in less developed nations. The poorest countries, especially African nations, stand out as having a relatively low morbidity coefficient for this type of tumor. However, this is caused by insufficient diagnosis and status of medical care [19]. Performance of some professions such as: butcher, farmer or fisherman predisposes one to an elevated risk of developing stomach cancer. This is associated with being exposed to herbicides or nitrates during work. Other professions exposed to a greater danger of carcinogenesis are: mechanic, manager, production supervisor as well as craftsmen, people working in stone quarries, metal industry, food industry, cooks, people working in laundries and cleaning personnel [19,31].

2.10. Migration

A reduction in the incidence of cancer is observed in an event of migration from an environment with a high risk coefficient to those having a lower coefficient, for example, migration of citizens of Japan to the United States. A significant fall in the occurrence of gastric cancer is observed in persons of Japanese origin born in the United States in comparison to recent immigrants [9]. Studies done on immigrants to the United States from countries with a high risk of gastric cancer occurrence, such as Japan or Poland, showed that subsequent generations of émigrés to the USA slowly become similar through following generations to native citizens of the country of settlement, meaning the risk of contracting the disease decreases [6].

2.11. Peptic ulcer

Patients suffering from gastric cancer often report having long lasting peptic ulcer disease of the stomach or the duodenum or gastrointestinal reflux disease. The symptoms of the diseases mentioned above and symptoms of early stages of gastric cancer are practically indistinguishable if correct forms of diagnostics are not utilized [32].

2.12. Family history of gastric cancer

Family history of gastric cancer has been studied in many regions including Eastern Asia, North America, Northern Europe and the nations of the Mediterranean region. Most cases of family history of gastric cancer have been recorded in the countries of the Mediterranean while the fewest cases of this type of disease have occurred in the countries of Western Europe. Additionally, it has been shown that family history of gastric cancer more often concerns women than men [33].

Occurrence of gastric cancer within a family significantly increases the risk of carcinogenesis. This is connected with similar environmental conditions in which a given family lives, genetic predispositions, habits, like smoking tobacco or a *Helicobacter pylori* infection [34,35]. Development of gastric cancer is observed in approximately 10 – 15% of people with the disease previously occurring among family members. Furthermore, the danger connected with the occurrence of gastric cancer in immediate family increases about 2 – 3 fold in families who are hereditarily degenerate [9,3]. Approximately 30% of gastric cancer cases connected to earlier occurrence of this tumor in family is linked to a mutation in the e-cadherine coding CDH1 gene [36].

Mutations in the e-cadherine coding gene (CDH1) lead to the inhibition of the reuptake of e-cadherine by the product of the APC gene as a result of which an intensification of the inflammatory response is observed. This results in an emergence of linitis plastica, a cancer which develops without the presence of *Helicobacter pylori* infection or chronic gastritis [4].

2.13. Level of pepsinogen in serum

Pepsinogen is a proenzyme of pepsin, a digestive enzyme produced in the mucous membrane of the stomach. Two subtypes of pepsinogen can be distinguished (sPG): pepsinogen I and pepsinogen II. Both subtypes are produced by chief cells, mucous neck cells and fundic glands. Pepsinogen II is also produced by the pyloric gland cells. When atrophy develops in the stomach, chief cells and fundic glands are replaced by pyloric gland cells, which leads to a decrease of the pepsinogen I level while the level of pepsinogen II remains unchanged. For this reason low levels of pepsinogen I and II are a good indicator of atrophic gastritis. Chronic atrophic gastritis is a precursor of gastric cancer, especially intestinal-type cancers. Hence designation of the level of pepsinogen in serum or the calculation of the coefficient of pepsinogen I/II is a good screening assay for gastric cancer. The ≤ 59 ng/ml level of pepsinogen I in serum and the ≤3.9 value of the coefficient of pepsinogen I/II have been regarded as the most predictive. The sensitivity of this test was 71% while the specificity reached 69.2% [37].

2.14. Single Nucleotide Polymorphisms (SNAPs)

2.14.1. Polymorphism of IL1B

Interleukin 1 beta (IL1B) is a proinflammatory cytokine which regulates the expression of some particles taking part in the inflammation process. It has been shown that the two functionally important polymorphisms in the promoter region, IL1B-31T/C and -511C/T, are connected to an increased risk of developing gastric cancer [38, 39].

2.14.2. Polymorphism of IL-8

IL-8 is a member of the α-chemokine family which acts as a strong chemoattractant and neurofilia activator. It has been suggested that this interleukin is strongly associated with the processes of carcinogenesis, angiogenesis, adhesion, invasion and metastasis. Hull et al. demonstrated the presence of a polymorphism of a single nucleotide in the -251 (A/T) position from the transcription starting place in a region closer to the promoter as well as a connection between the presence of the allele IL-8-251A and an increase in the production of IL-8 and an elevated risk of gastric cancer development in the cardia. The presence of the IL-8 251AA genotype was connected with increased risk of gastric cancer development in an Asian population, mainly Han Chinese as well as in intestinal-type cancer [41,42].

2.14.3. Polymorphism of IL-10

Interleukine-10 (IL-10) is an anti-inflammatory cytokine which regulates the cell immunological response. In the gene coding IL-10 three polymorphic promoter variants, located in positions -1082 (A>G), -819 (T>C) and -592 (A>C) have been discovered. These variants are connected with an elevated production of IL-10 and an increased risk of the occurrence of gastric cancer, especially the intestinal non-cardia gastric cancer. What is more, polymorphism of the gene coding IL-10 in combination with environmental factors, such as cigarette smoking or an *H. pylori* infection creates favorable conditions for the occurrence and progression of gastritis and carcinogenesis [43]. Additionally, polymorphism of IL-10 can influence the immune system by changing the activity of the NK, T cells and macrophages and in this manner influence the disease progression [44].

2.14.4. Polymorphism of IL-17A and IL-17F

Interleukin 17A and 17F are inflammatory cytokines, which play a critical role in inflammation and probably in cancer. An association has been found between IL-17F A7488G polymorphisms and the risk of intestinal-type gastric cancer. This polymorphism may influence the multi-steps of gastric carcinogenesis. Furthermore, patients having IL-17F 7488GA genotype had increased risk of large tumor size and lymph- node metastasis. Positive associations have been found between IL-17A 197AG genotype and elderly onset, early TNM stage and poorly differentiated gastric cancers [45].

2.14.5. Polymorphism of TLR2 and TRL4

TRLs are important innate immunity receptors. TRL2 and TRL4 promote transcription of genes involved in immune response activation including nuclear factor kappa B (NF-κB). TRL2 activates NF-κB in response to *H. pylori* infection, causing the expression of IL-8. TRL4 up regulated in gastric epithelial cell infected by *H. pylori*; expression of the TRL4 protein has been demonstrated in chronic active gastritis and in gastric tumor cells. It has been demonstrated that the presence of the TRL2-169 to -174del I TRL4+896G (Asp299Gly) polymorphic variant can increase the risk of gastric cancer development, especially the non-cardia intestinal-type [46-49].

2.14.6. Polymorphism of TP53

The TP53 gene is one of the most frequent targets for genetic mutations. The p53 pathway is crucial for effective prevention of genetically damaged cell propagation, either directly, by its participation in DNA repair mechanisms, or indirectly by induction of apoptosis. TP53 72ArgArg seems to be the survival factor for gastric cancer patients more advanced in years, while the TP53 Pro-A1 plays the same role in younger patients with this type of tumor. Additionally tumors at more advanced stages (III and IV) showed TP53 intron 3 A2A2 genotype carriers [50-52].

2.15. Gene mutations

2.15.1. CDH1 mutation

The germline CDH1 mutation is associated with the development of hereditary cancer syndrome, called hereditary diffuse gastric cancer (HDGC). Germline mutation of the CDH1 gene has also been discovered in patients with sporadic early onset gastric cancer (EOGC). Mutation of this gene has been described for the first time in 1998 in New Zealand in a Maori family with history of diffused gastric cancer. Various types of CDH1 gene mutations such as deletion, inertia, nonsense, and truncating have been described. The risk of developing gastric cancer with the occurrence of a non-missense mutation of the CDH1 gene is high at >80%, while with the occurrence of a missense mutation of this gene the risk has not been defined [53-55].

CDH1 gene (E-cadherin gene), is one of the most important tumor suppressor genes in gastric cancer. The mutations, chromosomal deletions, epigenetic modifications have been reported as a mechanisms, that cause CDH1 inactivation. Somatic CDH1 mutations have been found in about 50% of diffuse gastric cancer, germline mutations have been reported in familial gastric cancers.

http://dx.doi.org/10.5772/52136

CANCER SITE	CASES	(%) BOTH SEXES	ASR (world)
lip, oral cavity	263	2,1	3.9
Nosopharynx	84	0,7	1.2
other pharynx	135	1,1	0.2
Oesophagus	482	3,8	7.0
Stomach	**989**	**7,8**	**14.1**
Colorectum	1233	9,7	17.3
Liver	748	5,9	10.8
Gallbladder	145	1,1	2.0
Pancreas	277	2,2	3.9
Laryngx	151	1,2	2.3
Lung	1608	12,7	23.0
malanoma of skin	197	1,6	2.8
Kaposi sarcoma	34	0,3	0.5
Breast	1383	10,9	39.0
cervix uteri	529	4,2	15.2
corpus uteri	287	2,3	8.2
Ovary	225	1,8	6.3
Prostate	913	7,2	28.5
Testis	52	0,4	1.5
Kidney	271	2,1	3.9
Bladder	386	3	5.3
brain, nervous system	238	1,9	3.5
Thyroid	212	1,7	3.1
Hodkin lymphoma	67	0,5	1.0
non-Hodkin lymphoma	355	2,8	5.1
multiple myeloma	102	0,8	1.5
Leukemia	351	2,8	5.1

Table 1. Estimated new cancer cases (thousands), ASRs (per 100,000) and cumulative risks (percent) by sex and cancer site worldwide, 2008 [64].

CANCER SITE	**DEATHS**	**(%) BOTH SEXES**	**ASR (world)**
lip, oral cavity	127	1.7	1.9
Nosopharynx	51	0.7	0.8
other pharynx	95	1.3	1.4
Oesophagus	406	5.4	5.8
Stomach	**738**	**9.7**	**10.3**
Colorectum	608	8.0	8.2
Liver	695	9.2	10.0
Gallbladder	109	1.4	1.5
Pancreas	266	3.5	3.7
Laryngx	82	1.1	1.2
Lung	1378	18.2	19.4
malanoma of skin	46	0.6	0.6
Kaposi sarcoma	29	0.4	0.4
Breast	458	6.0	12.5
cervix uteri	274	3.6	7.8
corpus uteri	74	1.0	2.0
Ovary	140	1.8	3.8
Prostate	258	3.4	7.5
Testis	9	0.1	0.3
Kidney	116	1.5	1.6
Bladder	150	2.0	2.0
brain, nervous system	174	2.3	2.6
Thyroid	35	0.5	0.5
Hodkin lymphoma	30	0.4	0.4
non-Hodkin lymphoma	191	2.5	2.7
multiple myeloma	72	1.0	1.0
Leukemia	257	3.4	3.6

Table 2. Estimated cancer deaths (thousands), ASRs (per 100,000) and cumulative risks (percent) by sex and cancer site worldwide, 2008 [64].

REGION	MALE	FEMALE
Eastern Africa	4.0	3.3
Middle Africa	1.7	1.8
Northern Africa	2.9	1.9
Southern Africa	0.7	0.5
Western Africa	3.3	2.6
Caribbean	2.4	1.6
Central America	7.7	6.5
South America	29.3	17.9
Northen America	15.1	9.4
Eastern America	408.2	193.1
South-Eastern Asia	24.9	18.4
South-Central Asia	41.9	26.2
Western Asia	9.2	5.6
Cenral and Eastern Europe	43.3	30.6
Northern Europe	7.8	4.9
Southern Eutope	20.0	12.9
Western Europe	16.5	10.9
Australia/New Zealand	1.5	0.8
Melanesia	0.2	0.1
Micronesia/Polynesia	0.0	0.0

Table 3. Estimated numbers of new gastric cancer cases (thousands) by sex and regions, 2008 [64].

REGION	MALE	FEMALE
Eastern Africa	3.8	3.1
Middle Africa	1.6	1.7
Northern Africa	2.7	1.8
Southern Africa	0.6	0.5
Western Africa	3.1	2.5
Caribbean	1.8	1.2
Central America	6.4	5.6
South America	24.2	15.1
Northen America	7.6	5.2
Eastern America	274.3	144.2
South-Eastern Asia	20.1	15.3
South-Central Asia	39.5	24.1
Western Asia	8.1	4.9
Cenral and Eastern Europe	38.2	26.6
Northern Europe	5.4	3.6
Southern Eutope	14.6	9.8
Western Europe	11.1	7.9
Australia/New Zealand	0.9	0.6
Melanesia	0.2	0.1
Micronesia/Polynesia	0.0	0.0

Table 4. Estimated numbers of gastric cancer deaths (thousands) by sex and regions, 2008 [64].

2.15.2. DNA methylation

DNA methylation is an epigenetic mechanism regulating transcription which in cancer is attributed to the inappropriate silencing of tumor suppressor genes, or loss of oncogene repression. Methylation pattern of DNA can be useful in assessing the risk of cancer occurrence, prognosis and success of treatment. Aberrant DNA methylation appears in early stages of carcinogenesis, which makes it especially useful to predict the risk of contracting cancer. Methylated DNA is stable and has a high detectability (as much as 1:1000 particles) in biological fluids. What is more, in cancer patients DNA methylation can be an indicator of an answer for applied chemotherapy as well as can indicate a shorter time of post-operative survival [56-59].

2.15.3. RUNX3 promoter methylation

Runt-related transcription factor (RUNX3), a member of the runt domain family of transcription factors, plays an important role in the signaling path of the TGF-β (transforming growth factor β). In many reports not only the role of the RUNX3 in the correct development but also in the progression of cancer has been demonstrated. It has been shown that in younger gastric cancer patients the methylation of the RUNX3 promoter was associated with histological type and level of tumor differentiation. It has been suggested that RUNX3 promoter methylation or down-regulation of the RUNX3 gene may be related to a poor prognosis [60,61].

2.15.4. CHRF promoter methylation

CHRF (checkpoint with FHA and RING finger) is an important tumor suppressor gene. CHRF encodes a protein within the FHA and RING finger domain that governs transition from prophase to metaphase in the mitotic checkpoint pathway. Aberrant methylation of the CHRF gene is a frequent event in gastric cancer. The methylation rate of CHRF gene in stomach carcinoma was significantly higher than in paired normal gastric mucosa and it was associated with poorly differentiated tumor cells. Also, CHRF gene methylation was associated with the degree of malignancy of gastric cancer. The CHRF mRNA or protein expression level was down-regulated or loss [62,63].

3. Conclusion

Gastric carcinogenesis is a complex multistep process resulting from the interaction between genome and environmental factors. Many exogenous factors seem to contribute to the initiation of carcinogenesis in the stomach, including diet (especially high in salt, smoked or pickled foods, grilled meats or smoked fish), chronic a trophic gastritis with intestinal metaplasia, gastric ulcer, dysplasia, and partial resection of gastric polyps. Others risk factors for this cancer is chemical agents and infections, e. g. caused by Helicobacter pylori and Epstein- Barr virus. Also, genetic factors, such as blood group A, familial polyposis and the presence of gastric cancer among family members play a role in the development of this cancer. This group of factors also include radiation or pernicious anemia. Additionally, dysfunction of CDH1 gene (E-cadherin-coding gene) together with mutation have been found in diffuse-type gastric carcinoma. Mutation in CDH1 is a genetic defect found in approximately 1/3 of familial gastric cancers such as hereditary diffuse gastric cancers (HDGC). Also, the presence of single nucleotide polymorphisms (SNPs) in several genes can modulate the risk of gastric cancer.

Knowledge of various risk factors for stomach cancer can help to determined the risk of development this cancer. Also, a small change in diet or lifestyle can significantly reduce this risk.

Author details

Jolanta Czyzewska*

Address all correspondence to: czyzyk15@op.pl

Department of Clinical Laboratory Diagnostics Medical University of Bialystok, Bialystok, Poland

References

[1] Kelley, JR, & Duggon, JM. Gastric cancer epidemiology and risk factors. Commentary. J Clin Epidemiol 2003;56(1):1-9.

[2] Master SS. Gastric cancer. Dis Mon 2004;50(10):532-539.

[3] Leung WK, Wu M, Kakugawa Y, Kim JJ, Yeoh KG, Goh KL, Wu KC, Wu DC, Sollano J, Kachintorn U, Gotoda T, Lin JT, You WC, Ng EK, Sung JJ; Asia Pacific Working Group of Gastric Cancer. Screening for gastric cancer in Asia: current evidence and practice. Lancet Oncol 2008; 9(3):279-287.

[4] Crew KD, Neugut AL. Epidemiology of gastric cancer. World J Gastroenterol 2006; 12(3): 354-362.

[5] Robbins S, Olszewski WT. Patologia, Wrocław, 2010.

[6] Popiela T. Rakżołądka, Warszawa, 1987.

[7] Jee SH, Yun JE, Park EJ, Cho ER, Park IS, Sull JW, Ohrr H, Samet JM. Body mass index and cancer risk in Korean men and women. Int J Cancer 2008,123(8):1892-1896.

[8] Tsugane S, Sasazuki S. Diet and the risk of gastric cancer: review of epidemiological evidence. Gastric Cancer 2007:10(2):75-83.

[9] Catalono V, Labianca R, Beretta GD, Gatta G, de Braud F, Van Custem E. Gastric cancer. Crit Rev Oncol Hematol 2009;71(2):127-164.

[10] Moy KA, Fan Y, Wang R, Gao YT, Yu MC, Yuan JM. Alcohol and tobacco use in relation to gastric cancer: a prospective study of men in Shanghai, China. Cancer Epidemiol Biomarkers Prev. 2010, 19(9): 2287-2297.

[11] Sklyarov A, Yu. Mandryl: Wpływ alkoholu na funkcje wydzielnicze i barierę śluzową żołądka. Medycyna Ogólna 2004: 1-2.

[12] Tian W, Zhao Y, Liu S, Li X. Meta-analysis on the relationship between nonsteroidal anti-inflammatory drug use and gastric cancer. Eur J Gastric Prev 2010;19(4): 288-298.

[13] Watanabe M, Kawai T, Takata Y, Yamashina A. Gastric mucosal damage evaluated by transnasalendoskopy and QOL assessments in ischemic hart disease patients receiving low-dose aspiryn. Inter Med 2011;50(6):539-544.

[14] Oshima T, Miwa H, Joh T. Aspirin induces gastric epithelial barrier dysfunction by activating p28 MAPK via claudin-7. Am J Physiol Cell Physiol 2008;295(3):C800-806.

[15] Wang WH, Huang JQ, Zheng GF, Lam SK, Kerlberg J, Wong BC. Non-steroidal anti-inflammatory drug use and risk of gastric cancer: a systematic review and meta-analysis. J Natl Cancer Inst 2003;95(23):1784-1791.

[16] Kikuchi S. Epidemiology of Helicobacter pylori and gastric cancer. Gastric Cancer 2002;5(1):6-15.

[17] Miwa H, Go MF, Sato N. H. pylori and gastric cancer: the Asian enigma. Am J Gastroenterol 2002,97(5):1101-1112.

[18] O'Connor KG. Gastric cancer. Semi Oncol Nurs 1999;15(1):26-35.

[19] Clark CJ, Thirlby RC, Picozzi V Jr, Schembre DB, Cummings FP, Lin E. Current problems in surgery: gastric cancer. Cerr Probl Surg 2006;43(8-9):566-670.

[20] Zheng L, Wang L, Ajani J, Xie K. Molecular basis of gastric cancer development and progression. Gastric Cancer 2004,7(2):61-77.

[21] Correa P, Ruiz B, Shi TT, Janney A, Sobhan M, Torrado J, Hunter F. Helicobacter pylori and nucleolar organizer regions in gastric antral mucosa. Am J Clin Pathol 1994;101(5):656-660.

[22] Tamura G, Sakata K, Nishizuka S, Maesawa C, Suzuki Y, Iwaga T, Terashima M, Saito K, Satodate R. Analysis of the fragile histidine triad gene in the primary gastric carcinomas and gastric carcinoma cell lines. Genes Chromosomes Cancer 1997;20(1): 98-102.

[23] Ames BN, Gold LS. Too many rodent carcinogenesis: mitogenesis increases mutagenesis. Science 1990;249(4972):970-971.

[24] Feldman RA. Review article: Would eradication of Helicobacter pylori infection reduce the risk of gastric cancer? Aliment Pharmacol Ther 2001;1:2-5.

[25] Koneda A, Matsusaka K, Aburatani H, Fukayama M. Epstein- Barr virus infection as an epigenetic driver of tumorigenesis. Cancer Res 2012, 72(14):3445-3450.

[26] Lee JH, Kim SH, Han SH, An JS, Lee ES, Kim YS. Clinicopathological and molecular characteristics of Epstein-Barr virus-associated gastric carcinoma: a meta-analysis. J Gastroenterol Hepatol 2009,24(3):354-365.

[27] Osawa T, Chong JM, Sudo M, Sakuma K, Uozaki H, Shibahara J, Nagai H, Funata N, Fukayama M. Reduced expression and promoter methylation of p16 gene in Epstein-Barr virus-associated gastric carcinoma. Jpn J Cancer Res 2002,93(11):1195-1200.

[28] Ushiku T, Chong JM, Uozaki H, Hino R, Chang MS, Sudo M, Rani BR, Sakuma K, Nagai H, Fukayam M. p73 gene promoter methylation in Epstein-Barr virus-associated gastric carcinoma. Int J Cancer 2007;120(1):60-66.

[29] Sudo M, Chong JM, Sakuma K, Ushiku T, Uozaki H, Nagai H, Funata N, Matsumoto J, Fukayama M. Promoter hypermethylation of E-cadherin and its abnormal expression in Epstein-Barr virus-associated gastric carcinoma. Int J Cancer 2004;109(2): 194-199.

[30] van Beek J, zurHausen A, Klein Kranenbarg E, van de Velde CJ, Middeldorp JM, van de Brule AJ, Meijer CJ, Bloemena E. EBV-positive gastric adenocarcinomas: a distinct clinicopathologic entity with a low frequency of lymph node involvement. J Clin Oncol 2004;22(4):664-670.

[31] Bhattacharyya NK, Chatterjee U, Sarkar S, KunduAK. A study of proliferative activity, angiogenesis and nuclear grading in renal cell carcinoma. Indian J Pathol Microbiol 2008;51(1):17-21.

[32] Haglund U, Wallner B. Current management of gastric cancer. J Gastrointest Sur 2004;8(7):905-912.

[33] Zhou XF, He YL, Song W, Peng JJ, Zhang Ch, Li W, Wu H. Comparison of patients by family history with gastric and non-gastric cancer. World J Gastroenterol 2009;15(21): 2644-2650.

[34] Shin CM, Kim N, Yang HJ, Cho S, Lee HS, Kim JS, Jung HC, Song IS. Stomach cancer risk in gastric cancer relatives interaction between Helicobacter pylori infection and family history of gastric cancer for the risk of stomach cancer. J Clin Gastroenterol 2010;44(2):e34-39.

[35] Terry MB, Gaudet MM, Gammon MD. The epidemiology of gastric cancer. Semin Radiat Oncol 2002;12(2):111-127.

[36] Hartgrink HH, Jansen EP, van Grieken NC, van de Velde CJ. Gastric cancer. Lancet 2009;374(9688):447-490.

[37] Shikata K, Ninomiya T, Yonemoto K, Ikeda F, Hata J, Doi Y, Fukuhara M, Matsumoto T, Ilda M, Kitazono T, Kiyohara Y. Optimal cutoff value of the serum pepsinogen

level for prediction of gastric cancer incidence: the Hisayama study. Scand J Gastroenterol 2012;47(6):669-675.

[38] McColl KE, El-Omar E. How does H. pylori infection cause gastric cancer? Keio J Med 2002;51:53-56.

[39] El-Omar EM, Carrington M, Chow WH, McColl KE, Bream JH, Young HA, Herrera J, Lissowska J, Yuan CC, Rothman N, Lanyon G, Martin M, Fraumeni JF Jr, Rabkin CS. Interleukin-1 polymorphisms associated with increased risk of gastric cancer. Nature 2000;404(6776):398-402.

[40] Hull J, Thomson A, Kwiatkowski D. Association of respiratory syncytial virus bronchiolitis with the interleukin 8 gene region in UK families. Thorax 2000;55(12):1023-1027.

[41] Xue H, Liu J, Lin B, Wang Z, Sun J, Huang G. A meta-analysis of interleukin-8-251 promoter polymorphism associated with gastric cancer risk. PLoS One 2011;7(1):e28083-e28097.

[42] Savage SA, Abnet CC, Mark SD, Qiao LY, Dong ZW, Dawsey SM, Taylor PR, Chanock SJ. Variants of the IL8 and IL8RB genes and risk for gastric cardia adenocarcinoma and esophagel squamous cell carcinoma. Cancer Epidemiol Biomarkers Prev 2004;13(12):2251-2257.

[43] Kim J, Cho YA, Choi IJ, Lee Y-S, Kim S-Y, Shin A, Cho S-J, Kook M-Ch, Nam JH, Ryu KW, Lee JH, Kim YW. Effects of interleukin-10 polymorphisms, Helicobacter pylori infection, and smoking on the risk of noncardia gastric cancer. PLoS One 2012;7(1):e29643-e29650.

[44] Liu J, Song B, Bai X, Liu W, Li Z, Wang J, Zheng Y, Wang Z. Association of genetic polymorphisms on the interleukin-10 promoter with risk of prostate cancer in Chinese. BMC Cancer 2010;10:456.

[45] Wu X, Zeng Z, Chen B, Yu J, Xue L, Hao Y, Chen M, Sung JJ, Hu P. Association between polymorphisms in interleukin-17A and interleukin-17F genes and risks of gastric cancer. Int J Cancer 2010;127:86-92.

[46] Trejo- de la OA, Torres J, Perez-Rodriguez M, Camorlinga- Ponce M, Luna LF, Abdo-Francis JM, Lazcano E, Maldonado- Bernal C. TRL4 single-nucleotide polymorphisms alter mucosal cytokine and chemokine patterns in Mexican patients with Helicobacter pylori- associated gastroduodenal diseases. Clin Immunol 2008;129(2):333-340.

[47] Seya T, Shime H, Ebihara T, Oshiumi H, Matsumoto M. Pattern recognition receptors of innate immunity and their application to tumor immunotherapy. Cancer Sci 2010;101(2):313-320.

[48] Tahara T, Arisawa T, Wang F, Shibata T, Nakamura M, Sakata M, Hirata J, Nakano H. Toll-like receptor 2 (TRL)-196 to 174del polymorphism In gastro- duodenal diseases In Japanese population. Dig Dis Sci 2008;53(4):919-924.

[49] de Oliveira JG, Silva AE. Polymorphisms of the TRL2 and TRL4 genes are associated with risk of gastric cancer in a Brazilian population. World J Gastroenterol 2012;18(11):1235-1242.

[50] Andre AR, Ferreira MV, Mota RM, Ferrasi AC, Pardini MI, Rabenhorst SH. Gastric adenocarcinoma and Helicobacter pylori: correlation with p53mutation and p27 immunoexpression. Cancer Epidemiol 2010;34(5):618-625.

[51] Nayak A, Ralte AM, Sharma MC, Sinhg VP, Mahapatra AK, Mehta VS, Sarkar C. p53 protein alternations in adult astrocytic tumors and oligodendrogliomas. Neurol India 2004;52(2):228-232.

[52] Filho EHCN, Cordeiro DEF, Vieira APF, Rabenhorst SHB. TP53 codon 72 and intron 3 polymorphisms and mutational status in gastric cancer: an association with tumor onest and prognosis. Pathobiology 2012;79(6):323-328.

[53] Guiford P, Hopkins J, Harraway J, McLeod M, McLeod N, Harwira P, Taite H, Scoular R, Miller A, Reeve AE. E-cadherin germline mutations in familial gastric cancer. Nature 1998;392(6674):402-405.

[54] Fitzgerald RC, Hardwick R, Huntsman D, Carneiro F, Guilford P, Blair V, Chung DC, Norton J, Ragunath K, Van Krieken JH, Dwerryhouse S, Caldas C. International Gastric Cancer Linkage Consortium: hereditary diffuse gastric cancer: updated guidelines for clinical management and directions for future research. J Med Genet 2010;47(7):436-444.

[55] Corso G, Pedrazzani C, Pinheiro H, Fernandes E, Marrelli D, Rinnovati A, Pascale V, Seruca R, Oliveira C, Roviello F. E-cadherin genetic screening and clinico- pathologic characteristics of early onest gastric cancer. Eur J Cancer 2011;47(4):631-639.

[56] Laird PW. The power and the promise of DNA methylation markers. Nat Rev Cancer 2003;3(4):253-266.

[57] Nakajima T, Enomoto S, Ushijima T. DNA methylation: a marker for carcinogen exposure and cancer risk. Environ Health Prev Med 2008;13(1):8-15.

[58] Napieralski R, Ott K, Kremer M, Becker R, Boulesteix AL, Lordick F, Siewert JR, Höfler H, Keller G . Methylation of tumour-related genes in neoadjuvant-treated gastric cancer: relation to therapy response and clinicopathologic and molecular features. Clin Cancer Res 2007;13(17):5095-5102.

[59] Sapari NS, Loh M, Vaithilingam A, Soong R. Clinical potential of DNA methylation in gastric cancer: a meta-analysis. PLoS ONE 2012;7(4):e36275-e36283.

[60] Fan X, Hu XI, Han T, Wang N, Zhu Y, Hu W, MaZ, Zhang Ch, Xu X, Ye Z, Han Ch, Pan W. Association between RUNX3 promoter methylation and gastric cancer: a meta0analysis. BMC Gastroenterology 2011;11:92-101.

[61] Fukamachi H, Ito K. Growth regulation of gastric epithelial cells by RUNX3. Oncogene 2004;23(24):4330-4335.

[62] Scolnick DM, Halazonetis TD. Chrf defines a mitotic stress checkpoint that delays entry into metaphase. Nature 2000;406:430-435.

[63] Gao YJ, Xin Y, Zhang JJ, Zhou J. Mechanism and pathobiologic implications of CHRF promoter methylation in gastric carcinoma. World J Gastroenterol 2008,14(32): 5000-5007.

[64] Farley J, Shin HR, Bray F, Forman D, Mathers C, Parkin DM. Estimates of worldwide burden of cancer in 2008: GLOBOCAN 2008. Int J Cancer 2010;127(12):2893-2917.

Chapter 4

Relevance of Host Factors in Gastric Cancer Associated with *Helicobacter Pylori*

Elvira Garza-González and
Guillermo Ignacio Pérez-Pérez

Additional information is available at the end of the chapter

http://dx.doi.org/10.5772/51792

1. Introduction

In spite of a decline in incidence and mortality of gastric cancer over the last decades, it is still the fourth most common cancer and the second most common cause of cancer death in the world. The differences in prevalence of gastric cancer have been explained as a multifactorial process with an interaction involving both infection with *Helicobacter pylori* as a triggering factor and host genetic susceptibility as an important explanation for interindividual variation in gastric cancer risk. To discuss the genetic host polymorphisms, we classified them into first stage and second stage host genetic factors. In the first stage, *H. pylori* related inflammation seems to play a critical role in the development of gastric cancer; in the second stage, participation of tumor suppressor proteins and oncogenes appears to define the course of the disease. At present, there is no definitive host genetic risk marker, and evidence suggests that each proposed host risk factor should be evaluated in specific ethnic populations to define its importance. In this chapter, we present the most relevant up to date data on genetic polymorphisms that have been associated with an increased risk for the development of gastric cancer, its potential role in the development of this neoplasia, and its interplay with the virulence factors of the bacteria.

2. Epidemiology of gastric cancer

Stomach cancer is the fourth most common cancer worldwide with 930, 000 cases diagnosed in 2002 [1]. Despite a major decline in incidence and mortality over the last decades, stomach cancer is still the fourth most common cancer and the second most common cause of cancer death in the world, accounting for more than 803, 000 deaths each year.

It has been observed that there is a 10-fold variation in incidence between populations with the highest and lowest risk. For instance, the incidence of gastric adenocarcinoma is higher in East Asia, Central America, and South America than in most other parts of the world and is about twice as high among men [2]. This neoplasia is rare before the age of 40, and its incidence peaks in the seventh decade of life [3]. According to the National Cancer Institute, gastric cancer is more common in people over the age of 72 (National Cancer Institute) and the diagnosis of gastric cancers is frequently made based on dyspeptic and alarm symptoms. Unfortunately, sometimes alarm symptoms are not sufficiently sensitive to detect malignancies. Dysphagia, weight loss and a palpable abdominal mass appear to be major independent prognostic factors in gastric cancer, but when these symptoms appear, the patients are usually in advanced stages of cancer [4].

The difference in the prevalence of gastric cancer throughout the world has been described from different points of view. One of the most accepted explanations is that the development of gastric cancer is multifactorial with an interplay involving both infection with *Helicobacter pylori* and host polymorphisms in a process initiated by specific *H. pylori* genotypes and the host immune response [5].

3. Gastric cancer and *Helicobacter pylori*

H. pylori is a Gram-negative spiral-shaped bacterium that persistently colonizes the human stomach. It is the most common chronic bacterial infection worldwide and is associated with diverse clinical outcomes that range from asymptomatic gastritis to more serious conditions, such as peptic ulcer disease and gastric cancer [6, 7].

In general, countries with a high incidence of stomach cancer have a high prevalence of *H. pylori* infection but in Europe only a small fraction of those infected by *H. pylori* develop stomach cancer [8]. In Japan, the country with the highest incidence of stomach cancer in the world, it has been estimated that of the 60 million people infected by *H. pylori*, only 0.4% had stomach cancer [9].

The worldwide prevalence of *H. pylori* is more than 50% in the adult population and the incidence of *H. pylori* related diseases varies considerably throughout the world. After the discovery of *H. pylori*, it was reported that *H pylori*-positive subjects have a two to three-fold increased risk of developing gastric cancer when compared with H pylori-negative subjects. The risk was even higher in subjects infected with strains encoding the *H pylori cag*A, *vac*A s1 and *bab*A2, which are the main virulence genes related to this bacterium [10, 11].

One of the most prominent differences in gene content among *H. pylori* strains is the presence or absence of a 40-kb region of chromosomal DNA known as the cag pathogenicity island (PAI) [12, 13]. This island involves the cagA-encoded CagA protein, which is delivered into gastric epithelial cells via the bacterial type IV secretion system, where it undergoes tyrosine phosphorylation by Src and Abl kinases. Tyrosine-phosphorylated CagA then acquires the ability to interact with and deregulate SHP-2 phosphatase, the deregulation of this enzyme is involved in a variety of human malignancies (Figure 1). CagA also binds to and inhibits PAR1b/MARK2 polarity-regulating kinase to alter tight junctions and epithelial apical-basolateral polarity. These CagA activities may collectively contribute to the transformation of gastric epithelial cells [14].

Despite the overwhelming evidence that *H. pylori* infection is a risk factor for noncardia gastric cancer, accumulating evidence shows that although *H. pylori* eradication is relatively simple to accomplish. Impacting the global burden of gastric cancer will be a more difficult challenge.

H. pylori infection is a key risk factor for chronic atrophic gastritis, an established precursor of gastric cancer. There is increasing evidence of frequent elimination of the infection during progression of chronic atrophic gastritis and it has been proposed that there is a higher elimination of *H. pylori* during the development of the disease [15].

H. pylori,cagA+ strain, is an established risk factor for stomach cancer and *H. pylori* infection and cagA+ status have been inversely associated with a new diagnosis of Barrett's esophagus [16]. The findings are consistent with the hypothesis that *H. pylori* colonization protects against Barrett's esophagus and that the association may be at least partially mediated through Gastroesophageal Reflux Disease (GERD).

It has been recently proven that *H pylori* infection is associated with significantly reduced risks of esophageal adenocarcinoma and adenocarcinomas of the esophagogastric junction but not with squamous cell carcinomas [17].

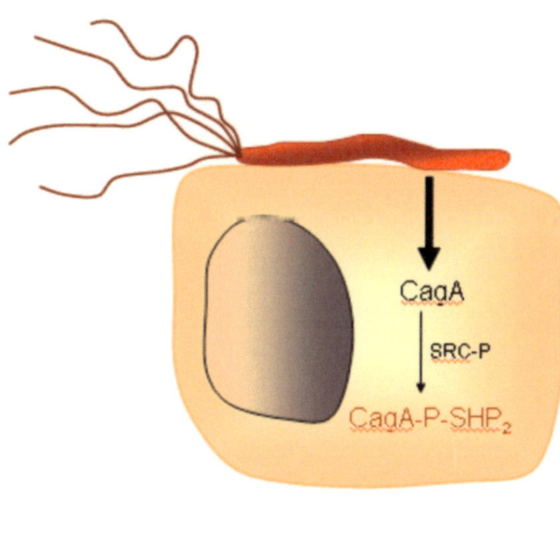

Figure 1. Cag A is translocated through a type IV secretion system. Once inside the cell, it is tyrosine-phosphorylated and binds to and activates Src homology 2-containing protein-tyrosine phosphatase-2 (SHP-2).

Infection with cagA-positive *H. pylori* seems to play an essential role in the development of gastric carcinoma [18], although the bacteria alone cannot be considered a unique factor in the promotion of gastric cancer. Host susceptibility has also been involved in this process, the interaction of some *H. pylori* genotypes, in relation to host polymorphisms can lead to gastric cancer. When *H. pylori* is eliminated in patients treated for early stage gastric cancer, the risk of developing a second gastric cancer decreases by two-thirds [19].

4. Host genetic polymorphisms and cancer susceptibility

Host genetic factors play an important role in influencing disease risk, but identifying candidate genes is a major challenge that requires a fundamental understanding of the disease [20]. The best-established risk factors for stomach cancer are *H. pylori* infection--by far the strongest established risk factor for distal stomach cancer--as well as male gender, a family history of stomach cancer, and smoking [21, 22].

5. Gastric carcinogenesis.

The precancerous process had been the subject of inquiry way before the scientific community was aware of *H. pylori* as a human pathogen. The histopathology of the precancerous stages has long been recognized: chronic gastritis, gland loss (atrophy), intestinal metaplasia (complete and incomplete), and epithelial dysplasia. Progression of the process in high-risk populations has been documented [23, 24].

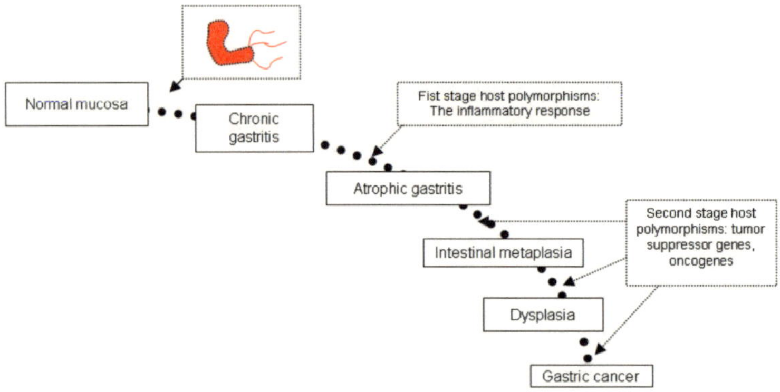

Figure 2. Modified model of carcinogenesis proposed by Correa Pelayo. *H. pylori* acts as a pivotal factor in the development of gastritis. Increased chronic inflammation is influenced by genetic susceptibility factors (fist stage genes) and progression of the disease is strongly influenced by second stage genes. Table 1 resumes both the first stage and second stage genes

The discovery of *H. pylori* strongly supported the carcinogenesis model triggering the response (Figure 2), with other factors having important roles in the progression thorough the carcinogenesis cascade. In the next paragraphs, some of the host factors involved will be discussed. The first group of genes related to host susceptibility is the "first stage genes", *i.e.*, which influence the first stage of the cascade and are related to a more intense inflammatory response after gastritis associated to *H. pylori* infection is clearly established in the stomach. "Second stage genes" seem to have an important role after atrophic gastritis has been established. The inflammatory process leads to *in situ* mutations and strong activity of antitumor genes such as p53 and oncogenes such as *c-fos, c-jun c-met, K-sam,* and *K-ras.*

Protein/Effectors	**Polymorphism or alleles**	**Effect**	**References**
First stage			
Interleukin-1 beta and its receptor antagonist	*IL-1B-31*C* *IL-1B-511*T* *IL-1RN*2*	High-level expression of IL-1B, reduction of acid output corpus and colonization by *H. pylori.* *IL-1B-31*C, IL-1B-511*T,* and *IL-1RN*2* alleles are associated to an increased risk of gastric cancer.	[25 - 32]
Interleukin-8	*IL-8-251*	High IL-8 levels are found in gastric cancer. *IL-8-251* *A allele is associated to a higher production of IL-8.	[33 - 37]
Nucleotide-binding oligomerization domain containing 2 (NOD2)	*NOD2 R702W*	NOD2 is upregulated in gastric epithelial cells of patients with chronic infection by H. pylori. NOD2 R702W has been associated to gastric lymphoma.	[38, 39]
Cyclooxygenase 2 (COX-2)	*PTGS2 5939C*	COX-2 is over-expressed in gastric cancer and in *H. pylori* infection. PTGS2 5939C allele carriers were at increased risk of gastric cancer.	[40 , 41]
Toll like receptor 4	*TLR4 Asp299Gly* *TLR4 Thr399Ile* *TLR4+3725 G/C*	TLR-4 is associated to hyporesponsiveness to LPS and therefore to H. pylori.	[22 , 42]
Interleukin-10	*IL-10 -1082 G/A* *IL-10 –819 C/T* *IL-10 –592 C/A* *IL-10 ATA* *IL-10 GCC* *IL-10 ACC*	Low secretion of IL-10 is associated to high inflammation and high risk to gastric cancer. Haplotype ATA is low IL-10 secreting and haplotype GCC is high IL-10 secreting.	[43]
Selenoprotein S	*SEPS1 -105 G/A*	Selenoprotein S participate in retro-translocation of misfolded proteins from the endoplasmic reticulum to the cytosol for their degradation.	[44 - 46]

Protein/Effectors	Polymorphism or alleles	Effect	References
		Association between the proximal promoter SEPS1 -105G/A polymorphism with circulating levels of pro-inflammatory IL-1β and TNF-α Selenoprotein S (SEPS1) gene -105G"/A promoter polymorphism influences the susceptibility to gastric cancer in the Japanese population.	
Reactive oxygen species (ROS) and reactive nitrogen species (RNS)		Production of ROS and RNS increase gastric inflammation and therefore carcinogenesis. *H. pylori*-induced ROS production affects gastric epithelial cell signal transduction, resulting in gastric carcinogenesis.	[47]
Survivin		Survivin downregulation correlate with apoptosis. Infection with *H. pylori* decreases survivin levels in the mucosa of patients with gastritis.	[48]
Second stage			
E-cadherin	*CDH1, OMIM +192090*	E-cadherin is a calcium dependent cell-cell adhesion glycoprotein. Heterozygous germline point or small frameshift mutations in the E-cadherin gene (*CDH1*, OMIM +192090) is associated with diffuse cancer.	[3, 49]
p53	*p53 codon 72* Two alleles encoding either arginine (CGC) or proline (CCC)	Repair of DNA. When *p53* mutates, DNA-damaged cells are not arrested in G_1 and DNA repair does not take place, allowing other mutations to accumulate and conduce to neoplasic transformation and cancer. p53 codon 72 polymorphism has been associated with gastric cancer.	[50 - 53]
Oncogene RAS		Down regulation of Ras proteins in cancer lead to increased invasion and decreased apoptosis. Mutations in the *RAS* family are common, and have been found in 20% to 30% of all human tumors	[54]
Oncogene MYC		Involved in cell cycle regulation, cell growth arrest, cell adhesion, metabolism, ribosome biogenesis, and protein synthesis	[55]

Table 1. First and second stage genes that have been associated to the development of gastric cancer

6. First stage genes

6.1. Interleukin 1 Family

The association of *IL-1* polymorphisms to gastric cancer has a deep principle: alleles *IL-1B-31*C*, *IL-1B-511*T*, and *IL-1RN*2*, lead to high-level expression of IL-1β, reduction of acid output, corpus-predominant colonization by *H. pylori*, pangastritis, atrophic gastritis, and increased risk of gastric cancer. The importance of the IL-1beta gene polymorphism with an increased risk of developing hypochlorhydria and gastric atrophy, which is considered a gastric cancer precursor, was first demonstrated in a Caucasian population [25] and later reported in other populations [26, 28-32, 56, 57]. El Omar et al. found that risk increases progressively and that individuals with three or four polymorphisms in IL-1, IL1-RN or IL10 and infected with *H. pylori* have a 27-fold increased risk of developing non-cardia cancer.

The interaction between a host's immunological defenses, and environmental and *H. pylori* virulence factors play an important role in the development of gastric cancer [58, 59]. Other researchers confirmed that the allelic variation in IL1-beta seems insufficient for the development of gastric cancer. Figueiredo et al. investigated combinations of bacterial and host genotypes in association with gastric cancer and found that a high proportion of gastric carcinoma patients were carriers of IL-1 beta-511*T (69%) allele. The results on the association between IL-1 β polymorphisms and gastric cancer risk remained inconclusive [60].

An association between these polymorphisms was not found in some populations [60, 61]; [62-67], suggesting that this divergence may reflect the different genetic background related to ethnicity and the potential confounding variables, such as *H. pylori* status and family history of malignancy.

6.2. Interleukin 8 and TNFA

Since the watershed publication of El-Omar et al. linking polymorphisms in genes regulating the gastric inflammatory responses to gastric cancer risk due to *H. pylori*, many groups have been investigating other susceptibility loci ruled by polymorphic alleles, particularly those of the innate immune response. One of the most studied is Interleukin-8 (*IL-8*), which is a potent chemokine that may play a role in gastric cancer pathogenesis.

Gastric cancer specimens have increased IL-8 protein levels, and many gastric cancer cell lines express high levels of *IL-8* mRNA and the protein [34-36]. The *IL-8-251* polymorphism might be a host susceptibility factor for gastric carcinoma development and angiogenesis in gastric carcinogenesis [37] but this association is likely to be ethnic-specific [68] because several studies have reported an association with gastric cancer [33, 69, 70]. This association has not been confirmed in studies of Caucasian populations [71, 72]. Another of the studied genes is TNFA. In relation to this gene, the TNFA-308 allele, which is thought to increase the production of TNF-alfa, confers an increased risk for the development of gastric cancer. This polymorphism increases the risk for non-cardia gastric cancer by approximately two-fold.

6.3. NOD1, NOD2, COX2, ROS and RNS

The pathogen-associated intracellular recognition molecules NOD1 and NOD2 are important regulators of chronic inflammation. NOD1 appears to be involved in the activation of a key transcription factor, NF-kB, by the Cag pathogenicity island [39]. Rosenstiel et al. reported that NOD1 and NOD2 were upregulated in the gastric epithelial cells of patients with chronic infection by *H. pylori, the* NOD2 variant R702W was more prevalent in patients with gastric lymphoma than in *H. pylori*-infected individuals with gastritis or gastric ulcers [38].

Cyclooxygenase2 (COX-2) has long been known to be over-expressed in gastric cancer and in *H. pylori* infection. Studies of gastric cancer cases and controls with preneoplastic lesions from China, showed an association between specific COX-2 genotypes with high level COX-2 expression and gastric cancer risk [40]. On the other hand, Reactive oxygen species (ROS) and reactive nitrogen species (RNS) have been implicated in increasing gastric inflammation and therefore carcinogenesis. The mechanism by which the bacteria induce gastric carcinogenesis is not defined. It has been reported that *H. pylori* produces ROS in addition to ROS/RNS by activated neutrophils. Some studies have revealed that *H. pylori*-induced ROS production affects gastric epithelial cell signal transduction, resulting in gastric carcinogenesis. ROS/RNS production in the stomach can damage DNA in gastric epithelial cells, thus increasing the risk of gastric carcinogenesis [47].

6.4. Survivin

The expression of the inhibitor-of-apoptosis protein survivin in adults is frequently linked to the development of cancer. Recently, it has been found that infection with *H. pylori* decreased survivin protein levels in the mucosa of patients with gastritis. Moreover, survivin downregulation correlated with apoptosis and a loss of cell viability in gastrointestinal cells infected with different *H. pylori*. Overexpression of survivin in gastric cells reducing cell death after infection with *H. pylori* [48] has also been reported. This may have some implications in gastric carcinogenesis.

6.5. Toll-like receptor 4

Recognition of pathogens is mediated by a set of germline-encoded receptors that are referred to as pattern-recognition receptors (PRRs). These receptors recognize conserved molecular patterns, which are found in many species of microorganisms. An important PRR is Toll-like receptor 4 (TLR4), a transmembrane receptor that recognizes a range of ligands, including lipopolysaccharide (LPS), which is found in Gram-negative bacteria like *H. pylori* [73]. TLR-4 polymorphisms have been associated with a variety of inflammatory conditions, where defective signaling through TLR-4 is thought to trigger an inappropriate inflammatory response.

Two single nucleotide polymorphisms (SNPs) in the *TLR4* gene, Asp299Gly and Thr399Ile transitions, have been shown to lead to hyporesponsiveness to LPS, reduced epithelial TLR4 density and reduced inflammatory cytokine response to LPS [42]. TLR4 Asp299Gly and Thr399Ile polymorphisms have been reported to be a risk factor for gastric carcinoma or its precursors in Caucasian and Indian populations. Also the TLR4+3725 G/C polymorphism has been described as a risk factor of severe gastric atrophy in *H. pylori* seropositive Japanese [22].

Hold et al. addressed the role of TLR with respect to *H. pylori* infection in gastric carcinogenesis by the study of patients previously investigated for cytokine polymorphisms and susceptibility to gastric cancer from Poland, Scotland, and the United States. An association between a polymorphism in TLR-4 and an increased risk of noncardia gastric cancer and its precursor lesions including achlorhydria was identified in that study [74]. This association was specific for noncardia gastric cancer as it was not observed in esophageal or gastric cardia cases and remained even after correcting for the polymorphic variations in IL-1β and the IL-1 receptor previously documented by this group.

6.6. Interleukin 10

Interleukin-10 (IL-10) is an anti-inflammatory cytokine that downregulates the production of Th1-derived cytokines [75] and seems to limit and terminate the inflammatory response by the blocking proinflammatory cytokine secretion. Some functional polymorphisms have been described for the IL-10 gene promoter. The single-nucleotide polymorphisms (SNP) at positions -1082 (G/A), −819 (C/T), and −592 (C/A) from the transcriptional start site are in linkage disequilibrium, and are responsible for three different haplotypes formed by the combination of ATA, GCC and ACC. The IL-10 haplotypes and cytokine production have been correlated with counterpointing results [46, 76, 77].

A higher prevalence of gastric cancer in patients with the proinflammatory (low IL-10 secreting) haplotype ATA has been reported, but contrasting results have also reported an association between carcinoma and the anti-inflammatory (high IL-10 secreting) haplotype GCC [43]. The study of Rad et al. showed that this contrastive observation might be explained by the finding that *cagA* $^{+}$ strains were more prevalent among GCC carriers [32]. Further studies are needed to clarify the role of *IL-10* polymorphisms in *H pylori* infection.

6.7. Selenoprotein S

Selenoprotein S participates in the retro-translocation of misfolded proteins from the endoplasmic reticulum to the cytosol for their degradation [44]. This membrane protein functions in stress responses to prevent the deleterious consequences of accumulation of misfolded proteins, accumulation that has been linked to immune and inflammatory processes.

A strong association between the proximal promoter SEPS1 polymorphism at -105G/A with circulating levels of pro-inflammatory IL-1β and TNF-α has been reported [45]. A regulatory loop has been recently proposed whereby cytokines stimulate the expression of SEPS1, which in turn diminishes cytokine production [15]. The -105G>A promoter polymorphism of SEPS1 has been associated with the intestinal type of gastric cancer [46]. In another report of stomach biopsies from 268 Japanese gastric cancer and 306 control patients found that carrying the SEPS1-105*A allele was associated with an increased risk of intestinal type gastric cancer (OR: 2.0, 95%CI 1.0–3.9, $p < 0.05$) as well as of gastric cancer located in the middle third of the stomach (OR: 2.0, 95% CI 1.0–3.9, $p < 0.05$).

7. Second stage genes

External environmental exposures play an important role. These can give rise to a number of different genetic changes, the most common of which include chromosomal changes such as loss of heterozygosity (LOH), rearrangements, deletions, gains, and translocations; gene mutations such as base substitutions, small insertions and deletions, allelic loss, amplification and rearrangements; and epigenetic events such as alteration in DNA methylation. Loss of tumor suppressor function leads to the initiation and progression of cancer [78, 79]. Inactivation of tumor suppressor genes can result from both genetic mechanisms, such as mutation, and epigenetic mechanisms, such as DNA hypermethylation.

7.1. E-cadherin

E-cadherin is a calcium dependent cell-cell adhesion glycoprotein. Mutations in this gene are associated with gastric, breast, colorectal, thyroid and ovarian cancer [80]. It has been reported that promoter hypermethylation of E-cadherin plays an important role in gastric carcinogenesis [49]. Evidence shows that a heterozygous germline point or small frameshift mutations in the E-cadherin gene (*CDH1*, OMIM +192090) are associated with diffuse cancer [81]. Carriers of *CDH1* germline mutations have an accumulative GC risk, before age 75, of 40–67% for men and 63–83% for women [82].

7.2. P53

The p53 gene has been called the genome guard is critical in maintaining orderly proliferation of cells. Normally, damage to cellular DNA initiates increased expression of *p53* that may lead to the arrest of the cell cycle. This interruption allows DNA repair to occur before abnormal proliferation is produced. If DNA repair is not successful, then the cell undergoes apoptosis to avoid proliferation of mutated cells. When *p53* mutates, DNA-damaged cells are not arrested in G_1 and DNA repair does not take place, allowing other mutations to accumulate and conduce to neoplasic transformation and cancer. Mutation of *p53* is probably the most significant genetic change characterizing the transformation of cells from normal to malignant [83]. With this principle, one of the most known polymorphisms in p53 have been studied in relation to gastric cancer and some polymorphisms in this gene have been associated with the development of distal GC in Mexican, Chinese, Korean and Japanese populations [51, 53]. A meta-analysis suggests that the p53 codon 72 polymorphism may be associated with gastric cancer particularly among Asians, and that the difference in genotype distribution may be associated with the location, stage, and histological differentiation of gastric cancer.

7.3. Oncogenes

Once activated, a proto-oncogene or its product is a tumor-inducing protein [84]. Some of the well-known oncogenes are *RAS, WNT, MYC, ERK,* and *TRK.* Among these, one of the most studied is MYC, which is involved in multiple cellular functions, such as cell cycle regulation, cell growth arrest, cell adhesion, metabolism, ribosome biogenesis, protein synthesis, and mitochondrial function. It has a main role in several carcinogenesis processes in humans [55].

The *RAS* family is responsible for cell proliferation and functions. They act as a switch that controls intracellular signaling networks in processes such as actin cytoskeleton integrity, proliferation, differentiation, cell adhesion, apoptosis and cell migration. Ras proteins are often deregulated in cancers, leading to increased invasion and decreased apoptosis. Mutations in the *RAS* family are common, and have been found in 20% to 30% of all human tumors [54], but no specific mutation has been consistently related to gastric cancer.

8. Conclusions

Host genetic susceptibility has been suggested as one of the most important possible explanations for interindividual differences in gastric cancer risk and even to tumor invasion. In the first stage, inflammation seems to play a critical role in the development of many types of cancer, including gastric cancer and genetic changes in gene coding some crucial mediators in the inflammatory response may play an essential role in *Helicobacter pylori*-infected individuals. In the second stage, participation of tumor suppressor proteins and oncogenes seems to define the course of the disease.

In conclusion, there are currently no definitive genetic risk markers for gastric cancer risk that can be applied to all populations. We need to recognize that distal gastric cancer is a multifactorial event. We do not discuss the effect of the environment that may influence both bacteria and the host factors.

Author details

Elvira Garza-González[1*] and Guillermo Ignacio Pérez-Pérez[2]

*Address all correspondence to: elvira_garza_gzz@yahoo.com

1 Servicio de Gastroenterología, Hospital Universitario "Dr. José Eleuterio González" Universidad Autónoma de Nuevo León, Mexico

2 Departments of Medicine and Microbiology, New York University School of Medicine, USA

References

[1] Parkin, D. M., Bray, F., Ferlay, J., & Pisani, P. (2005). Global cancer statistics, 2002. *CA: a cancer journal for clinicians.*, 55(2), 74-108.

[2] Fuchs, C. S., & Mayer, R. J. (1995). Gastric carcinoma. *New England Journal of Medicine Engl J Med*, 333(1), 32-41.

[3] Gore, R. M. (1997). Colorectal cancer. *Clinical and pathologic features. Radiologic clinics of North America.*, 35(2), 403-29.

[4] Maconi, G., Manes, G., & Porro, G. B. (2008). Role of symptoms in diagnosis and outcome of gastric cancer. *World Journal of Gastroenterology.*, 14(8), 1149-55.

[5] Wroblewski, L. E., Peek, R. M., & Wilson, K. T. (2010). Helicobacter pylori and gastric cancer: factors that modulate disease risk. *Clinical Microbioliology Revew.*, 23(4), 713-39.

[6] Peek, R. M., & Blaser, M. J. (2002). Helicobacter pylori and gastrointestinal tract adenocarcinomas. *Nature reviews Cancer.*, 2(1), 28-37.

[7] Suerbaum, S., & Michetti, P. (2002). Helicobacter pylori infection. *New England Journal of Medicine*, 347(15), 1175-86.

[8] An international association between Helicobacter pylori infection and gastric cancer. (1993). The EUROGAST Study Group. *Lancet.*, 341(8857), 1359-62.

[9] Asaka, M., Kudo, M., Kato, M., Sugiyama, T., & Takeda, H. (1998). Review article: Long-term Helicobacter pylori infection--from gastritis to gastric cancer. *Alimentary pharmacology & therapeutics*, 1, 9-15.

[10] Yamaoka, Y., Kodama, T., Gutierrez, O., Kim, J. G., Kashima, K., & Graham, D. Y. (1999). Relationship between Helicobacter pylori iceA, cagA, and vacA status and clinical outcome: studies in four different countries. *Journal of Clinical Microbiology*, 37(7), 2274-9.

[11] Zambon, C. F., Basso, D., Navaglia, F., Germano, G., Gallo, N., Milazzo, M., et al. (2002). Helicobacter pylori virulence genes and host IL-1RN and IL-1beta genes interplay in favouring the development of peptic ulcer and intestinal metaplasia. *Cytokine*, 18(5), 242-51.

[12] Bourzac, K. M., & Guillemin, K. (2005). Helicobacter pylori-host cell interactions mediated by type IV secretion. *Cellular microbiology*, 7(7), 911-9.

[13] Censini, S., Lange, C., Xiang, Z., Crabtre,e, J. E., Ghiara, P., Borodovsky, M., et al. (1996). Cag, a pathogenicity island of Helicobacter pylori, encodes type I-specific and disease-associated virulence factors. *Proceedings of the National Academy of Sciences of the United States of America*, 93(25), 14648-53.

[14] Hatakeyama, M. (2009). Helicobacter pylori and gastric carcinogenesis. *Journal of Gastroenterology*, 44(4), 239-48.

[15] Gao, Y., Hannan, N. R., Wanyonyi, S., Konstantopolous, N., Pagnon, J., Feng, H. C., et al. (2006). Activation of the selenoprotein SEPS1 gene expression by pro-inflammatory cytokines in HepG2 cells. *Cytokine.*, 33(5), 246-51.

[16] Corley, D. A., Kubo, A., Levin, T. R., Bloc,k, G., Habel, L., Zhao, W., et al. (2008). Helicobacter pylori infection and the risk of Barrett's oesophagus: a community-based study. *Gut.*, 57(6), 727-33.

[17] Whiteman, D. C., Parmar, P., Fahey, P., Moore, S. P., Stark, M., Zhao, Z. Z., et al. (2010). Association of Helicobacter pylori infection with reduced risk for esophageal cancer is independent of environmental and genetic modifiers. Gastroenterology quiz e11-2., 139(1), 73-83.

[18] Azuma, T., Ohtani, M., Yamazaki, Y., Higashi, H., & Hatakeyama, M. (2004). Meta-analysis of the relationship between CagA seropositivity and gastric cancer. *Gastroenterology*, 126(7), 1926-7.

[19] Fukase, K., Kato, M., Kikuchi, S., Inoue, K., Uemura, N., Okamoto, S., et al. (2008). Effect of eradication of Helicobacter pylori on incidence of metachronous gastric carcinoma after endoscopic resection of early gastric cancer: an open-label, randomised controlled trial. *Lancet.*, 372(9636), 392-7.

[20] El -Omar, E. M., Oien, K., Murray, L. S., El -Nujumi, A., Wirz, A., Gillen, D., et al. (2000). Increased prevalence of precancerous changes in relatives of gastric cancer patients: critical role of H. pylori. *Gastroenterology*, 118(1), 22-30.

[21] Brenner, H., Rothenbacher, D., & Arndt, V. (2009). Epidemiology of stomach cancer. Methods in molecular biologyClifton, N.J. , 472, 467-77.

[22] Hishida, A., Matsuo, K., Goto, Y., & Hamajima, N. (2010). Genetic predisposition to Helicobacter pylori-induced gastric precancerous conditions. *World J Gastrointest Oncol.*, 2(10), 369-79.

[23] Correa, P. (1995). Helicobacter pylori and gastric carcinogenesis. *The American journal of surgical pathology*, (1), 37-43.

[24] Correa, P., Haenszel, W., Cuello, C., Zavala, D., Fontham, E., Zarama, G., et al. (1990). Gastric precancerous process in a high risk population: cohort follow-up. *Cancer Research.*, 50(15), 4737-40.

[25] El -Omar, E. M., Carrington, M., Chow, W. H., Mc Coll, K. E., Bream, J. H., Young, H. A., et al. (2000). Interleukin-1 polymorphisms associated with increased risk of gastric cancer. *Nature.*, 404(6776), 398-402.

[26] El -Omar, E. M. (2001). The importance of interleukin 1beta in Helicobacter pylori associated disease. *Gut*, 48(6), 743-7.

[27] Figueiredo, C., Machado, J. C., Pharoah, P., Seruca, R., Sousa, S., Carvalho, R., et al. (2002). Helicobacter pylori and interleukin 1 genotyping: an opportunity to identify high-risk individuals for gastric carcinoma. *Journal of the National Cancer Institute*, 94(22), 1680-7.

[28] Furuta, T., El -Omar, E. M., Xiao, F., Shirai, N., Takashima, M., Sugimura, H., et al. (2002). Interleukin 1beta polymorphisms increase risk of hypochlorhydria and atrophic gastritis and reduce risk of duodenal ulcer recurrence in Japan. *Gastroenterology*, 123(1), 92-105.

[29] Garza-González, E., Bosques-Padilla, F. J., El -Omar, E., Hold, G., Tijerina-Menchaca, R., Maldonado-Garza, H. J., et al. (2005). Role of the polymorphic IL-1B, IL-1RN and TNF-A genes in distal gastric cancer in Mexico. *International Journal of Cancer*, 114(2), 237-41.

[30] Hwang, I. R., Kodama, T., Kikuchi, S., Sakai, K., Peterson, L. E., Graham, D. Y., et al. (2002). Effect of interleukin 1 polymorphisms on gastric mucosal interleukin 1beta production in Helicobacter pylori infection. *Gastroenterology*, 123(6), 1793-803.

[31] Machado, J. C., Figueiredo, C., Canedo, P., Pharoah, P., Carvalho, R., Nabais, S., et al. (2003). A proinflammatory genetic profile increases the risk for chronic atrophic gastritis and gastric carcinoma. *Gastroenterology*, 125(2), 364-71.

[32] Rad, R., Dossumbekova, A., Neu, B., Lang, R., Bauer, S., Saur, D., et al. (2004). Cytokine gene polymorphisms influence mucosal cytokine expression, gastric inflammation, and host specific colonisation during Helicobacter pylori infection. *Gut.*, 53(8), 1082-9.

[33] Garza-Gonzalez, E., Bosques-Padilla, F. J., Mendoza-Ibarra, S. I., Flores-Gutierrez, J. P., Maldonado-Garza, H. J., & Perez-Perez, G. I. (2007). Assessment of the toll-like receptor 4 Asp299Gly, Thr399Ile and interleukin-8-251 polymorphisms in the risk for the development of distal gastric cancer. BMC Cancer. , 7, 70.

[34] Kido, S., Kitadai, Y., Hattori, N., Haruma, K., Kido, T., Ohta, M., et al. (2001). Interleukin 8 and vascular endothelial growth factor-- prognostic factors in human gastric carcinomas? *European journal of cancer*, 37(12), 1482-7.

[35] Kitadai, Y., Haruma, K., Mukaida, N., Ohmoto, Y., Matsutani, N., Yasui, W., et al. (2000). Regulation of disease-progression genes in human gastric carcinoma cells by interleukin 8. *Clinical Cancer Research.*, 6(7), 2735-40.

[36] Yamaoka, Y., Kodama, T., Kita, M., Imanishi, J., Kashima, K., & Graham, D. Y. (2001). Relation between cytokines and Helicobacter pylori in gastric cancer. *Helicobacter.*, 6(2), 116-24.

[37] Song, J. H., Kim, S. G., Jung, S. A., Lee, M. K., Jung, H. C., & Song, I. S. (2010). The interleukin-8-251 AA genotype is associated with angiogenesis in gastric carcinogenesis in Helicobacter pylori-infected Koreans. *Cytokine*, 51(2), 158-65.

[38] Rosenstiel, P., Hellmig, S., Hampe, J., Ott, S., Till, A., Fischbach, W., et al. (2006). Influence of polymorphisms in the NOD1/CARD4 and NOD2/CARD15 genes on the clinical outcome of Helicobacter pylori infection. *Cellular microbiology*, 8(7), 1188-98.

[39] Viala, J., Chaput, C., Boneca, I. G., Cardona, A., Girardin, S. E., Moran, A. P., et al. (2004). Nod1 responds to peptidoglycan delivered by the Helicobacter pylori cag pathogenicity island. *Nature immunology.*, 5(11), 1166-74.

[40] Liu, F., Pan, K., Zhang, X., Zhang, Y., Zhang, L., Ma, J., et al. (2006). Genetic variants in cyclooxygenase-2: Expression and risk of gastric cancer and its precursors in a Chinese population. *Gastroenterology*, 130(7), 975-84.

[41] Li, Y., He, W., Liu, T., & Zhang, Q. (2010). A new cyclo-oxygenase-2 gene variant in the Han Chinese population is associated with an increased risk of gastric carcinoma. *Molecular diagnosis & therapy*, 14(6), 351-5.

[42] Schröder, N. W., & Schumann, R. R. (2005). Single nucleotide polymorphisms of Toll-like receptors and susceptibility to infectious disease. *The Lancet infectious diseases.*, 5(3), 156-64.

[43] Wu, M. S., Wu, C. Y., Chen, C. J., Lin, M. T., Shun, C. T., & Lin, J. T. (2003). Interleukin-10 genotypes associate with the risk of gastric carcinoma in Taiwanese Chinese. *International Journal of Cancer*, 104(5), 617-23.

[44] Ye, Y., Shibata, Y., Yun, C., Ron, D., & Rapopor,t, T. A. (2004). A membrane protein complex mediates retro-translocation from the ER lumen into the cytosol. *Nature*, 429(6994), 841-7.

[45] Curran, J. E., Jowett, J. B., Elliott, K. S., Gao, Y., Gluschenko, K., Wang, J., et al. (2005). Genetic variation in selenoprotein S influences inflammatory response. *Nature Genetics.*, 37(11), 1234-41.

[46] Shibata, T., Arisawa, T., Tahara, T., Ohkubo, M., Yoshioka, D., Maruyama, N., et al. (2009). Selenoprotein S (SEPS1) gene-105G>A promoter polymorphism influences the susceptibility to gastric cancer in the Japanese population. BMC Gastroenterology. , 9, 2.

[47] Handa, O., Naito, Y., & Yoshikawa, T. (2010). Helicobacter pylori: a ROS-inducing bacterial species in the stomach. *Inflammation Research*, 59(12), 997-1003.

[48] Valenzuela, M., Pérez-Pérez, G., Corvalán, A. H., Carrasc,o, G., Urra, H., Bravo, D., et al. (2010). Helicobacter pylori-induced loss of the inhibitor-of-apoptosis protein survivin is linked to gastritis and death of human gastric cells. *Journal of Infectious Diseases*, 202(7), 1021-30.

[49] Miyazaki, T., Murayama, Y., Shinomura, Y., Yamamoto, T., Watabe, K., Tsutsui, S., et al. (2007). E-cadherin gene promoter hypermethylation in H. pylori-induced enlarged fold gastritis. *Helicobacter*, 12, 523-31.

[50] Lane, D. P. (1992). Cancer. p53,guardian of the genome. *Nature.*, 358(6381), 15-6.

[51] Hiyama, T., Tanaka, S., Kitadai, Y., Ito, M., Sumii, M., Yoshihara, M., et al. (2002). P53 Codon 72 polymorphism in gastric cancer susceptibility in patients with Helicobacter pylori-associated chronic gastritis. *International Journal of Cancer*, 100(3), 304-8.

[52] Pérez-Pérez, G. I., Bosques-Padilla, F. J., Crosatti, M. L., Tijerina-Menchaca, R., & Garza-González, E. (2005). Role of p53 codon 72 polymorphism in the risk of development of distal gastric cancer. *Scandinavian Journal of Gastroenterology*, 40(1), 56-60.

[53] Yi, S. Y., & Lee, W. J. (2006). A p53 genetic polymorphism of gastric cancer: difference between early gastric cancer and advanced gastric cancer. *World Journal of Gastroenterology.*, 12(40), 6536-9.

[54] Bos, J. L. (1989). Ras oncogenes in human cancer: a review. *Cancer Research*, 49(17), 4682-9.

[55] Oster, S. K., Ho, C. S., Soucie, E. L., & Penn, L. Z. (2002). The myc oncogene: MarvelouslY Complex. *Advances in Cancer Research*, 84, 81-154.

[56] Calam, J. (1999). Helicobacter pylori modulation of gastric acid. *The Yale Journal of Biology and Medicine*, 72(2-3), 195-202.

[57] Chiurillo, M. A., Moran, Y., Cañas, M., Valderrama, E., Alvarez, A., & Armanie, E. (2010). Combination of Helicobacter pylori-iceA2 and proinflammatory interleukin-1 polymorphisms is associated with the severity of histological changes in Venezuelan chronic gastritis patients. *FEMS Immunology and Medical Microbiology*, 59(2), 170-6.

[58] Akopyanz, N., Bukanov, N. O., Westblom, T. U., Kresovich, S., & Berg, D. E. (1992). DNA diversity among clinical isolates of Helicobacter pylori detected by PCR-based RAPD fingerprinting. *Nucleic Acids Res.*, 20(19), 5137-42.

[59] Marshall, D. G., Coleman, D. C., Sullivan, D. J., Xia, H., O'Moráin, C. A., & Smyth, C. J. (1996). Genomic DNA fingerprinting of clinical isolates of Helicobacter pylori using short oligonucleotide probes containing repetitive sequences. *The Journal of Applied Bacteriology*, 81(5), 509-17.

[60] Perri, F., Piepoli, A., Bonvicini, C., Gentile, A., Quitadamo, M., Di Candia, M., et al. (2005). Cytokine gene polymorphisms in gastric cancer patients from two Italian areas at high and low cancer prevalence. *Cytokine*, 30(5), 293-302.

[61] Kim, N., Cho, S. I., Yim, J. Y., Kim, J. M., Lee, D. H., Park, J. H., et al. (2006). The effects of genetic polymorphisms of IL-1 and TNF-A on Helicobacter pylori-induced gastroduodenal diseases in Korea. *Helicobacter*, 11(2), 105-12.

[62] Ruzzo, A., Graziano, F., Pizzagalli, F., Santini, D., Battistelli, V., Panunzi, S., et al. (2005). Interleukin 1B gene (IL-1B) and interleukin 1 receptor antagonist gene (IL-1RN) polymorphisms in Helicobacter pylori-negative gastric cancer of intestinal and diffuse histotype. *Annals of Oncology*, 16(6), 887-92.

[63] Sakuma, K., Uozaki, H., Chong, J. M., Hironaka, M., Sudo, M., Ushiku, T., et al. (2005). Cancer risk to the gastric corpus in Japanese, its correlation with interleu-

kin-1beta gene polymorphism (+3953*T) and Epstein-Barr virus infection. *International Journal of Cancer*, 115(1), 93-7.

[64] Sicinschi, L. A., Lopez-Carrillo, L., Camargo, M. C., Correa, P., Sierra, R. A., Henry, R. R., et al. (2006). Gastric cancer risk in a Mexican population: role of Helicobacter pylori CagA positive infection and polymorphisms in interleukin-1 and-10 genes. *International Journal of Cancer.*, 118(3), 649-57.

[65] Starzyńska, T., Ferenc, K., Wex, T., Kähne, T., Lubiński, J., Lawniczak, M., et al. (2006). The association between the interleukin-1 polymorphisms and gastric cancer risk depends on the family history of gastric carcinoma in the study population. *American Journal of Gastroenterology.*, 101(2), 248-54.

[66] Zambon, C. F., Basso, D., Navaglia, F., Belluco, C., Falda, A., Fogar, P., et al. (2005). Pro- and anti-inflammatory cytokines gene polymorphisms and Helicobacter pylori infection: interactions influence outcome. *Cytokine*, 29(4), 141-52.

[67] Zhang, K., Mc Clure, J., Elsayed, S., Louie, T., & Conly, J. (2005). Novel multiplex PCR assay for characterization and concomitant subtyping of staphylococcal cassette chromosome mec types I to V in methicillin-resistant Staphylococcus aureus. *Journal of Clinical Microbiology*, 43(10), 5026-33.

[68] Canedo, P., Castanheira-Vale, A. J., Lunet, N., Pereira, F., Figueiredo, C., Gioia-Patricola, L., et al. (2008). The interleukin-8-251*T/*A polymorphism is not associated with risk for gastric carcinoma development in a Portuguese population. *European Journal of Cancer Prevention*, 17(1), 28-32.

[69] Lu, W., Pan, K., Zhang, L., Lin, D., Miao, X., & You, W. (2005). Genetic polymorphisms of interleukin (IL)-1B, IL-1RN, IL-8, IL-10 and tumor necrosis factor {alpha} and risk of gastric cancer in a Chinese population. *Carcinogenesis*, 26(3), 631-6.

[70] Ohyauchi, M., Imatani, A., Yonechi, M., Asano, N., Miura, A., Iijima, K., et al. (2005). The polymorphism interleukin 8-251 A/T influences the susceptibility of Helicobacter pylori related gastric diseases in the Japanese population. *Gut.*, 54(3), 330-5.

[71] Kamangar, F., Abnet, C. C., Hutchinson, A. A., Newschaffer, C. J., Helzlsouer, K., Shugart, Y. Y., et al. (2006). Polymorphisms in inflammation-related genes and risk of gastric cancer (Finland). *Cancer Causes Control.*, 17(1), 117-25.

[72] Savage, S. A., Hou, L., Lissowska, J., Chow, W. H., Zatonski, W., Chanock, S. J., et al. (2006). Interleukin-8 polymorphisms are not associated with gastric cancer risk in a Polish population. *Cancer Epidemiology Biomarkers & Prevention*, 15(3), 589-91.

[73] Ferrero, R. L. (2005). Innate immune recognition of the extracellular mucosal pathogen, Helicobacter pylori. *Molecular immunology*, 42(8), 879-85.

[74] Hold, G. L., Rabkin, C. S., Chow, W. H., Smith, M. G., Gammon, M. D., Risch, H. A., et al. (2007). A functional polymorphism of toll-like receptor 4 gene increases risk of gastric carcinoma and its precursors. *Gastroenterology*, 132(3), 905-12.

[75] Podolsky, D. K. (2002). Inflammatory bowel disease. *New England Journal of Medicine*, 347(6), 417-29.

[76] Crawley, E., Kay, R., Sillibourne, J., Patel, P., Hutchinson, I., & Woo, P. (1999). Polymorphic haplotypes of the interleukin-10 5′ flanking region determine variable interleukin-10 transcription and are associated with particular phenotypes of juvenile rheumatoid arthritis. *Arthritis and Rheumatism*, 42(6), 1101-8.

[77] Turner, D. M., Williams, D. M., Sankaran, D., Lazarus, M., Sinnott, P. J., & Hutchinson, I. V. (1997). An investigation of polymorphism in the interleukin-10 gene promoter. *European Journal of Immunogenetics*, 24(1), 1-8.

[78] Futreal, P. A., Coin, L., Marshall, M., Down, T., Hubbard, T., Wooster, R., et al. (2004). A census of human cancer genes. *Nat Rev Cancer*, 4(3), 177-83.

[79] Vogelstein, B., & Kinzler, K. W. (2004). Cancer genes and the pathways they control. *Nature Medicine*, 10(8), 789-99.

[80] Semb, H., & Christofori, G. (1998). The tumor-suppressor function of E-cadherin. *American Journal of Human Genetics*, 63(6), 1588-93.

[81] Guilford, P., Hopkins, J., Harraway, J., Mc Leod, M., Mc Leod, N., Harawira, P., et al. (1998). E-cadherin germline mutations in familial gastric cancer. *Nature.*, 392(6674), 402-5.

[82] Kaurah, P., Mac, Millan. A., Boyd, N., Senz, J., De Luca, A., Chun, N., et al. (2007). Founder and recurrent CDH1 mutations in families with hereditary diffuse gastric cancer. *JAMA : the journal of the American Medical Association*, 297(21), 2360-72.

[83] Wynford-Thomas, D., & Blaydes, J. (1998). The influence of cell context on the selection pressure for p53 mutation in human cancer. *Carcinogenesis*, 19(1), 29-36.

[84] Todd, R., & Wong, D. T. (1999). Oncogenes. *Anticancer Research*, 19(6A), 4729-46.

Chapter 5

Fetal-type Glycogen Phosphorylase (FGP)Expression in Intestinal Metaplasia as a High Risk Factor of the Development of Gastric Carcinoma

Masafumi Kuramoto, Shinya Shimada, Satoshi Ikeshima, Kenichiro Yamamoto, Toshiro Masuda, Tatsunori Miyata, Shinichi Yoshimatsu, Masayuki Urata and Hideo Baba

Additional information is available at the end of the chapter

http://dx.doi.org/10.5772/51793

1. Introduction

It has been reported that an enzyme-glycogen phosphorylase [EC 2.4.1.1] histochemical reaction is observed in differentiated hepatic or muscular tissues and in some proliferating tissues including fetus and carcinoma [1,2]. In the human stomach, a phosphorylase reaction appears in the undifferentiated gastric epithelium at the midpoint of fetal life, and is not detected in gastric epithelium after birth.

In our previous study we hitochemically demonstrated intense glycogen phosphorylase (GP) activity in gastric cancer cells, especially well-differentiated adenocarcinoma, and in the proliferative zone of some intestinal metaplasia (IM), despite phosphorelase being negative in normal gastric epithelium, even in its proliferative zone. Detailed histochemical observations of the enzyme activity were undertaken on the whole mucous membrane of surgically resected stomachs. A positive reaction was observed in all of the well-differentiated adenocarcinomas, whereas only a few poorly differentiated adenocarcinomas reacted positively. A positive reaction of the proliferative zone was observed in 69.5% of all metaplastic glands of the stomachs with well-differentiated adenocarcinoma, in 25.7% with poorly differentiated adenocarcinoma, and only rarely in glands from patients with peptic ulcer. Moreover, there was an apparent coincidence between the location of well-differentiated adenocarcinoma and the distribution of IM with the proliferative zone showing a positive reaction for GP.

GP plays a central role in the mobilization of carbohydrate reserves in a wide variety of organs and tissues [3,4]. Mammalian GPs are found in three major isoforms, i. e., muscle, liver and brain that can be distinguished by functional and structural properties, as well as by the tissues in which they are predominantly expressed [4-6]. cDNAs encoding the three human GP isoforms have been cloned and sequenced, and the tissue and organism-specific expression patterns and chromosomal localization of GP genes has been clarified [4,7]. Chromosome mapping analyses have revealed that the genes encoding muscle, liver and brain GP are assigned to chromosomes 11, 14, and 20, respectively, suggesting that distinct *cis*-acting elements govern the differential expression of the phosphorylase isoforms in various tissues. The physiological role of muscle and liver GP is to provide fuel for the energy production required for muscle contraction and to ensure a constant supply of glucose for extrahepatic tissues, respectively. However, the physiological role of brain GP is poorly understood, although brain GP is generally thought to induce an emergency glucose supply during a stressful and/or ischemic period [4,6,8,9]. In addition, it has been proven that the major isoform of GP found in fetal tissue and tumor tissue is brain GP, and brain GP is identical to fetal-type GP (FGP) [8,9].

We developed an immunohistochemical method of detecting GP isoforms in human tissues by using specific antibodies raised against highly purified GP isoforms from rat brain, muscle and liver, and immunohistochemical staining of GP isoforms was undertaken to define the type of GP present in well-differentiated adenocarcinoma and in the proliferative zone of IM of the human stomach. Both the malignant cells of well-differentiated adenocarcinoma and the proliferative zone of some IM of the stomach were stained when the anti-FGP antibody was used, but not when the other two types were used. The results suggested that the newly appearing GP in gastric carcinoma was FGP, and it could be one example of fetal protein expression in cancer, like α-fetoprotain or carcinoembryonic antigen. Moreover, the proliferative zone of some IM having FGP (FGP-positive IM) might histogenetically relate to well-differentiated adenocarcinoma, i. e., FGP-positive IM could be regarded as a precursor of well-differentiated adenocarcinoma [10].

2. Novel subtyping of IM according to FGP expression

It is generally accepted that IM in the stomach increases the risk of gastric carcinoma [11-15]. A paucity of gene rearrangements is common to IM and carcinoma, which makes it difficult to establish a direct carcinogenic link between them. IM has been classified into subtypes with the aim of clarification of gastric carcinogenesis according to different definitions of the subtypes from the viewpoints of morphologic, enzymatic, and mucin-secreting patterns [16-19]. In such a classification, the subtyping is complicated and subjective, resulting in the existence of many variants within it. And also, some studies suggested that IM was a good marker for high risk of gastric cancer but the subclassification of IM was not important

http://dx.doi.org/10.5772/51793

[13,20]. A better classification of IM related to carcinogenesis that resolved the discrepancy between these two opinions would contribute to studying the direct link between gastric cancer and IM and to follow-up of the high-risk group.

To establish a noble classification of IM from a carcinogenic viewpoint, we studied 136 specimens with gastric carcinoma and the adjacent IM, that were obtained from gastric cancer patients (intestinal type, 72 patients; diffuse type, 64 patients), using specific anti-FGP antibody, and assessed how FGP expression correlates with subtypes of IM, proliferating cell nuclear antigen-labeling index, and various oncogene products.

	Intestinal-Type Carcinoma (n = 72)		*IM (n =64)*	
	No. (%) BGP Positive	***No. (%) BGP Negative***	***No. (%) BGP Positive***	***No. (%) BGP Negative***
	58 (80)*	14 (19)	56 (88)*	8 (12)
p53 Positivity (%)	42 (72.4)	8 (57.1)	10 (17.9)	0 (0.0)
	Diffuse-Type Carcinoma (n = 64)		*IM (n = 24)*	
	No. (%) BGP Positive	***No. (%) BGP Negative***	***No. (%) BGP Positive***	***No. (%) BGP Negative***
	12 (19)*	52 (81)	10 (42)*	14 (58)
p53 Positivity (%)	2 (16.7)	10 (19.2)	0 (0.0)	0 (0.0)

BBGP = brain-type glycogen phosphorylase; IM = intestinal metaplasia.

*P < .001.

Table 1. Incidence of FGP and p53 positivity in gastric carcinoma and IM.

2.1. FGP expression in gastric carcinoma and IM

As shown in Table 1, 80% (58/72) of the intestinal type carcinoma expressed FGP, while 19% (12/64) of the diffuse type showed positive staining for FGP. The percentage of the immunohistochemical positivity for anti-FGP was significantly greater in intestinal type than in diffuse type carcinoma (P < 0.001). The IM adjacent to carcinoma was found in 88% (64/72) and 38% (24/64) of intestinal and diffuse type carcinoma cases, respectively. In the intestinal type, 88% (56/64) of the adjacent IM showed FGP positivity, on the other hand, 42% (10/24) of the adjacent IM showed anti-FGP antibody reactivity in the diffuse type. The expression of FGP in the IM adjacent to intestinal carcinoma was significantly higher than in the diffuse type (P < 0.001).

2.2. Relationship between complete and incomplete IM and expression of FGP in the generative cells

The expressions of FGP in the generative zone of IM were compared with the type of complete or incomplete IM. We selected 64 cases in which the adjacent mucosa to intestinal-type carcinoma was IM. The morphologic and mucin-histochemical examination revealed that 23 (36%) and 41 (64%) cases of the adjacent IM were complete and incomplete, respectively.

The incidence of incomplete-type IM adjacent to the intestinal type of cancer was significantly higher than that of complete-type IM. However, there was no significant relationship between the conventional subtyping of IM and the expressions of FGP. The FGP expressions in complete and incomplete IM adjacent to the carcinoma were high in both of them (19/23, 82.6%; 37/41, 90.6%; respectively).

2.3. Proliferating state and FGP-positive IM

The proliferative compartment measured by proliferating cell nuclear antigen (PCNA) staining in the FGP-negative IM tend to be confined to the lower layer. In the FGP-positive IM, however, the PCNA labeling was frequently expanded to the upper layer. The labeling index analysis revealed that the index of the FGP-positive IM was significantly higher than that of the FGP-negative IM, although there was not a significant difference between PCNA labeling index of FGP-positive carcinoma and that of FGP-negative carcinoma (Figure 1).

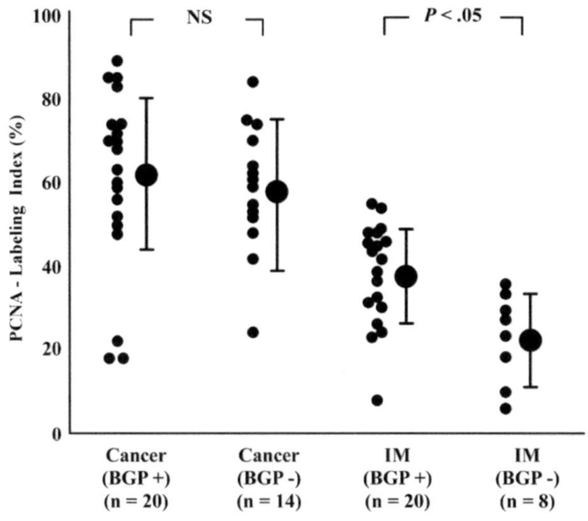

Figure 1. Distribution of PCNA labeling index in intestinal-type gastric cancer and adjacent IM with or without FGP expression. NS: not significant

2.4. Relevance of p53 expression with FGP-positive IM

Abnormal p53 accumulation was observed in 10 of 56 (17.9%) of the FGP-positive IM adjacent to intestinal carcinoma (Table 1). The staining of p53 was restricted to the FGP-positive IM mainly in their generative zone (Figure 2), and none of the staining was detected in the FGP-negative IM. In cancer foci, the overexpression of p53 was observed in 42 of 58 (72.4%), 8 of 14 (57.1%), 2 of 12 (16.7%), and 10 of 52 (19.2%) in the intestinal-type carcinomas with or without FGP or the diffuse-type with or without FGP, respectively. The percentage of p53 staining of intestinal-type carcinoma was significantly higher than that of the diffuse-type (P

< 0.001), and the intestinal-type carcinoma with FGP tend to be stained with p53 more frequently than that without FGP. The immunohistochemical staining of APC and c-K-ras was consistently negative in IM.

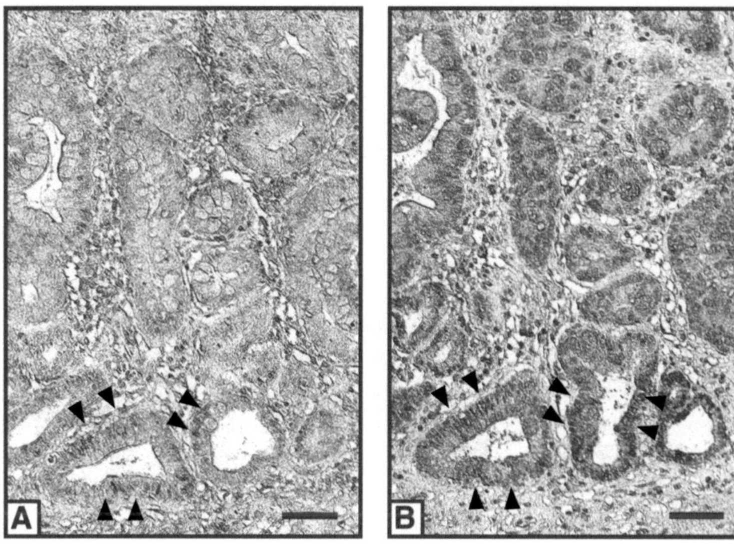

Figure 2. Overexpression of p53 protein in FGP-positive IM (arrows).A, p53 staining; B, FGP staining; Bar-100μm

In this study, FGP was expressed in 80% of the intestinal-type carcinoma and in 88% in the generative zone of IM adjacent to the cancer foci, whereas no positive staining was observed in the normal gastric mucosa, including its generative zone. The proportion of FGP positivity in cancer and IM was significantly greater in intestinal-type carcinoma than in the diffuse-type (P < 0.001). Thus, these results indicate an apparently close association between FGP-positive IM and intestinal-type gastric carcinoma. Interestingly, morphologic and mucin characterization revealed that there was no significant correlation between the subtypes of IM (i.e., complete or incomplete) and the expression of FGP in the generative cells of IM adjacent to intestinal-type carcinoma

The characterization of FGP-positive IM was also conducted in this study, using the PCNA labeling index and the expression of oncogene products. PCNA staining revealed that there was an expansion of proliferative compartment in FGP-positive IM and it was significantly higher in a proliferating state than FGP-negative IM. A comparison of the PCNA labeling index of FGP-positive IM with that of FGP-negative IM indicated that the labeling index might predict more than 40% of the FGP positivity. Furthermore, some of the FGP-positive IMs were coexpressed accumulated p53 in the generative cells, although other oncogene products (APC and c-K-ras) that are common in the adenoma-carcinoma sequence in the colon [21] were detected in none of the generative cells of IM. PCNA and p53 have been considered to be crucial markers for the demonstration of cell proliferation in the cell cycle phase [22]. The timing of the genetic alteration of p53 has been investigated in the chain of chronic gastritis, IM, dysplasia, and early carcinoma and reported to be an early event in stomach carcinogenesis [23-25]. Abnormal protein accumulation of p53, however, has not been well demonstrated in IM. In this study, we detected p53 accumulation in the generative cell zone of FGP-positive IM despite sporadic expression. These observations suggest that the generative cells of FGP-positive IM may deviate from the differentiation and be blocked from apoptotic cell death. Thus, this novel classification of IM based on the linkage between the generative cell zone of IM and gastric carcinoma using FGP expression may open new vistas in research of the carcinogenesis of gastric carcinoma.

3. Gastric and intestinal phenotypes of gastric carcinoma with reference to expression of FGP

Characterization of differentiated gastric carcinoma, i.e., gastric- and intestinal-phenotypic classification, has been advocated, mainly from the carcinogenic point of view, using analysis of the expression of gastric and/or intestinal mucin [26-29]. Carcinoma of the stomach has long been classified into differentiated type and undifferentiated types according to its histological morphologic characteristics [30]. Because the differentiated type is closely related to IM, and the tumor cells often have intestinal properties, the differentiated type is called intestinal type, while the undifferentiated type is called diffuse type [31]. Some differentiated-type carcinoma, however, are composed of cells resembling foveolar epithelium or pyloric gland cells, indicating that these carcinomas may arise from the proper gastric epithelium. In recent years, immunohistochemical staining with various mucins has been shown to discriminate mucins with characteristics of gastric and colonic epithelium, leading to a better understanding of the background of gastric tumorigenesis [32,33]. However, differentiated gastric carcinoma is classified into five subtypes, i.e., gastric type, gastric type-dominant mixed type, intestinal type-dominant mixed type, intestinal type, and null type according to the relative amount of gastric and intestinal mucins, and this classification is complicated and may be confusing [29].

In this section, we focused on the relationship between the expression of FGP and gastric and intestinal mucin in gastric carcinoma, and we propose that FGP expression is a simple marker for discriminating carcinomas with intestinal phenotype from those with gastric phenotype. Ninety-six tissues of gastric carcinoma surgically resected from the patients (differentiated type: 46, undifferentiated type: 50) were studied regarding correlation of FGP expression with intestinal and gastric phenotypes, determined histologically and immunohistochemically with the various anti-mucin antibodies (HGM, CD10, MUC2).

3.1. Proportions of gastric and intestinal phenotypes in gastric carcinoma

The FGP expression in gastric carcinoma was seen in 82.6% (38/46) of the differentiated type and 24.0% (12/50) of the undifferentiated type, and which corresponded well with the results of our previous study. Both differentiated and undifferentiated gastric carcinomas were classified into three subtypes, i.e., gastric, mixed and intestinal types, according to the relative amount of gastric (HGM-positive) and intestinal (MUC2 and/or CD10-positive) mucins and the histological morphology. The proportions of gastric, mixed and intestinal types in differentiated gastric carcinoma were 13.0%, 47.8% and 39.2%, respectively, while hand, these proportions in undifferentiated gastric carcinoma were 56.0%, 32.0% and 12.0%, respectively [Table 2].

Histological type	Gastric type	Mixed type	Intestinal type	Total
Differentiated (%)	6 (13.0)	22 (47.8)	18 (39.2)	46 (100.0)
Undifferentiated (%)	28 (56.0)	16 (32.0)	6 (12.0)	50 (100.0)
Total (%)	34 (35.4)	38 (39.6)	24 (25.0)	96 (100.0)

Table 2. Incidence of gastric and intestinal phenotypes in gastric carcinoma.

3.2. Relationship between phenotype and FGP expression

Figure 3 shows combination graphs for the mucin phenotypes of gastric carcinoma and FGP expression in differentiated adenocarcinoma (A) and undifferentiated adenocarcinoma (B). In both differentiated and undifferentiated types, the phenotype of gastric and intestinal mucin expression corresponded very well with FGP expression, that is, almost all carcinomas with gastric type (92.3% and 97.1%, respectively) did not express FGP, whereas almost all with intestinal type (90.9% and 83.3%, respectively) expressed FGP. However, 97.3% of the mixed type of differentiated adenocarcinoma expressed FGP, while only 33.3% of the mixed type of undifferentiated carcinoma expressed FGP.

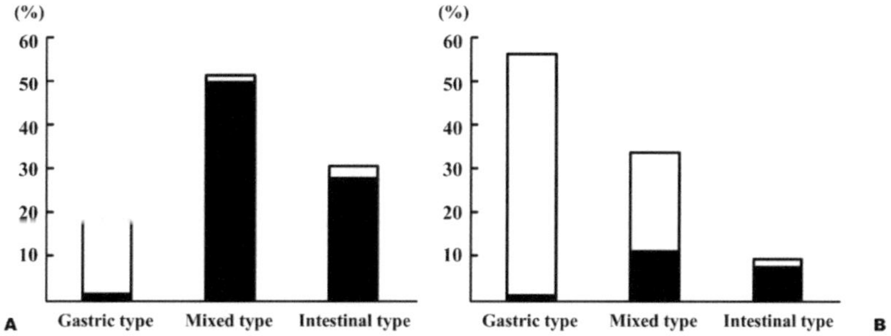

Figure 3. Combination graphs for mucin phenotype and FGP expression in A differentiated and B undifferentiated gastric carcinoma. *Open bars*, FGP-negative; *closed bars*, FGP-positive.

Recent progress in mucin histochemistry and immunohistochemistry has enabled us to differentiate the gastric and intestinal phenotypic properties of gastric carcinoma [C4, 7, 8]. However, in considerable numbers of gastric carcinomas that do not have typical and/or sufficient mucins (47.8% of the differentiated carcinomas in our study), it is difficult to decide the phenotype, and this leaves an equivocal group in this classification. Our study revealed that almost all the phenotypes decided on by FGP expression corresponded with the results obtained with mucin immunohistochemistry and H&E staining, suggesting that FGP expression can discriminate the gastric and intestinal phenotypes in gastric carcinoma. We assume that this is not because FGP directly contributes to mucin carbohydrate expression, but probably because FGP-positive gastric carcinoma has intestinal-type lineage, leading to concordance with intestinal-type mucin expression findings. Accordingly, the mixed type carcinomas determined by mucin analysis were divided into two groups (gastric and intestinal types) according to FGP expression. Classification due to FGP expression can be achieved more easily, objectively, and simply than classification via the combined analysis of mucin immunohistochemistry.

Of note, this study also showed that the undifferentiated type of gastric cancer had gastric and intestinal phenotypes. Furthermore, in undifferentiated adenocarcinoma, the phenotype determined via mucin analysis corresponded with that determined via FGP expression. These results suggest that undifferentiated adenocarcinoma with FGP expression may arise from IM, while those without FGP expression arise from proper gastric epithelium, as has long been indicated [C5, 6].

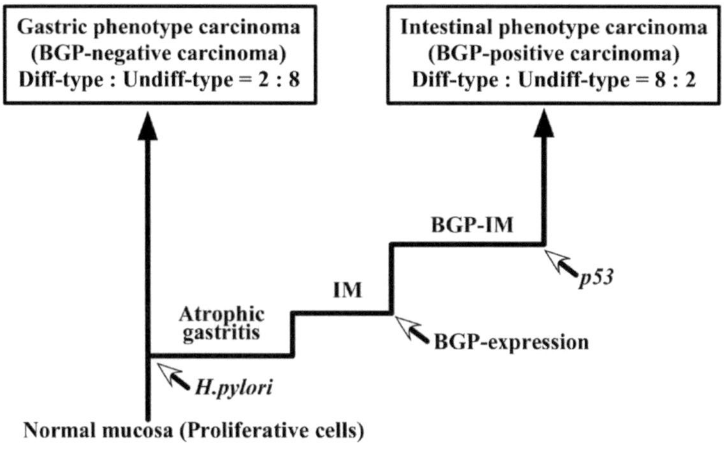

Figure 4. Relevance of FGP expression in the carcinogenesis of gastric and intestinal phenotypes of gastric carcinoma. *Diff-type*: Differentiated type, *Undiff-type*: Undifferentiated type, *IM*: intestinal metaplasia

A schema for our hypothesis derived from this study is shown in Figure 4. The ratios of differentiated and undifferentiated gastric cancers in FGP-positive and FGP-negative carcinomas were around 8:2 and 2:8, respectively. In a previous investigation, we found that FGP-positive proliferating cells in the IM appeared to be premalignant cells of intestinal-type carcinoma of the stomach. Therefore, it is suggested that approximately 80% and 20% of the differentiated and undifferentiated cancers, respectively, arise from FGP-positive proliferating cells of IM. On the other hand, approximately 20% and 80% of the differentiated and un-

http://dx.doi.org/10.5772/51793

differentiated cancers, respectively, arise from proper gastric mucosa, but candidates for the premalignant cells in proper gastric mucosa have not yet been suggested.

4. FGP expression in stomachs as a predictive risk factor for the synchronous and/or metachronous multiple gastric cancer

The recent advantage of endoscopic and laparoscopic local treatments has offered a better quality of life to patients with early gastric cancer involving no lymph node metastasis [34-38]. These treatments, however, incur increasing risks of missing the coexistence of accessory or microscopic carcinomas and/or developing new cancers in the remnant stomach [39-42]. The incidence of multiple primary gastric carcinomas has been reported to be from 5% to 10% in patients who had gastrectomy for gastric cancer [43-47]. The incidence is elevated with age and male sex, and with intestinal-type tumors; frequent occurrence in the lower third, and mucosal cancers, were significantly correlated with multiple early gastric cancer. However, these accessory lesions were missed preoperatively in approximately 30%-40% of the patients with multifocal early gastric cancers. Furthermore, considerable numbers of microscopic cancers could have been overlooked. Therefore, we should always remember that other lesions may also be present and/or grow when we are treating patients with gastric cancer by local treatment such as endoscopic treatment or laparoscopic wedge resection.

Local treatment for early gastric cancer is currently indicated mainly for intestinal-type carcinoma. If there were some indicators that predict the frequent coexistence of multiple gastric cancers and/or the metachronous growth of another gastric cancer of the intestinal-type, these would be very useful to identify the high-risk group and would contribute to the follow-up examinations after local treatment of gastric cancer patients. Our previous studies have demonstrated the significant role of the generative cells of FGP-positive IM as a premalignant lesion of intestinal-type gastric carcinoma.

Then, we designed the study to investigate the incidence of FGP-positive IM in gastric biopsy specimens and to establish FGP-positive IM as a predictor of the coexistence of accessory carcinoma and/or metachronous cancers before and after local treatment for early gastric cancer. Fifty-nine patients with intestinal-type early gastric cancer and endoscopic atrophic gastritis were analyzed. Of these patients, 14 had synchronous multiple gastric carcinomas, 25 had a single cancer, 20 had endoscopic atrophic gastritis without any localized lesions. During endoscopic examination, the lower two-thirds of the stomach was dyed with methylene blue and eight endoscopic biopsies were made from the stained mucosa in the anterior, posterior, greater and lesser curvature wall of the antrum and lower body of the stomach, respectively. Clinicopathological features of the patients showed that the patients with multiple early gastric carcinomas were significantly older than those with single early gastric carcinoma. However, there was no significant difference with the other parameters among the three groups.

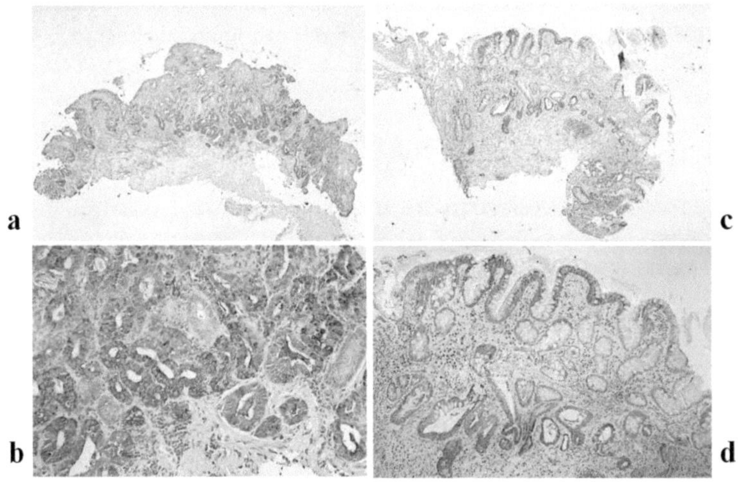

Figure 5. Immunohistochemical staining of biopsy specimens with anti-FGP antibody.**a** FGP-positive carcinoma, ×60; **b** high-power view, ×260; **c** FGP-positive IM, ×60; **d** high-power view, ×260

4.1. FGP expression in endoscopic biopsy specimens of gastric carcinoma and IM

Strongly positive reactivity was observed in the cytoplasm of cancer cells. In 93.3% (28/30) of the multiple carcinomas and 80.0% (20/25) of the single carcinomas, the biopsy specimens showed positive staining for FGP. The percentage of immunohistochemical positivity for anti-FGP antibody in the intestinal-type carcinoma corresponded well with previous our reports. The IM glands had structural deformity to a slight degree, but no cellular atypia. The generative cell zone of IM showed positive reactivity. Strong reactivity, similar to that in the cancer cells, was observed in the cytoplasm of the generative cells of IM (Figure 5).

4.2. Incidence of FGP-positive IM in stomachs with multiple carcinoma, single carcinoma and atrophic gastritis

Incidence of FGP-positive IM is shown in Figure 6. The distribution of the plots showing FGP-positive IM in the stomach was extremely characteristic in each group. The distribution was almost symmetrical in the multiple carcinoma and the atrophic gastritis groups. Although almost all stomachs with atrophic gastritis had no FGP-positive IM in any biopsy specimens, all the stomachs with multiple carcinomas had FGP-positive IM in each of the biopsy specimens. Furthermore, all the carcinomas in the multiple carcinoma group had high percentages of FGP-positive IM appearance, except for two in which FGP was negative in the cancer foci. On the other hand, a bipolarized distribution of the plots was observed in the single-carcinoma group; that is, about a quarter of the group had FGP-positive IM at high percentages, but about half of the group did not have it at all. The incidences of FGP-positive IM in the stomachs with multiple carcinomas, single carcinoma and atrophic gastritis were 83.2% ± 22.8%, 36.5% ± 41.3% and 7.1% ± 18.0%, respectively. The incidence of FGP-positive IM in the stomachs with multiple carcinomas was significantly higher than that in those with a single carcinoma or those with atrophic gastritis. The incidence in stomachs with a single carcinoma was significantly higher than that in those with atrophic gastritis.

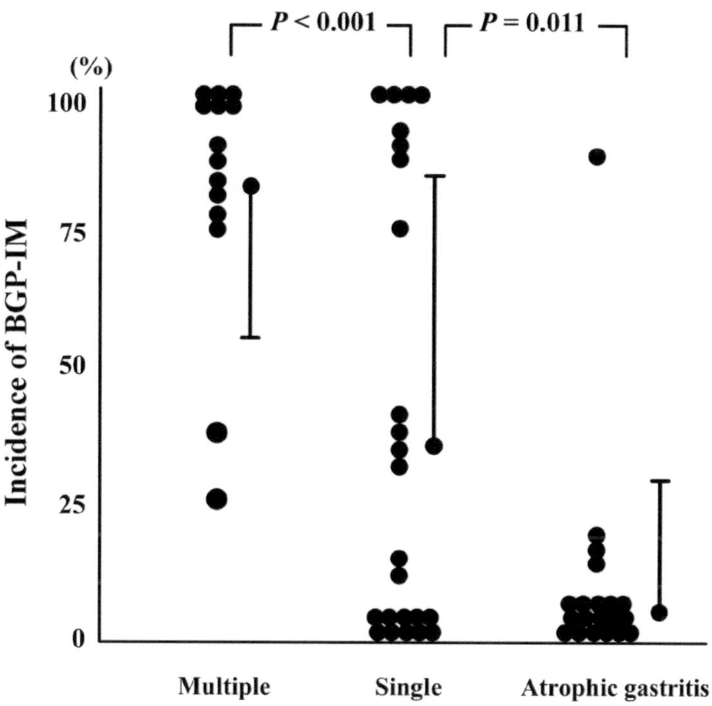

Figure 6. Distribution of incidence of FGP-positive IM in multiple carcinomas, single-carcinoma and atrophic gastritis groups.

4.3. Useful predictor for the development of new lesions after local treatment for early gastric cancer

One of the major problems with the local treatment of gastric cancer is that of the metachronous carcinomas in other parts of the stomach being different from the initial site of the carcinoma. A recent molecular biological study has suggested that high microsatellite instability in gastric tumors had a relationship with synchronous and/or metachronous gastric cancer compared with single carcinoma, whereas there was no difference in proliferative ability, carcinogenic pathway through p53 or K-ras, and various mismatch repair genes, although the mechanism was unclear [48]. However, the application of molecular genetics in the screening and surveillance of the patients with gastric cancer is still in its infancy. Arima et al. reported that metachronous recurrence was found in 6 of 76 endoscopically treated patients, and it was detected significantly more frequently in patients whose synchronous multiple lesions were found during the initial treatment; they stressed the importance of the detection of gastric mucosal recurrence by frequent periodic endoscopic examinations during the follow-up period after the endoscopic treatment [41]. Early detection of the metachronous cancer is beneficial for the subsequent treatment of the new lesion, for which minimally invasive therapy, including endoscopic treatment, can be used. The necessity for frequent endoscopic follow-up, however, affects the quality of life for the patients and increases the overall medical cost. Therefore, a reliable predictive indicator of patients with a high risk of metachronous recurrence is very important for determining the schedule of endoscopic follow-up after the initial endoscopic treatment. Because metachronous recurrence was detected significantly more frequently in patients with synchronous multiple lesions [35,36,41], a predictive indicator for metachronous recurrence would correspond with the indicator for synchronous multiple gastric carcinoma.

Wittekind et al. analyzed 61 patients with synchronous gastric carcinoma from among 1664 patients, and suggested that multiple primary tumors arose from precancerous conditions leading to similar genetic alterations [47]. It is generally accepted that IM in the stomach increases the risk of gastric cancer [11-14]. However, it has been suggested that only 0.1-0.2% of IM is related to the carcinogenesis of intestinal-type gastric cancer worldwide [49]. Therefore, the IM significantly correlated with carcinogenesis of intestinal-type cancer should be selected for use as an appropriate marker. Our previous consecutive studies revealed that the proportion of FGP positivity in both cancer and IM was significantly greater in the intestinal-type carcinoma than in the diffuse-type; also, we found that FGP-positive IM had a much stronger correlation with gastric carcinoma than the conventional typing of IM, and FGP-positive IM was significantly higher in proliferating state than in those samples without FGP, and p53 mutation occurred only in FGP-positive IM, suggesting that FGP-positive IM is a precancerous condition for intestinal-type carcinoma [10,50-53]. Thus, our findings indicate that FGP-positive IM is an excellent marker of the early stage of gastric carcinogenesis.

We also clearly demonstrated that the incidence of FGP-positive IM appearance was significantly more frequent in the stomachs with multiple gastric carcinomas than in those with single carcinoma or those with atrophic gastritis. The finding that some of the stomachs with a single carcinoma had a high incidence of FGP-positive IM may suggest the coexistence of microscopic intestinal-type carcinomas or the possibility of metachronous recurrence in the future. Assay of FGP in IM by immunohistochemistry in endoscopic biopsy specimens is an easy and reliable technique to assess FGP-positive IM status in the stomach, and thus could serve as a predictor of the high potential of a stomach in which synchronous gastric carcinoma coexists for generating metachronous gastric carcinoma. These results suggest that the analysis of FGP expression in IM in biopsy specimens will contribute to the pre- and postoperative assessment of multiple and metachronous gastric cancer.

Most gastric cancers of the intestinal type are known to occur on the distal side of the endoscopic atrophic border [54,55]. We agree with both the opinion that "the surgeon is required to resect the area including the F-line at the time of distal gastrectomy so as not to leave another cancer in the gastric remnant" [54] and the opinion that "the treatment of multiple gastric cancer does not require extended operative procedure, and endoscopic resection may be indicated if each lesion fits the criteria for treatment and careful follow-up is ensured" [56].

http://dx.doi.org/10.5772/51793

The important thing is to have a good predictor for metachronous recurrence after local treatment [41,48]. Our study demonstrated that FGP-positive IM was detected even in the stomachs with endoscopic atrophic gastritis without any malignant lesion, suggesting that FGP-positive IM was not a pathological entity which was associated with the change of a carcinogenic microenvironment in the gastric mucosa. Therefore, FGP can serve as a potential predictor for the risk-assessment of the development of multiple and/or metachronous carcinomas. It may be possible to follow-up new lesions by this method, and follow-up studies will give better information on whether FGP-positive IM positivity could be a good predictor for metachronous recurrence after local treatment.

5. Conclusion

We have proposed that the novel classification of IM based on the linkage between the generative cell zone of IM and gastric carcinoma using FGP expression. And also, the classification of gastric and intestinal phenotypes of gastric carcinoma is simpler and clearer when FGP expression is used than when mucin immunohistochemical analysis is used. It is suggested that FGP is a useful biomarker for the classification of intestinal and gastric types of carcinoma of the stomach, including classification from the carcinogenic point of view. And lastly we demonstrated the importance of FGP-positive IM as a predictor for the metachronous recurrence of gastric carcinoma, and we propose immunohistochemical staining of FGP in multiple endoscopic biopsy specimens as a predictive indicator of synchronous cancer and/or metachronous recurrence.

Author details

Masafumi Kuramoto[1*], Shinya Shimada[1], Satoshi Ikeshima[1], Kenichiro Yamamoto[1], Toshiro Masuda[1], Tatsunori Miyata[1], Shinichi Yoshimatsu[2], Masayuki Urata[2] and Hideo Baba[3]

*Address all correspondence to: kuramoto@yatsushiro-gh.jp

1 Department of Surgery, Yatsushiro Social Insurance General Hospital, Yatsushiro, Japan

2 Department of Gastroenterology and Hepatology, Yatsushiro Social Insurance General Hospital, Yatsushiro, Japan

3 Department of Gastroenterological Surgery, Graduate School of Medical Sciences, Kumamoto University, Kumamoto, Japan

References

[1] Takeuchi, T., & Kuriaki, H. (1955). Histochemical detection of phosphorylase in animal tissues. *The Journal of histochemistry and cytochemistry*, 3(3), 153-160.

[2] Takeuchi, T., Miyayama, H., & Iwamasa, T. (1978). Histochemical demonstration of total phosphorylase activity for diagnosis of carcinoma cells in human stomach and intestines. *Stain technology*, 53(5), 257-260.

[3] Cori, C. F., & Cori, G. T. (1936). Mechanism and formation of hexosemonophosphate in muscle and isolation of a new phosphate ester. *Proceedings of the Society for Experimental Biology and Medicine*, 34, 702-712.

[4] Newgard, C. B., Hwang, P. K., & Fletterick, R. J. (1989). The family of glycogen phosphorylases: structure and function. *Critical reviews in biochemistry and molecular biology*, 24(1), 69-99.

[5] Shimada, S., Maeno, M., Akagi, M., Hatayama, I., Sato, T., & Sato, K. (1986). Immunohistochemical detection of glycogen phosphorylase isoenzymes in rat and human tissues. *The Histochemical journal*, 18(6), 334-338.

[6] Newgard, C. B., Littman, D. R., Genderen, C. V., Smith, M., & Fletterick, R. J. (1988). Human brain glycogen phosphorylase. Cloning, sequence analysis, chromosomal mapping, tissue expression, and comparison with the human liver and muscle isozymes. *The Journal of biological chemistry*, 263(8), 3850-3857.

[7] Nakano, K., Hwang, P. K., & Fletterick, R. J. (1986). Complete cDNA sequence for rabbit muscle glycogen phosphorylase. *FEBS letters*, 204(2), 283-287.

[8] Sato, K., Morris, H. P., & Weinhouse, S. (1972). Phosphorylase: a new isozyme in rat hepatic tumors and fetal liver. *Science*, 178(4063), 879-881.

[9] Gelinas, R. P., Froman, B. E., Mc Elroy, F., Tait, R. C., & Gorin, F. A. (1989). Human brain glycogen phosphorylase: characterization of fetal cDNA and genomic sequences. *Molecular brain research*, 6(2-3), 177-85.

[10] Shimada, S., Maeno, M., Misumi, A., Takano, S., & Akagi, M. (1987). Antigen reversion of glycogen phosphorylase isoenzyme in carcinoma and proliferative zone of intestinal metaplasia of the human stomach. An immunohistochemical study. *Gastroenterology*, 93(1), 35-40.

[11] Morson, B. C. (1955). Intestinal metaplasia of the gastric mucosa. *British journal of cancer*, 9(3), 365-376.

[12] Ming, S. C., Goldman, H., & Freiman, D. G. (1967). Intestinal metaplasia and histogenesis of carcinoma in human stomach. Light and electron microscopic study. *Cancer*, 20(9), 1418-1429.

[13] Stemmermann, G. N. (1994). Intestinal metaplasia of the stomach. A status report. *Cancer*, 74(2), 556-564.

[14] Correa, P., & Shiao, Y. H. (1994). Phenotypic and genotypic events in gastric carcinogenesis. *Cancer research*, 54(7), 1941-1943.

[15] Hill, M. J. (1994). Mechanisms of gastric carcinogenesis. *European journal of cancer prevention*, 3(2), 25-9.

[16] Tosi, P., Filipe, M. I., Baak, J. P., Luzi, P., Santopietro, R., Miracco, C., Sforza, V., & Megha, T. (1990). Morphometric definition and grading of gastric intestinal metaplasia. *The Journal of pathology*, 161(3), 201-208.

[17] Filipe, M. I., Muñoz, N., Matko, I., Kato, I., Pompe-Kirn, V., Jutersek, A., Teuchmann, S., Benz, M., & Prijon, T. (1994). Intestinal metaplasia types and the risk of gastric cancer: a cohort study in Slovenia. *International journal of cancer*, 57(3), 324-329.

[18] Iida, F., Murata, F., & Nagata, T. (1978). Histochemical studies of mucosubstances in metaplastic epithelium of the stomach, with special reference to the development of intestinal metaplasia. *Histochemistry*, 56(3-4), 229-37.

[19] Matsukura, N., Suzuki, K., Kawachi, T., Aoyagi, M., Sugimura, T., Kitaoka, H., Numajiri, H., Shirota, A., Itabashi, M., & Hirota, T. (1980). Distribution of marker enzymes and mucin in intestinal metaplasia in human stomach and relation to complete and incomplete types of intestinal metaplasia to minute gastric carcinomas. *Journal of the National Cancer Institute*, 65(2), 231-240.

[20] Kato, Y., Kitagawa, T., Yanagisawa, A., Kubo, K., Utsude, T., Hiratsuka, H., Tamaki, M., & Sugano, H. (1992). Site-dependent development of complete and incomplete intestinal metaplasia types in the human stomach. *Japanese journal of cancer research*, 83(2), 178-183.

[21] Fearon, E. R., & Vogelstein, B. (1990). A genetic model for colorectal tumorigenesis. *Cell*, 61(5), 759-767.

[22] Brito, M. J., Filipe, M. I., & Morris, R. W. (1992). Cell proliferation study on gastric carcinoma and non-involved gastric mucosa using a bromodeoxyuridine (BrdU) labelling technique. *European journal of cancer prevention*, 1(6), 429-435.

[23] Ranzani, G. N., Luinetti, O., Padovan, L. S., Calistri, D., Renault, B., Burrel, M., Amadori, D., Fiocca, R., & Solcia, E. (1995). p53 gene mutations and protein nuclear accumulation are early events in intestinal type gastric cancer but late events in diffuse type. *Cancer epidemiology biomarkers & prevention*, 4(3), 223-231.

[24] Tahara, E. (1993). Molecular mechanism of stomach carcinogenesis. *Journal of cancer research and clinical oncology*, 119(5), 265-272.

[25] Shiao, Y. H., Rugge, M., Correa, P., Lehmann, H. P., & Scheer, W. D. (1994). p53 alteration in gastric precancerous lesions. *The American journal of pathology*, 144(3), 511-517.

[26] Tatematsu, M., Ichinose, M., Miki, K., Hasegawa, R., Kato, T., & Ito, N. (1990). Gastric and intestinal phenotypic expression of human stomach cancers as revealed by pep-

sinogen immunohistochemistry and mucin histochemistry. *Acta pathologica japonica*, 40(7), 494-504.

[27] Kushima, R., & Hattori, T. (1993). Histogenesis and characteristics of gastric-type adenocarcinomas in the stomach. *Journal of cancer research and clinical oncology*, 120(1-2), 103-11.

[28] Akashi, H., Hinoda, Y., Itoh, F., Adachi, M., Endo, T., & Imai, K. (1997). A novel gastric-cancer-associated mucin antigen defined by a monoclonal antibody A3D4. *International journal of cancer*, 73(6), 795-801.

[29] Egashira, Y., Shimoda, T., & Ikegami, M. (1999). Mucin histochemical analysis of minute gastric differentiated adenocarcinoma. *Pathology international*, 49(1), 55-61.

[30] Nakamura, K., Sugano, H., & Takagi, K. (1968). Carcinoma of the stomach in incipient phase: its histogenesis and histological appearances. *Gann*, 59(3), 251-258.

[31] Lauren, P. (1965). The two histological main types of gastric carcinoma: diffuse and so-called intestinal-type carcinoma. An attempt at a histo- clinical classification. *Acta pathologica et microbiologica Scandinavica*, 64, 31-49.

[32] Bara, J., Gautier, R., Mouradian, P., Decaens, C., & Daher, N. (1991). Oncofetal mucin M1 epitope family: characterization and expression during colonic carcinogenesis. *International journal of cancer*, 47(2), 304-310.

[33] Tytgat, K. M., Büller, H. A., Opdam, F. J., Kim, Y. S., Einerhand, A. W., & Dekker, J. (1994). Biosynthesis of human colonic mucin: Muc2 is the prominent secretory mucin. *Gastroenterology*, 107(5), 1352-63.

[34] Tada, M., Murakami, A., Karita, M., Yanai, H., & Okita, K. (1993). Endoscopic resection of early gastric cancer. *Endoscopy*, 25(7), 445-450.

[35] Takekoshi, T., Baba, Y., Ota, H., Kato, Y., Yanagisawa, A., Takagi, K., & Noguchi, Y. (1994). Endoscopic resection of early gastric carcinoma: results of a retrospective analysis of 308 cases. *Endoscopy*, 26(4), 352-358.

[36] Kojima, T., Parra-Blanco, A., Takahashi, H., & Fujita, R. (1998). Outcome of endoscopic mucosal resection for early gastric cancer: review of the Japanese literature. *Gastrointestinal endoscopy*, 48(5), 550-554.

[37] Ohgami, M., Kumai, K., Otani, Y., Wakabayashi, G., Kubota, T., & Kitajima, M. (1994). Laparoscopic wedge resection of the stomach for early gastric cancer using a lesion-lifting method. *Digestive surgery*, 11, 64-67.

[38] Roukos, D. H. (1999). Current advances and changes in treatment strategy may improve survival and quality of life in patients with potentially curable gastric cancer. *Annals of surgical oncology*, 6(1), 46-56.

[39] Janssen, C. W., Jr, Lie, R. T., Maartmann-Moe, H., & Matre, R. (1990). Who gets a second primary cancer after gastric cancer surgery? *European journal of surgical oncology*, 16(3), 195-199.

[40] Seto, Y., Nagawa, H., & Muto, T. (1996). Treatment of multiple early gastric cancer. *Japanese journal of clinical oncology*, 26(3), 134-138.

[41] Arima, N., Adachi, K., Katsube, T., Amano, K., Ishihara, S., Watanabe, M., & Kinoshita, Y. (1999). Predictive factors for metachronous recurrence of early gastric cancer after endoscopic treatment. *Journal of clinical gastroenterology*, 29(1), 44-47.

[42] El -Zimaity, H. M., & Ota, H. (1999). Endoscopic resection for early gastric cancer: possibilities and limitations. *Journal of clinical gastroenterology*, 29(1), 5-6.

[43] Honmyo, U., Misumi, A., Murakami, A., Haga, Y., & Akagi, M. (1989). Clinicopathological analysis of synchronous multiple gastric carcinoma. *European journal of surgical oncology*, 15(4), 316-321.

[44] Kosaka, T., Miwa, K., Yonemura, Y., Urade, M., Ishida, T., Takegawa, S., Kamata, T., Ooyama, S., Maeda, K., Sugiyama, K., et al. (1990). A clinicopathologic study on multiple gastric cancers with special reference to distal gastrectomy. *Cancer*, 65(11), 2602-2605.

[45] Brandt, D., Muramatsu, Y., Ushio, K., Mizuguchi, Y., Itabashi, M., Yoshida, S., Moriyama, N., Nawano, S., Ishikawa, T., Yamada, T., et al. (1989). Synchronous early gastric cancer. *Radiology*, 173(3), 649-652.

[46] Kodera, Y., Yamamura, Y., Torii, A., Uesaka, K., Hirai, T., Yasui, K., Morimoto, T., Kato, T., & Kito, T. (1995). Incidence, diagnosis and significance of multiple gastric cancer. *The British journal of surgery*, 82(11), 1540-1543.

[47] Wittekind, C., Klimpfinger, M., Hermanek, P., & Tannapfel, A. (1997). Multiple simultaneous gastric carcinomas. *British journal of cancer*, 76(12), 1604-1609.

[48] Kawamura, A., Adachi, K., Ishihara, S., Katsube, T., Takashima, T., Yuki, M., Amano, K., Fukuda, R., Yamashita, Y., & Kinoshita, Y. (2001). Correlation between microsatellite instability and metachronous disease recurrence after endoscopic mucosal resection in patients with early stage gastric carcinoma. *Cancer*, 91(2), 339-345.

[49] Kubo, T. (1981). Etiology of intestinal metaplasia. *In: Takemoto T, Kawai K, Ida K, Suzuku S (eds). Intestinal metaplasia of the human stomach (in Japanese). Tokyo: Igaku-Tosho-Shuppan*, 27-31.

[50] Shimada, S., Maeno, M., Misumi, A., & Akagi, M. (1984). Histochemical study of phosphorylase in proliferating cells of intestinal metaplasia and carcinoma of the human stomach. *Scandinavian journal of gastroenterology*, 19(7), 965-970.

[51] Shimada, S., Honmyo, U., Yagi, Y., Ikeda, T., Ogawa, M., & Yokota, T. (1992). Expression of glycogen phosphorylase activity in minute gastric carcinoma. *The American journal of gastroenterology*, 87(9), 1230-1231.

[52] Matsuzaki, H., Shimada, S., Uno, K., Tsuruta, J., & Ogawa, M. (1998). Novel subtyping of intestinal metaplasia in the human stomach: brain-type glycogen phosphory-

lase expression in the proliferative zone and its relationship with carcinogenesis. *American journal of clinical pathology*, 109(2), 181-189.

[53] Shimada, S., Tashima, S., Yamaguchi, K., Matsuzaki, H., & Ogawa, M. (1999). Carcinogenesis of intestinal-type gastric cancer and colorectal cancer is commonly accompanied by expression of brain (fetal)-type glycogen phosphorylase. *Journal of experimental & clinical cancer research*, 18(1), 111-118.

[54] Kimura, K., & Takemoto, T. (1969). An endoscopic recognition of the atrophic border and its significance in chronic gastritis. *Endoscopy*, 1, 87-97.

[55] Yoshimura, T., Shimoyama, T., Fukuda, S., Tanaka, M., Axon, A. T., & Munakata, A. (1999). Most gastric cancer occurs on the distal side of the endoscopic atrophic border. *Scandinavian journal of gastroenterology*, 34(11), 1077-1081.

[56] Takeshita, K., Tani, M., Honda, T., Saeki, I., Kando, F., Saito, N., & Endo, M. (1997). Treatment of primary multiple early gastric cancer: from the viewpoint of clinicopathologic features. *World journal of surgery*, 21(8), 832-836.

Chapter 6

Naringenin Inhibits Oxidative Stress Induced Macromolecular Damage in N-methyl N-nitro N-nitrosoguanidine Induced Gastric Carcinogenesis in Wistar Rats

Ekambaram Ganapathy, Devaraja Rajasekaran,
Murugan Sivalingam, Muhammed Farooq Shukkur,
Ebrahim Abdul Shukkur and
Sakthisekaran Dhanapal

Additional information is available at the end of the chapter

http://dx.doi.org/10.5772/45896

1. Introduction

Neoplasia of the stomach represents the second most recurrent cause of cancer mortality in the world [1]. Despite major efforts, the number of deaths from gastric cancer has not decreased in recent years. There have also been major efforts to better understand the mechanisms responsible for oncogenesis and a number of animal models of have been developed to study the correlates of gastric carcinoma in recent years [2, 3]. Among these, the 1-methyl 3 nitro 1 nitrosoguanidine (MNNG) model has proven to be very useful. Evidences suggest that MNNG administration results in oncogenesis as a result of increased free radical synthesis in the gastric mucosa [4, 5]. DNA damage induced by oxidative stress and/or deficient DNA-repair is reported to have an etiological or prognostic role in cancer [4].

Research also suggests that electrophiles could play a key role in chemical carcinogenesis. The oxidative inactivation of enzymes by free radicals and accumulation of oxidized proteins may play a critical role in the alteration of cellular function and cell death. Oxidative damage can generate large amounts of carbonyl products and hence measurement of these components could reflect oxidative protein damage [6]. Synthesis of certain polyamines notably histamine, putrescine, spermine and spermidine is essential for the regulation of protein, RNA and DNA synthesis. In addition, the ability of polyamines to alter DNA–protein interactions could disrupt certain cellular functions under cancerous conditions [7]. These biomarkers are biological and molecular end-points that are quantitatively modulated by chemopreventive agents and as such could indicate the efficacy of the dietary agents.

Dietary antioxidants are important health-protecting factor. Studies have convincingly stated that frequent consumption of fruits and vegetables rich in antioxidants could decrease the risk of cancer [8]. Naringenin, a flavanone compound highly enriched in grapefruits, has been identified as a possible inhibitor of cell proliferation and potential to act as an antitumorigenic agent [9-11]. We recently reported that naringenin could reduce tumor size, ROS levels and enhance antioxidant status [12]. However, the mechanism of action of naringenin to suppress cell growth is still ambiguous since this compound appears to have multiple cellular targets including cytochrome P450 enzymes [13]. We analyzed gastric cancer induced by MNNG, which reportedly induce cellular oxidative damage through DNA strand breaks [14] and explored the possible protective role of naringenin by measuring the levels of protein damage and polyamine synthesis in MNNG-induced gastric carcinogenesis in experimental rats.

2. Materials and methods

2.1. Drugs and chemicals

MNNG, Naringenin [~95%, $C_{15}H_{12}O_5$; (±)-2,3-Dihydro-5,7-dihydroxy-2-(4-hydroxy phenyl) -4*H*-1-benzopyran-4-one 4′,5,7-Trihydroxyflavanone, Molecular Weight: 272.25, CAS Number 67604-48-2] Histopaque 1077, RPMI 1640 and BSA were purchased from Sigma (St.Louis, MO, USA), Hanks Balanced Salt Solution from Himedia (Mumbai, India), LMPA and other chemicals of analytical grade were purchased from SRL, Mumbai, India.

2.2. Animals

All the experiments were carried out with male Wistar rats 6–8 weeks old (80-90g) obtained from the Central Animal House, University of Madras, Dr. ALM PG IBMS, Taramani, Chennai, Tamilnadu, India. The rats were housed six in a polypropylene cage and provided food and water *ad libitum*. The animals were maintained under standard conditions of temperature (23 ± 2ºC) and humidity (50-70%) with an alternating 12-hour light/dark cycle with free access to standard pellet diet (Mysore Snack Feed Ltd, Mysore, India) and maintained in accordance with the guidelines of the National Institute of Nutrition, Indian Council of Medical Research (ICMR), Hyderabad, India and approved by the ethical committee of University of Madras (IAEC no. 02/055/05).

2.3. Treatment schedule

Rats in Group I served as control and was given oral corn oil for 20 weeks. Group II animals were induced with MNNG 200 mg/kg b. wt, by oral gavage at days 0 and 14 and saturated NaCl (1ml/rat) was given 3 days once for four weeks and maintained till the end of the experimental period. Group III animals were induced with MNNG + NaCl (as in group II) and treated with naringenin (200 mg/kg b.wt, dissolved in corn oil, orally) simultaneously for 20 weeks from the first dose of MNNG + NaCl. Group IV animals were post-treated with naringenin (200 mg/kg b.wt, dissolved in corn oil, orally) from the 6th week of MNNG (as in group II) induction up to end of experimental period. Group V animals were treated with naringenin (200 mg/kg b.wt, dissolved in corn oil, orally) alone for 20 weeks. The experiment was terminated at the end of 20 weeks and all the animals were sacrificed by cervical dislocation after an overnight fasting.

2.4. Tumour weight

Tumour weight was estimated according to the method of Geren et al.,[15]. The resultant solid tumour was considered to be prelate ellipsoid with one long axis and two short axes. The two short axes were measured using a vernier caliper. The tumour weight was calculated by multiplying the length of the tumour with the square of the width and dividing the product by 2.

2.5. Analysis of ROS

To examine the *in vivo* generation of ROS, we used the cell permeable probe 2′, 7′-dichlorodihydrofluorescin diacetate (CM-H_2DCFH-DA; Molecular Probes, Eugene, OR, USA) according to the method described by Parsons et al.,[16]

2.6. Biochemical analysis

The oxidative protein damage was determined by the estimation of carbonyl content by the method of Levins et al., [17]. Protein content was estimated by the method of Lowry et al., [18]. The DNA and RNA contents were estimated in the homogenate by the method of Burton [19] and Rawal et al., [20]. Lipid peroxidation (LPO) was estimated by the method of Ohkawa et al., [21].

2.7. DNA fragementation

The extent of DNA fragmentation was measured by the method of Sellins and Cohen [22]. The isolated DNA was visualized for fragmentation by electrophoresis in a 1.2% agarose gel containing ethidium bromide.

2.8. Assessment of DNA damage

DNA damage was assessed with alkaline single cell gel electrophoresis (comet assay) according to the method described by Singh et al., [23].

2.9. Polyamine analysis

Separation of various polyamine fractions such as histamine, putrescine, spermine and spermidine and their subsequent estimation was done by the method of Endo [24]. CM-cellulose column chromatography: Rat tissues (stomach-100 mg) were homogenized in ice-cold 0.4 M $HClO_4$ containing 2 mM ethylenediaminetetracetic acid. The homogenate was centrifuged at 1000 g for 5 min. The neutralized supernatant was applied to a CM cellulose column. Each sample solution (0.5 – 3 mL) was applied to a CM-cellulose column (0.6×10 cm) equilibrated with 0.01 M phosphate buffer (pH 6.2). After the column was washed with 15 mL of 0.01 M phosphate buffer (pH 6.2) and 15 mL of 0.03 M phosphate buffer (pH 6.2), histamine, putrescine, spermidine and spermine were eluted out from the column with borate buffer without NaCl (30 mL), borate buffer containing 0.03 M NaCl (20 mL), borate buffer containing 0.075 M NaCl (20 mL), and borate buffer containing 0.15 M NaCl (20 mL), respectively. Fractions (3 mL) were collected at a flow rate of approximately 3 mL/min. Trinitrobenzenesulphonate (TNBS) reagent (1 mL) was added to the elute (3 mL) from the CM-cellulose column. The reaction was carried out at 50°C for 10 min and terminated by cooling the reaction mixture in water. Absorbance at 420 nm was measured within 20 min.

2.10. Statistical analysis

The data are presented as mean ± SD for six rats in each group. Significance of the differences between mean values was determined by one-way analysis of variance (ANOVA) followed by the Duncan test for multiple comparison. P values 0.001, 0.01, 0.05 were considered to reveal significance.

3. Results

The mean body weights were decreased and tumor weights increased in group II (MNNG + S-NaCl) animals as compared with all the other groups (Table 1). A 100% incidence in gastric cancer was noticed among group II animals. Importantly, naringenin treatment significantly increased the body weight and decreased the tumor weights among group III ($p<0.05$) and IV animals as compared to group II animals. Furthermore, a progressive increase in the mean body weight was observed among group V animals during the experimental period. Conceptually, the increase in body weight after the administration of naringenin in Group III and Group IV rats highlights the protective efficacy of the flavonoid.

A significant increase in ROS generation was observed in stomach and liver tissue of MNNG induced groups II animals as compared with control animal group I (Fig. 1). However, there was significantly decreased activity in group III and group IV naringenin treated animals. The results were suggested that the antioxidant effect of naringenin in MNNG induced animals could be due to its free radical scavenging action.

Figure 2a and 2b shows the levels of LPO and protein carbonyl content in stomach and liver tissues of various experimental groups. A significant ($p<0.001$) increase in the extent of LPO and protein carbonyl content was observed in the stomach and liver of carcinoma bearing group II animals as compared to the control animals (group I). Naringenin significantly decreased the LPO and protein carbonyls of group III and group IV animals ($p<0.001$, $p<0.01$) as compared to carcinogen-induced group II rats. However, naringenin alone treated ani-

http://dx.doi.org/10.5772/45896

mals (group V) did not show any significant change as compared with the control animals (group I).

Groups	Group I (Control)	Group II (MNNG + NaCl Induced)	Group III (Naringenin simultaneous treatment)	Group IV (Naringenin post treatment)	Group V (Naringenin alone)
Body Weight (g)	310.17 ± 15.78	166.41± 16.80a#	270.18 ± 17.99b@	230.75 ± 15.18b@c@	330.23 ± 16.08
Tumor weight (g)	-	0.72 ± 0.05	0.31±0.03 a#	0.51±0.04a@ b#	-
No. of rats with gastric cancer (%)	0 (0%)	6/6 (100%)	0/6 (0%)	2 (33.3%)	0 (%)

Values are expressed as mean ± SD (n=6) for each group. Different letters represent significant variations as calculated by 1-way analysis of variance and the Duncan test. Body weight: a, as compared with group I; b, as compared with group II; c, as compared with group III. Tumor weight: a, as compared with group II. @ - $p<0.05$; # - $p<0.01$; * - $p<0.001$.

Table 1. Effect of naringenin on body and tumor weight and incidence of gastric cancer of control and experimental rats.

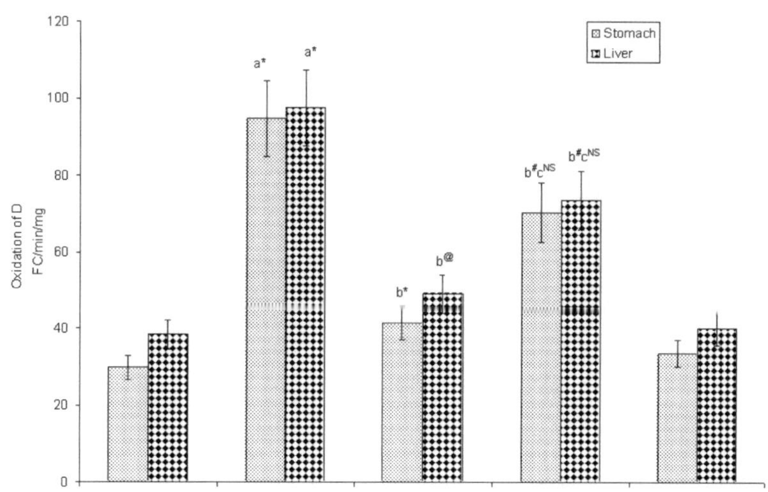

Figure 1. Effect of naringenin on ROS generation in control and experimental animals. ROS production estimated by oxidation of the fluorescent probe, DCFDA. Groups (I-V) are Control, MNNG induced, naringenin simultaneous treatment, naringenin post treated and naringenin alone respectively. The details are described under materials and methods. Values are the mean ± SD of six rats in each group. (a-c) represent (a) as compared with Group I; (b) as compared with Group II; (c) as compared with group III (*$p<0.001$,@$p<0.01$, #$p<0.05$).

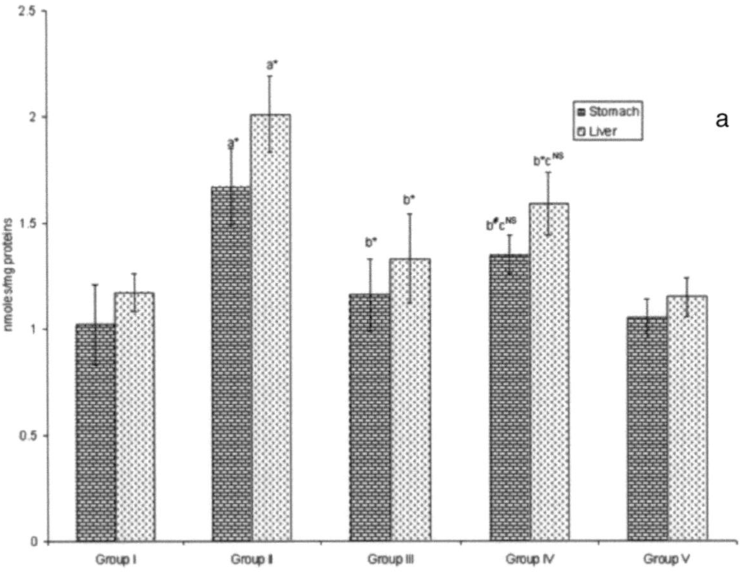

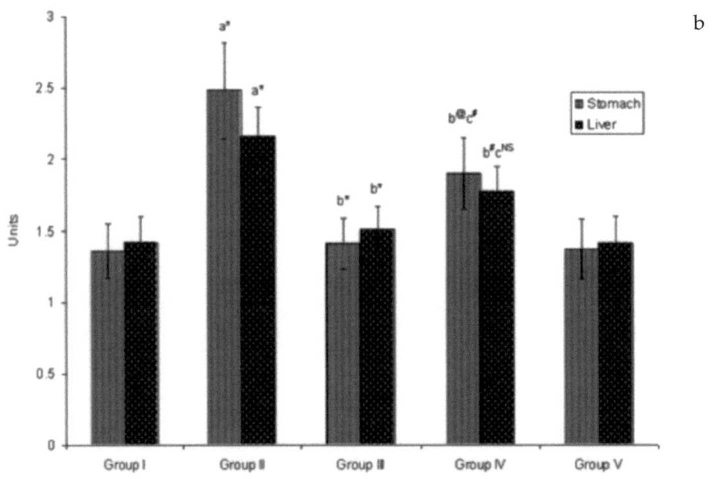

Figure 2. a. Effect of naringenin on lipidperoxidation in stomach and liver of control and experimental animals. Formation of lipid peroxidation product was determined in terms of MDA as described under materials and methods. Groups (I-V) are Control, MNNG induced, naringenin simultaneous treatment, naringenin post treated and naringenin alone respectively. Units: nmoles of MDA release/mg protein. Values are the mean ± SD of six rats in each group. (a-c) represent (a) as compared with Group I; (b) as compared with Group II; (c) as compared with group III (*p<0.001,@p<0.01, #p<0.05). b. Effect of naringenin on protein carbonyl formation in control and experimental animals. Oxidation of Stomach and liver proteins of all animals were determined in terms of protein carbonyl formation. Groups (I-V) are Control, MNNG induced, naringenin simultaneous treatment, naringenin post treated and naringenin alone respectively. The details are described under materials and methods. Units: nmoles/mg protein. Values are the mean ± SD of six rats in each group. (a-c) represent (a) as compared with Group I; (b) as compared with Group II; (c) as compared with group III (*p<0.001,@p<0.01, #p<0.05).

http://dx.doi.org/10.5772/45896

Fig. 3 shows the agarose gel electrophoretic pattern of DNA isolated from the stomach tissue of control and experimental animals. In group I control and group II cancer bearing animals, there was no significant DNA fragmentation. Naringenin treated (group III) animals exhibited a significant DNA fragmentation. In group IV animals was shown less DNA fragmentation when compared with group III. However, a significant fragmentation of DNA was observed in animals treated with naringenin alone (group V).

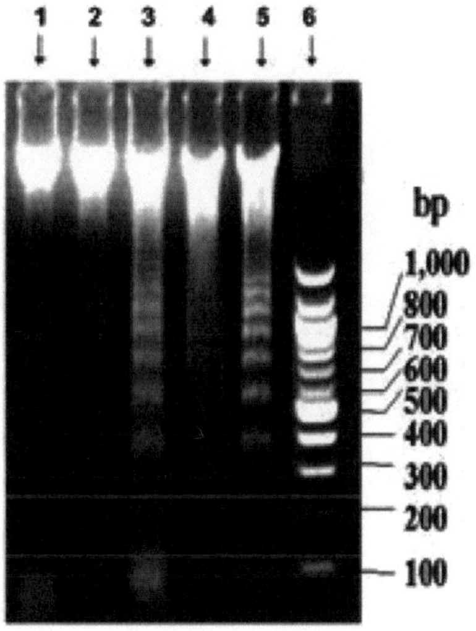

Figure 3. Effect of naringenin on DNA fragmentation in control and experimental animals. Groups (I-VI) are Control, MNNG induced, naringenin simultaneous treatment, naringenin post treated, naringenin alone and DNA marker respectively. The details are described under materials and methods. DNA was isolated by agarose gel electrophoresis and visualized by ethidium bromide staining.

Fig. 4 shows the level of DNA damage measured using single cell gel electrophoresis in stomach tissue of control and experimental animals. There was a significant increase in DNA tail length (3.21- fold) in cancer bearing animals (group II) as compared with group I control animals and significant decrease (2.27 - fold) in Group III and Group IV in (1.84-fold) (naringenin treated) animals when compared with group II animals. In addition, there was no comparable difference between rats treated with naringenin alone (group V) and the control animals.

Figure 5 and 6 shows the levels of nucleic acids and polyamines in the stomach of control and experimental animals. Cancer induced animals (group II) showed a significant increase ($p<0.001$) in nucleic acid and polyamine contents in stomach tissue when compared with the control animals (group I). On treatment with naringenin (group III and group IV), there was found to be a significant ($p<0.001$, $p<0.01$) decrease in the levels of nucleic acids and polyamines in stomach tissue when compared with cancer-induced animals (group II). However, naringenin alone treated animals (group V) did not show any significant changes when compared with control animals (group I).

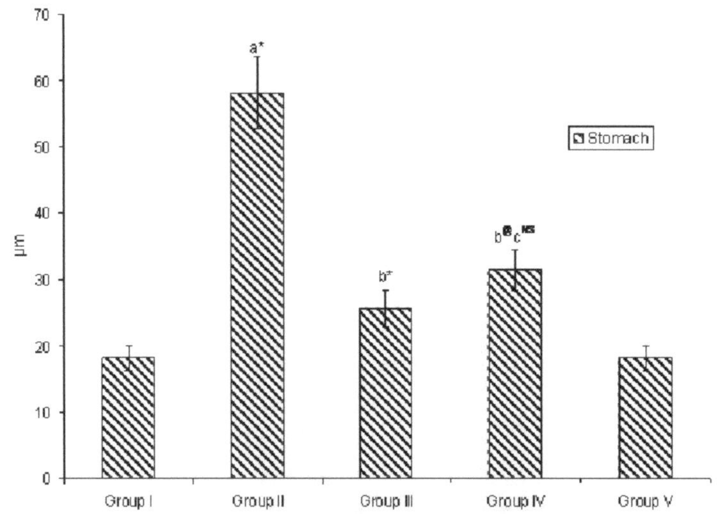

Figure 4. Effect of naringenin on DNA single strand breaks in control experimental animals. Oxidative DNA damage in stomach of control and experimental animals were determined by comet assay. Groups (I-V) are Control, MNNG induced, naringenin simultaneous treatment, naringenin post treated and naringenin alone respectively. The details are described under materials and methods. DNA tail length was expressed in µm. Values are the mean ± SD of six rats in each group. (a-c) represent (a) as compared with Group I; (b) as compared with Group II; (c) as compared with group III (*p<0.001,@p<0.01, #p<0.05).

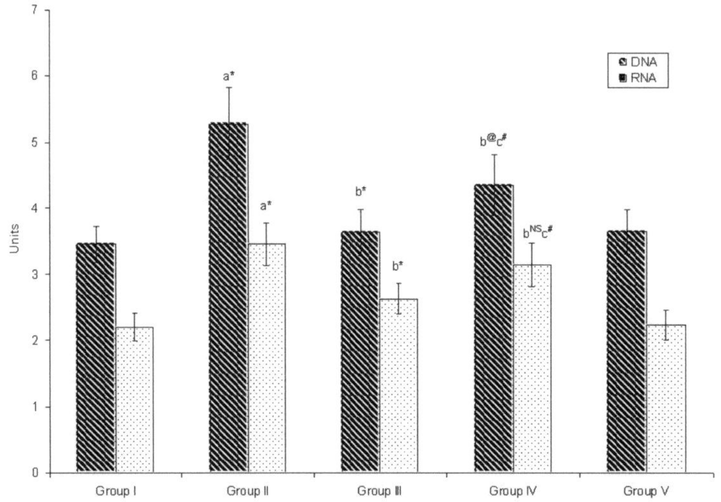

Figure 5. Effect of naringenin on the levels of nucleic acid content in stomach of control and experimental animals. Groups (I-V) are Control, MNNG induced, naringenin simultaneous treatment, naringenin post treated and naringenin alone respectively. The details are described under materials and methods. Units: mg/g wet tissue. Values are the mean ± SD of six rats in each group. (a-c) represent (a) as compared with Group I; (b) as compared with Group II; (c) as compared with group III (*p<0.001,@p<0.01, #p<0.05).

http://dx.doi.org/10.5772/45896

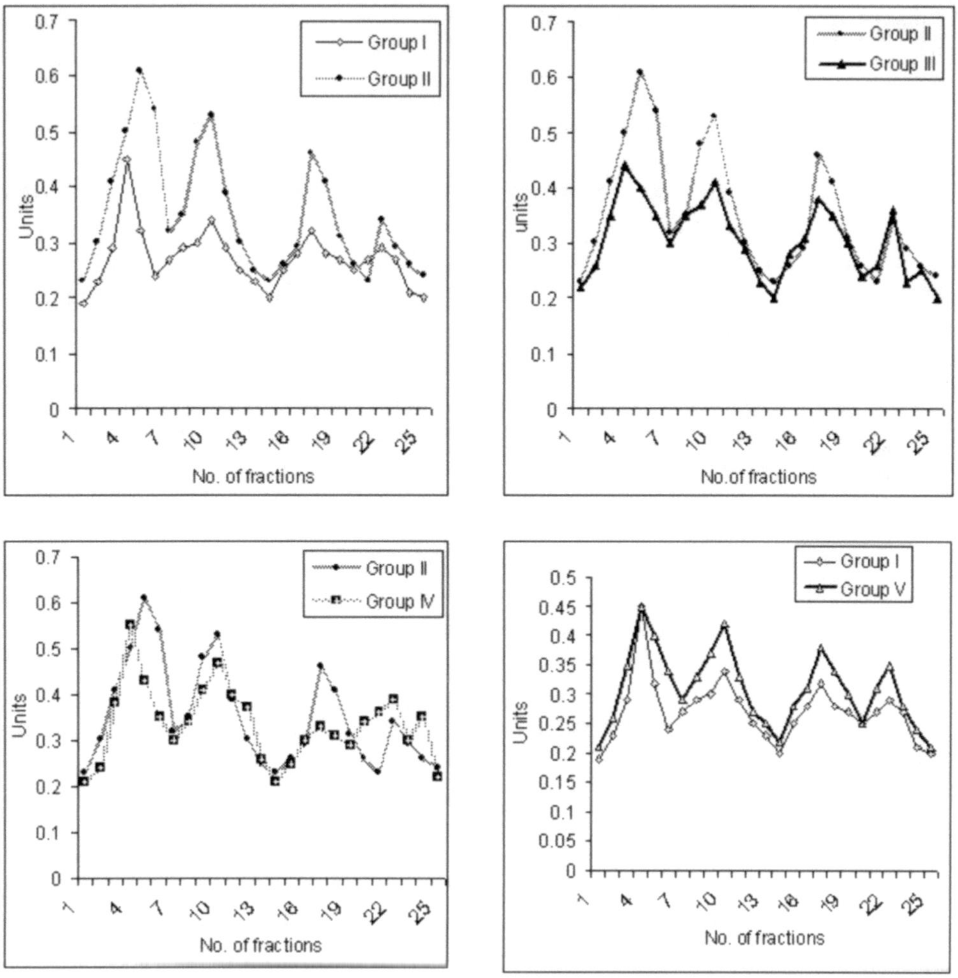

Figure 6. Effect of naringenin on the levels of polyamines in stomach of control and experimental animals. 25 fractions were collected from each group. Groups (I-V) are Control, MNNG induced, naringenin simultaneous treatment, naringenin post treated and naringenin alone respectively. The details are described under materials and methods.

4. Discussion

Development of a diet that provides adequate nutrition and effective cancer prevention is an important goal in nutrition and cancer research [8]. We suggest that naringenin could be an effective chemopreventive agent in MNNG induced gastric carcinoma. ROS and organic free radical intermediates formed from carcinogens reportedly initiate carcinogenic transformation [25]. Consequently, the accumulation of free radical mediated damage may be a possible mechanism of cancer development [26]. MNNG is an effective carcinogen with a capability to induce enormous amounts of free radicals, which in turn reacts with lipids causing release of lipid peroxides [27]. Naringenin significantly reduced the lipid peroxides and increased free radicals scavenging capabilities in cancer bearing animals, which could be due to its capability to enhance antioxidant enzymes [28,29]. This has been supported by our recent report that administration of naringenin to gastric carcinoma-induced rats largely upregulated the redox status to decrease the risk of cancer [12]. The antioxidant enzymes may reduce the carcinogen-DNA interaction by providing a large nucleophilic pool for the electrophilic carcinogens such as MNNG [30], and it causes oxidative protein damage in gastric carcinogenesis-induced animals [31]. Among the various oxidative modifications in protein, carbonyl formation may be an early marker for protein oxidation [32]. Protein carbonyls have been used as a biomarker of oxidative stress because of the relative stability of carbonylated proteins and the high protein concentration in blood. However, we found that tissue carbonyl levels in naringenin treated groups were decreased when compared with MNNG induced with cancer.

A number of flavonoids have been shown to suppress carcinogenesis in various animal models [33]. There is currently considerable interest in these compounds as they appear to exert a beneficial effect on several key mechanisms involved in the pathogenesis of cancer. DNA fragmentation is generally considered to be the hallmark of apoptosis. Indeed the nuclear DNA of apoptotic cells shows a characteristic laddering pattern of oligonucleosomal fragments. Several studies have demonstrated a positive correlation between DNA fragmentation and apoptosis. Medicinal plants and natural dietary constituents such as naringenin have been reported to induce apoptosis in malignant cells *in vitro* [34]. Our present study we observed DNA fragmentation induced by naringenin, which possess, prevention of MNNG.

Additionally, we have also observed an induction of apoptosis on naringenin in stomach cancer bearing animals as revealed by the enhancement of LPO and oxidative DNA damage. The absence of intranucleosomal DNA-fragmentation in MNNG induced animals reflects the prevention of apoptotic mechanisms in malignant cells. Our report has shown that intranucleosomal DNA fragmentation during chemoprevention of naringenin treated rats. The results support that the findings of key changes in cell death can occur without DNA fragmentation and it alone should not be considered as a criterion for assessing apoptotic cell death [35].

Feng et al., [36] reported natural antioxidants are capable of inhibiting the ROS production and thereby reducing the associated intra-cellular oxidative stress. Importantly, ROS, damaging almost all classes of subcellular components, are produced in numerous pathophysiological states and have been recognized as participating in the development of multistage carcinogenesis [37]. Oxidative stress is associated with damage to a wide range of macromolecular species including lipids, proteins, and nucleic acids thereby producing major interrelated derangements of cellular metabolism including peroxidation of lipids, formation of protein carbonyls, and single strand breaks in DNA [38]. Previous report from our laboratory, dietary agent could effectively inhibited B(a)P induced lung carcinogenesis by offering protection from protein damage and also by suppressing cell proliferation [39]. Our result demonstrated that naringenin; MNNG induced intracellular ROS and oxidized protein carbonyl accumulation dependent on the hydroxyl group presents in the structure [40,41].

LPO is the most studied biologically relevant free radical chain reaction. It is regarded as one of the basic mechanisms of tissue damage caused by free radicals [42]. Increased level of LPO was reported during DEN induced and Phenobarbital promoted hepatocellular carcinogenesis [26]. In this result, an increased level of tail length was observed in carcinogen induced rats (Group II). The OH- radical is implicated to the oxidation of DNA bases, the most studied, product being 8-oxo-7, 8-dihydroguanine. Oxygen radicals attack DNA bases and deoxyribose residues producing damaged bases and single stand breaks. This radical induced oxidative stress generated a large number of modifications in DNA including strand breaks [36]. Contrary to this, the diets rich in fruits and vegetables can decrease both DNA damage and cancer incidence [43].

Polyamines are essential for the growth of cells and rapidly proliferating cells have higher levels of polyamines than do slowly growing or quiescent cells [44]. Earlier studies with different carcinoma tissues have demonstrated a marked increase in the levels of polyamines and ornithine decarboxylase (ODC) activity, confirming their correlation with neoplastic growth and high rate of cell proliferation [45]. Others cited the importance of polyamines in chemotherapy by demonstrating depleted levels of polyamines upon treatment with anticancer agents [39, 46]. Earlier reports demonstrate the potential of flavonoids and alkaloids to inhibit ODC in various cancer conditions [47]. Hence, naringenin, one of the flavonoids, may inhibit ODC activity and reduce cell proliferation in stomach carcinogenesis through depleting the levels of polyamines.

One or more independent/interdependent pathways such as the inhibition of activation of MNNG to the ultimate carcinogen, it's antioxidative and free radical scavenging properties may be responsible for the anticancer potential of naringenin [48]. Our study strongly displays the protective effect of naringenin against MNNG induced gastric carcinogenesis, which may be due to its inhibitory effect on cell proliferation. Therefore, naringenin may be explored as a chemopreventive agent for humans at high risk of gastric cancer.

Acknowledgments

Ganapathy. Ekambaram gratefully acknowledges the Indian Council of Medical Research (ICMR), Ministry of Human Resources and Manpower Development, Government of India, New Delhi, India for the financial assistance awarded in the form of a senior research fellowship (Grant No: 3/2/2/96/2006/NCD-III; dt 20/9/06).

Author details

Ekambaram Ganapathy[1], Devaraja Rajasekaran[2], Murugan Sivalingam[2],
Muhammed Farooq Shukkur[3], Ebrahim Abdul Shukkur[4] and Sakthisekaran Dhanapal[2*]

*Address all correspondence to: g_ekambaram@yahoo.co.in

1 Department of Pathology and Lab Medicine, David Geffen School of Medicine, University of California, Los Angeles, California, USA

2 Department of Medical Biochemistry, Dr. ALM PG Institute of Basic Medical Sciences, University of Madras, Taramani Campus, Chenna, India

3 Internal Medicine, Wayne State University, School of Medicine, Detroit, Michigan, USA

4 Pharmacy Practice, Wayne State University, Detroit, Michigan, USA

References

[1] Chen, J., Rocken, C., Malfertheiner, P. and Ebert, M.P. (2004) Recent advances in molecular diagnosis and therapy of gastric cancer. *Dig. Dis*, 22, 380 – 5.

[2] Su, Y.P., Tang, J.M., Tang, Y. and Gao, H.Y. (2005) Histological and ultrastructural changes induced by selenium in early experimental gastric carcinogenesis. *World J Gastroenterol*, 11, 4457-60.

[3] Kodama, M., Murakami, K., Sato, R., Okimoto, T., Nishizono, A. and Fujioka, T. (2005) Helicobacter pylori-infected animal models are extremely suitable for the investigation of gastric carcinogenesis. *World J Gastroenterol*, 11: 7063-71.

[4] Lin, C.T., Lin, W.H., Lee, K.D. and Tzeng, P.Y. (2006) DNA mismatch repair as an effector for promoting phorbol ester-induced apoptotic DNA damage and cell killing: implications in tumor promotion. *Int. J. Cancer*, 119, 1776-84.

[5] Fiaschi, A.I., Cozzolino, A., Ruggiero, G. and Giorgi, G. (2005) Glutathione, ascorbic acid and antioxidant enzymes in the tumor tissue and blood of patients with oral squamous cell carcinoma. *Eur. Rev. Med. Pharmacol Sci.* 9, 361-7.

[6] Sundari, P.N., Wilfred, G.J. and Ramakrishna, B. (1997) Oxidative protein damage plays a role in pathogenesis of carbon tetrachloride induced liver injury in the rat. *Biochim. Biophys. Acta*, 1362, 169 – 76.

[7] Thomas, T. and Thomas, T.J. (2001) Polyamines in cell growth and cell death: molecular mechanisms and therapeutic applications. *Cell Mol. Life Sci*, 58, 244 – 58.

[8] Sauer, L.A., Blask, D.E. and Dauchy, R.T. (2007) Dietary factors and growth and metabolism in experimental tumors. *J. Nutr. Biochem*. 18, 637-49.

[9] Moon, Y.J., Wang, X. and Morris, M.E. (2006) Dietary flavonoids: effects on xenobiotic and carcinogen metabolism. *Toxicol In Vitro* 20, 187 - 210.

[10] Russ, M., Martinez, R., Ali, H. and Steimle, P.A. (2006) Naringenin is a novel inhibitor of Dictyostelium cell proliferation and cell migration. *Biochem. and Biophy. Res. Commun.* 345, 516 – 22.

[11] Silberberg, M., Gil-Izquierdo, A., Combaret, L., Remesy, C., Scalbert, A. and Morand, C. (2006) Flavanone metabolism in healthy and tumor-bearing rats. *Biomed Pharmacother.* 60, 529 - 35.

[12] Ekambaram, G., Rajendran, P., Magesh, V. and Sakthisekaran. (2008) Antioxidant and free radical scavenging effect of naringenin reduces tumor size and weight loss in N-Methyl-N'-Nitro-N-Nitrosoguanidine induced gastric carcinogenesis. *Nutr. Res.*, 28; 106-112

[13] Ross, J.A. and Kasum, C.M. (2002) Dietary flavonoids: bioavailability, metabolic effects, and safety. *Annu. Rev. Nutr.* 22, 19 – 34.

[14] Oshima, H., Yoshie, Y., Auriol, S. and Gilibert, I. (1998) Antioxidant and pro-oxidant actions of flavonoids: effects on DNA damage induced by nitric oxide, peroxynitrite and nitroxyl anion. *Free Radical Biol. Med.* 25, 1057 – 65.

[15] Geren, R.J., Greenberg, N.H., Mcdonald, M.M. and Schumacher, A.M. (1972) Protocols for screening chemical agents and natural products against animal tumours and other biological systems. *Cancer Chemotherapy Report.* 3, 1-103.

[16] Parsons, H.L., Yip, J.Y.H. and Vanlerberge, G.C. (1999) Increased respiratory restriction during phosphate-limited growth in transgenic tobacco cells lacking alternative oxidase. *Plant Physiol.* 121, 1309 – 20.

[17] Levins, R.L., Garland, D., Oliver, C.N., et al. (1990) Determination of carbonyl contents in oxidative modified proteins. *Methods Enzymol*, 186, 464 – 78.

[18] Lowry, O.H., Rosebrough, N.J., Farr, A.L. and Randall, R.J. (1951) Protein measurement with the Folin phenol reagent. *J. Biol. Chem.* 193, 265 – 75.

[19] Burton, K. (1956) A study of the conditions and mechanism of the diphenylamine reaction for the colorimetric estimation of deoxyribonucleic acid. *Biochem. J.* 62, 315 - 23.

[20] Rawal, V.M., Patel, V.S., Rao, G.N. and Desai G.R. (1977) Chemical and biochemical studies on characters of human lenses: III. Quantitative study of protein, RNA and DNA. *Arogya J Health Sci* 3, 315 - 9.

[21] Ohkawa, H., Ohishi, N. and Yagi, K.Y. (1979) Assay of lipid peroxides in animal tissues by thiobarbituric acid reaction. *Anal. Biochem*, 95, 351–8.

[22] Sellins, K.S. and Cohen, J.J. (1987) Gene induction by γ-irradiation leads to DNA fragmentation in lymphocytes. *J. Immunol.* 139, 3199 - 3206.

[23] Singh, J. and Roscher, E. (1991) Induction of DNA damage by N-nitrosodiethylamine in rat hepatoma cells: correlation with cytochrome P450-mediated aldrin epoxidase activity. *Mutagenesis*. 6, 117 - 21.

[24] Endo, Y. (1978) A simple and sensitive method of analysis of histamine, putrescine and polyamines without the use of an amino acid analyser. *Anal. Biochem*. 89, 235 – 46.

[25] Panandiker, A., Maru, G.B. and Rao, K.V.K. (1994) Dose response effects of malachite green on free radical formation, lipid peroxidation and DNA damage in hamster embryo cells and their modulation by antioxidants. *Carcinogenesis*. 15, 2445 – 8.

[26] Thirunavukkarasu, C. and Sakthisekaran, D. (2001) Effect of selenium on N-nitrosodiethylamine induced multistage hepatocarcinogenesis with reference to lipid peroxidation and enzymic antioxidants. *Cell Biochem. Funct*. 19, 27 - 35.

[27] Tandon, R., Khanna, H.D., Dorababu, M. and Goel, R.K. (2004) Oxidative stress and antioxidants status in peptic ulcer and gastric carcinoma. *Indian J. Physiol. Pharmacol.* 48, 115 - 8.

[28] Mildred, K., Richerd, L., Joseph, G., Alexander, W. and Conney, A. (1981) Activation and inhibition of benzo(a)pyrene and aflatoxinB1 metabolism in human liver microsomes by naturally accruing flavonoids. *Cancer Res.* 41, 67 – 72.

[29] Yao, H., Liao, Z.X., Wu, Q., Lei, G.Q., Liu, Z.J., Chen. D.F., Chen, J.K. and Zhou, T.S. (2006) Antioxidative flavanone glycosides from the branches and leaves of Viscum coloratum. *Chem. Pharm. Bull.* 54, 133 - 5.

[30] Wyatt, M.D. and Pittman, D.L. (2006) Methylating agents and DNA repair responses: Methylated bases and sources of strand breaks. *Chem. Res. Toxicol*. 19, 1580 - 94.

[31] Izzotti, A., De Flora, S., Cartiglia, C., Are, B.M., Longobardi, M., Camoirano, A., Mura, I., Dore, M.P., Scanu, A.M., Rocca, P.C., Maida, A. and Piana, A. (2007) Interplay between Helicobacter pylori and host gene polymorphisms in inducing oxidative DNA damage in the gastric mucosa. Carcinogenesis, 28, 892 - 8.

[32] Liggins, J. and Furth, A.J. (1997) Role of protein carbonyl groups in the formation of advanced glycation end products. *Biochim. Biophys. Acta,* 1361, 123 – 30.

[33] Yang, C.S., Landau, J.M., Huang, M.T. and Newmark, H.L. (2001) Inhibition of Carcinogenesis by dietary polyphenolic compounds. *Annu. Rev. Nutr.* 21, 381 – 406.

[34] Traphdar, A.K., ROY, M. and Bhattacharya, R.K. (2001) Natural products as inducers of apoptosis: implication for cancer therapy and prevention. *Curr. Science,* 80, 1387 - 95.

[35] Cohn, S.M., Sun, X.M., Snowden, R.T., Dinsdale, D. and Skillter, D.N. (1992) Morphological features of apoptosis may occur in the absences of micronucleosomal DNA fragmentation. *Biochem. J,* 286, 331 - 4.

[36] Feng, Q., Kumagai, T., Torii, Y., Nakamura, Y., Osawa, T. and Uchida, K. (2001) Anti-carcinogenic antioxidants as inhibitors against intracellular oxidative stress. *Free Radic Res*, 35, 779 – 88.

[37] Jeyabal, P.V., Syed, M.B., Venkataraman, M., Sambandham, J.K. and Sakthisekaran, D. (2005) Apigenin inhibits oxidative stress-induced macromolecular damage in N-nitrosodiethylamine (NDEA)-induced hepatocellular carcinogenesis in Wistar albino rats. *Mol. Carcino*, 44, 11 - 20.

[38] Young, I.S. and Woodside, J.V. (2001) Antioxidants in health and disease. *J. Clin. Pathol*, 154, 176 - 86.

[39] Selvendiran, K., Mumtaz Banu, S. and Sakthisekaran, D. (2004) Protective effect of piperine on benzo(a)pyrene-induced lung carcinogenesis in Swiss albino mice. *Clinica Chimica Acta*, 350, 73-78.

[40] Miyoshi, N., Naniwa, K., Yamada, T., Osawa, T. and Nakamura, Y. (2007) Dietary flavonoid apigenin is a potential inducer of intracellular oxidative stress: The role in the interruptive apoptotic signal. Arch. Biochem. Biophys, 466, 274 – 82.

[41] Rice-Evans, C. (2004) Flavonoids and isoflavones: absorption, metabolism, and bioactivity. *Free Radic. Biol. Med*, 36, 827–828.

[42] Esterbauer, H., Schaur, R.J. and Zollner, H. (1991) Chemistry and biochemistry of 4-hydroxynonenal, malonaldehyde and related aldehydes. *Free Radic. Biol. Med*, 11, 81 - 128.

[43] Welch, R.W., Turley, E., Sweetman, S.F., Kennedy, G., Collins, A.R., Dunne, A., Livingstone, M.B., McKenna, P.G., McKelvey-Martin, V.J. and Strain, J.J. (1999) Dietary antioxidant supplementation and DNA damage in smokers and nonsmokers. *Nutr. Cancer*, 34, 167 - 72.

[44] Milovica, V., Turchanowa, L., Khomutov, R.M., Caspary, W.F. and Stein, J. (2001) Hydroxylamine-containing inhibitors of polyamine biosynthesis and important of colon cancer cell growth. *Biochem. Pharmacol.* 61, 199 – 206.

[45] Farriol, M., Segovia, S.T., Venero, Y. and Orta, X. (2001) Role of polyamines in cell proliferation in a colon carcinoma cell line. *Nutrition*, 17, 934 – 8.

[46] Pegg, A. (1988) Polyamine metabolism and its importance in neoplastic growth and as a target for chemotherapy. *Cancer Res*, 48, 759 – 74.

[47] Edurdo, D.S., Paolo, B. and Hugo, D. (1999) Dietary antioxidants and lung cancer risk. *Nutr. Cancer.* 34, 100 – 10.

[48] Kuo, S.M. (1996) Antiproliferative potency of structurally distinct dietary flavonoids on human colon cancer cells. *Cancer Lett.* 110, 41 – 8.

Section 3

Morphological and Molecular Aspects

Chapter 7

Gastric Carcinoma: Morphologic Classifications and Molecular Changes

Sun-Mi Lee, Kyoung-Mee Kim and Jae Y. Ro

Additional information is available at the end of the chapter

http://dx.doi.org/10.5772/54617

1. Introduction

Gastric cancer is the second leading cause of cancer death and the fourth most prevalent malignancy worldwide, affecting about one million people per year [1]. In the United States, an estimated 21,320 cases of gastric cancer (13,020 men and 8,300 women) will be diagnosed and 10,540 patients will die from this disease in 2012 [2]. The overall incidence of gastric cancer in the United States has been steadily declined over the past 75 years. Based on National Cancer Institute's Surveillance, Epidemiology, and End Results (SEER) cancer statistic data from 2005 to 2009, it is estimated approximately 1/114 men and women will be diagnosed with gastric cancer during their life; most people diagnosed with gastric cancer are over 65 years of age and men have higher gastric cancer incidence and mortality rates than women [3]. Asians/Pacific Islanders have the highest incidence as well as high mortality rates. The incidence of gastric cancer is exceptionally high in Northeast Asia, including Japan and South Korea, probably as a consequence of genetic factors and active screening policies [4]. Central Europe and South America also show a higher incidence rate of gastric cancer than the United States and Northern and Western European countries [5]. In addition to the geographic, ethnic, racial and genetic differences on the incidence of gastric cancer, environmental factors such as a high infection rate of Helicobacter pylori in Northeast Asia, also play an important role [6].

The significant improvement and widespread use of upper gastrointestinal endoscopy have led to early detection of gastric cancer. Early gastric cancer represents approximately 20% of all newly diagnosed cancer in the United States and up to 60% in Japan and South Korea [7, 8]. Marked advances in endoscopic procedures such as endoscopic mucosal resection (EMR) and submucosal dissection enhance a dramatic clinical therapeutic impact on the mortality rate and quality of life after procedures. Now gastric cancer is considered as a potentially curable cancer at an early stage. Moreover, modern targeted therapies for gastric cancer using trastuzumab suggest a promising progress in treatment and clinical outcome even in an advanced stage.

Data on topographic distribution of esophageal and gastric cancers since 1976 indicate that cancers of distal esophagus, gastroesophageal junction (GEJ), and gastric cardia have been increased in incidence with the reverse in incidence of the distal gastric cancers [9]. Now, adenocarcinomas of proximal stomach (upper third) account for approximately 30% of all gastric cancers and its clinical impact becomes more important. Although active and vivid clinical trials have been ongoing on to seek effective therapeutic modalities for GEJ and gastric cardia adenocarcinomas, there has been no universal consensus classification of these disease entities into one over the other, gastric carcinoma vs. esophageal carcinoma, due to lack of standard definition of GEJ and cardia as an anatomic site [10]. The International Classification of Diseases and Siewert classification system have shown different categorizations of the origins of these tumors into esophageal or gastric cancer. In the recently published seventh edition of the Cancer Staging Manual of the American Joint Commission of Cancer, however, tumors of the GEJ and gastric cardia are included under the esophageal carcinoma [11]. The debate on this categorization is still ongoing, especially for general surgeons [12, 13].

2. Adenocarcinoma of gastroesophageal junction

Despite dramatic decrease in incidence of distal gastric cancer with a better clinical outcome, the incidence of adenocarcinomas of the distal esophagus, GEJ, and gastric cardia has been increased from 4% to 10% per year in the United States, predominantly in men since 1976 [9, 14-16]. In Japan, the proportion of these tumors has also increased among men over last 15 years [17]. This epidemiologic trend has an important clinical influence because adenocarcinomas of the GEJ and gastric cardia showed much worse prognosis than that of distal gastric cancer, with 5-year survival rates in the range of 14% to 22%, and minimal chemotherapeutic response in an advance stage [18, 19]. Moreover, there has been no established consensus for the classification of these tumors and therapeutic modalities including lymphadenectomy, the extent of surgical resection, and chemotherapy [20, 21]. In addition, some studies have demonstrated that adenocarcinomas of the cardia have different clinicopathologic characteristics compared to adenocarcinomas of distal stomach such as a higher male to female ratio, different ethnic background, a history of chronic heartburn or duodenal ulcer, and association with smoking and alcohol drinking [22, 23]. Furthermore, adenocarcinoma of the gastric cardia shows a greater tendency to invade deeply into the gastric wall and frequent lymph node metastasis with a worse prognosis [24-26].

Although the main cause of the increasing rate of GEJ cancer is controversial, previous studies demonstrated that these tumors were significantly associated with symptomatic reflux disease and suggested that GEJ cancers are more likely arising from the distal esophagus than from the stomach [27, 28]. In addition to symptomatic reflux disease as a risk factor, recent studies from Japan demonstrated that Helicobacter pylori infection appeared to be also correlated with GEJ cancers in the Helicobacter pylori infection endemic areas [29].

In 1998, Siewert and Stein have proposed the new classification of GEJ cancers based on their anatomic sites with estimated origins. This system divides these tumors into three types as follows: type I, distal esophageal adenocarcinoma with the epicenter of the tumor lying 2.5 cm above the cardia; type II, cardiac adenocarcinoma that the tumor straddles the GEJ with the epicenter in the region 1 cm above or 2 cm below the cardia (Fig.1); and type III, subcardiac adenocarcinoma with its epicenter 2-5 cm below the cardia [30].

In the International Classification of Disease recently, however, adenocarcinomas arising in the distal third of the esophagus and those that straddle the GEJ are grouped with tumors of the gastric cardia and all these tumors assign under the category of gastric adenocarcinoma [31].

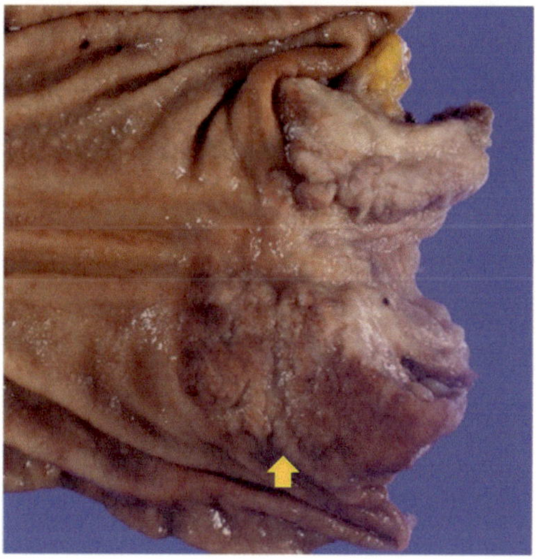

Figure 1. Siewert type II gastroesophageal junction carcinoma. The tumor is ill defined and irregularly elevated (yellow arrow). It involves cardia and distal esophagus, which exactly straddles the gastroesophageal junction.

The current 7th edition of the AJCC TNM classification of malignant tumors provided rules for classifying adenocarcinomas of distal esophagus, GEJ, and gastric cardia [11]. According to this system, any tumors with an epicenter within 5 cm of the GEJ and tumors which extend into the distal esophagus are to be classified as esophageal carcinomas and staged as such. It means that all other tumors at the GEJ with an epicenter in the stomach > 5 cm from the GEJ or those within 5 cm of the GEJ without extension into the esophagus are to be classified and staged as gastric carcinomas. Therefore, most of type II cardiac and type III subcardiac adenocarcinomas by Siewert are now staged as esophageal adenocarcinomas (Fig.2). In a recent clinical study, the prevalence and distribution of lymph node metastasis in patients with adenocarcinoma of the distal esophagus and GEJ cancers were similar after esophagectomy and there was no difference in overall survival or recurrence between these two groups of cancers. Based on this study, they reported that an effort to separate these two groups of the tumors is not required, and both are effectively treated with esophagectomy [32]. However, in the series by Gertler et al, 1141 patients with type II cardiac and type III subcardiac adenocarcinoma were reclassified following the current TNM system and compared two different categorization schemes of cardiac and subcardiac adenocarcinoma as esophageal or gastric cancer and concluded that neither of the two staging systems proved to be clearly superior over the other [33]. Thus, the categorization of cardiac and subcardiac adenocarcinoma (type II and III by Siewert) into esophageal or gastric cancers, respectively or independent disease entity needs to be evaluated further in the near future.

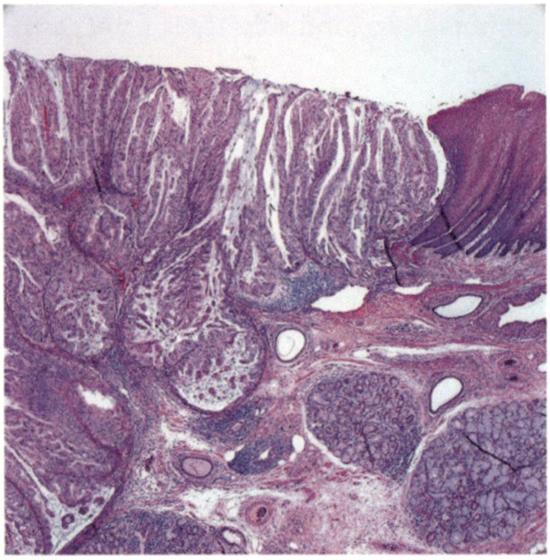

Figure 2. Gastroesophageal junction carcinoma without Barrett's esophagus. Well differentiated papillary adenocarcinoma infiltrates into the submucosa of the esophagus without evidence of Barrett's esophagus in the overlying mucosa.

3. Early gastric carcinoma

3.1. Definition, epidemiology and clinical manifestation

Early gastric carcinoma (EGC) is defined as an invasive adenocarcinoma that involves only the mucosa or submucosa but not the muscularis propria, independent of lymph node status [34]. The term, EGC, implies not only the limited extent of the disease but also an early stage in development and a less aggressive neoplasm, which carries an excellent prognosis if the lesion is completely removed [35]. Nowadays EGC represents approximately 20% of all newly diagnosed gastric cancers in Western countries, whereas in Northeast Asia (Japan and Korea), it accounts for over 50% of cases [36]. The difference in incidence between Northeast Asia and Western countries may be due to a higher prevalence of gastric cancer with mass screening test, and widely adapted use of magnifying upper endoscopy with high-resolution images and chromoendoscopy in Northeast Asia.

Most patients with EGC are diagnosed at a median age of 63 (range 21-89) years and men are affected more than women like other types of gastric cancer (male to female ratio, 1.4 - 2.4:1) [37-40]. The majority of patients with EGC are asymptomatic, but some may present with non-specific upper abdominal symptoms such as heartburn or epigastric pain, so-called dyspeptic symptoms. Weight loss, anorexia, anemia, and hypoalbuminemia frequently found in patients with advanced gastric cancer are not commonly seen [41]. Dyspeptic symptoms may occur in up to 40% of the patients with EGC [42]. Sometimes, dyspeptic symptoms may be an important clue for the detection of EGCs [39]. However, dyspeptic symptoms related with EGC can be easily masked by the use of anti-acid drugs such as cimetidine or proton pump inhibitors [43, 44]. Many EGCs are believed to go through a cycle consisting of ulceration, followed by healing, and re-ulceration [45]. It suggests that EGC can be partially healed by acid suppression, which makes difficult to diagnose EGC endoscopically because it mimics a benign peptic ulcer. Therefore, it is strongly recommended that patients with dyspeptic symptoms should undergo an endoscopic procedure with biopsy at least once after the symptoms are relieved by medication.

EGC is regarded as an early stage lesion in development that can progress to an advanced lesion [35]. One prospective study on EGCs reported that the median duration for tumor progression is approximately 3.7 years [46]. However, some EGCs can show a rapid progression into advanced lesions within a year [47]. Generally, EGCs are considered to be curable if the lesion is completely removed by endoscopic resection or surgery. Most of Japanese series have reported more than 90% of 5 and 10 year survival rates for the patients with EGC [48, 49]. In the Western series, 5-year survival rates are variable, ranging from 68% to 92% [8, 38-40, 50]. EGCs can recur at least 1.9 % of cases after resection with intervals ranging from 4 months to more than 10 years, with important risk factors for the recurrence including the presence of submucosal invasion, nodal metastasis, and undifferentiated histology [51].

3.2. Methods for evaluation and staging of EGC

Double-contrast barium upper gastrointestinal series have been used to detect gastric cancer over the past two decades. However, this study has a limitation to detect small EGCs. For the lesions of EGC between 5 and 10 mm in diameter, false negative rates are as high as 25% [52]. Endoscopy is the procedure of choice and should be performed on all patients in whom the diagnosis of gastric carcinoma is suspected. The endoscopic findings favoring an EGC associated ulcer include: (1) disruption and clubbing of the surrounding mucosal folds, (2) a dirty appearance of the surrounding mucosa with adherent mucus or exudates, (3) irregular margins of the ulcer itself, and (4) island-like residues of intact mucosa within the depressed area [53].

EGCs can be divided into two subtypes depend on the depth of invasion; intramucosal and submucosal invasive adenocarcinomas. The status of submucosal invasion in EGC is critical for determining the treatment option, surgery vs. endoscopic resection and estimating a risk of lymph node metastasis that is directly related with a clinical outcome. The 5-year survival rate for intramucosal invasive EGC is close to 100%, whereas for submucosal invasive EGC is from 80% to 90% [54, 55]. Therefore, active trials are ongoing in Japan and South Korea to detect the submucosal invasion in EGCs preoperatively by endoscopy and endoscopic ultrasonography (EUS). Different endoscopic features of intramucosal and submucosal gastric carcinoma have been investigated for an accurate local staging. Choi et al demonstrated that intramucosal gastric carcinoma was endoscopically characterized by smooth surface protrusion or depression, erosion, or marginal elevation [56]. In contrast, submucosal gastric carcinomas usually showed distinct endoscopic features with fold convergence (clubbing, fusion, abrupt cutting) and nodular protrusion/depression [57]. EUS is now widely used for substaging of EGCs. The overall accuracy rates for staging the depth of invasion of EGCs by endoscopy and EUS were reported 72.2% and 64.8%, respectively [58]. The diagnostic accuracy of EUS for the depth of invasion can be significantly affected by EGC with undifferentiated histology and large tumor size [59].

3.3. Gross features

EGCs vary greatly in size raging from microscopic foci to 5 cm, but larger lesions up to 7 cm in diameter are not unusual [38, 60, 61]. These large tumors are typically located in the antrum, around the angle, with predominance in the lesser curvature [40, 60]. The larger EGCs have a tendency to frequently invade into the submucosal layer, however, some studies demonstrated minute EGCs can also invade into the submucosa in 3.3% to 9% of cases [62-64]. EGCs can be found as multiple lesions in the background of intestinal metaplasia. In recent series, more than half of synchronous gastric carcinomas were EGCs, frequently in elderly patients, with the incidence of multiple synchronous EGC ranges from 3.7 % to 7.7% [65, 66]. Oohara et al and Hirota et al demonstrated that synchronous EGCs are macroscopically flat and small lesions, rarely infiltrate into submucosa and can be easily missed in preoperative endoscopic or intraoperative evaluation (Fig. 3) [67, 68]. Although it is well known that EGCs rarely metastasize to other organs, Ishida et al reported that 15 (0.6 %) of 2,707 patients with EGC developed liver metastasis, especially in patients with submucosal invasion, macroscopically elevated type, and with vascular invasion [69].

The endoscopic or macroscopic classification of gastric cancer established by the Japanese Gastric Cancer Association has now been accepted worldwide and was endorsed at an international workshop in Paris in 2002 [70]. Particularly, this Japanese classification system based on endoscopic findings of EGCs has been known to be useful to be employed for the endoscopic procedures. EGCs are classified into three different subtypes according to the morphologic appearance of the lesion on the mucosal surface as follows: type I (protruding type, polypoid tumors), type II (superficial tumors with or without minimal elevation or depression) and, type III (excavated type, tumors with deep depression) (Fig 4). Type I EGC is a tumor that protrudes above the mucosal surface more than 2.5 mm in height. Tumors with type II are further subdivided into three subtypes depend on the degree of elevation or depression compared to the imaginary horizontal line from both ends of the normal surrounding mucosa as follow: type IIa (superficial elevated), type IIb (superficial flat), and type IIc (superficial depressed) (Fig 5). Type IIa EGCS is defined as a lesion that is twice as thick as normal mucosa, but less than or equal to 2.5 mm in height [71]. The distinction between type I from IIa EGC depends on the extent of elevation: if the height of the lesion > 2.5 mm, it is regarded as type I, and if ≤ 2.5 mm, then it is type IIa [42]. Type IIb lesions represent 58% of minute EGCs measuring < 5 mm in size and are the most difficult type to diagnose endoscopically [52, 72]. Therefore, multiple sampling is highly recommended for an accurate histopathologic diagnosis when the lesion is suspicious for type IIb EGC. Type III lesions are characterized by prominent depression and, ulcer-like excavation (Fig. 6). Many EGCs may have a combination of different macroscopic types, i.e., IIc+III and IIa+III. Type II EGCs account for approximately 80% of cases with type IIc being the most common macroscopic subtype [73]. In the series by Craanen et al, types I and IIa lesions are likely to represent the intestinal type, whereas diffuse-type EGCs are likely to be types of IIc or III lesions [74]. They also described that specific endoscopic types of EGCs are associated with a risk of lymph node metastasis, with the lowest rates reported in type I or IIa EGC.

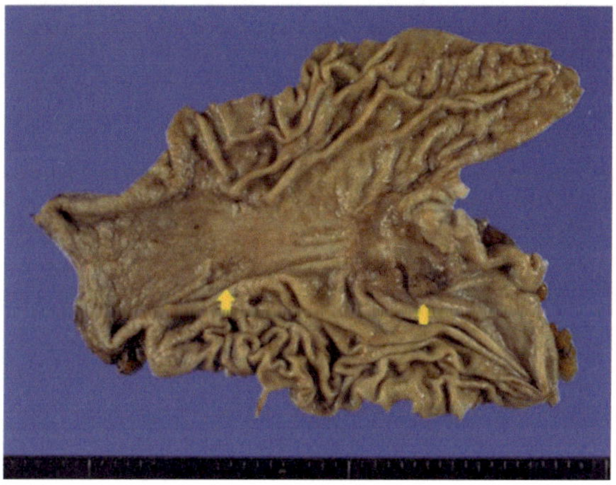

Figure 3. Multiple gastric carcinomas case. An ulceroinfiltrating Bormann type 3 gastric carcinoma is located in the subcardia (right yellow arrow). In the antrum of lesser curvature, additional small type IIa+IIc early gastric carcinoma (left yellow arrow) is found. The surrounding gastric mucosa shows diffuse atrophic changes.

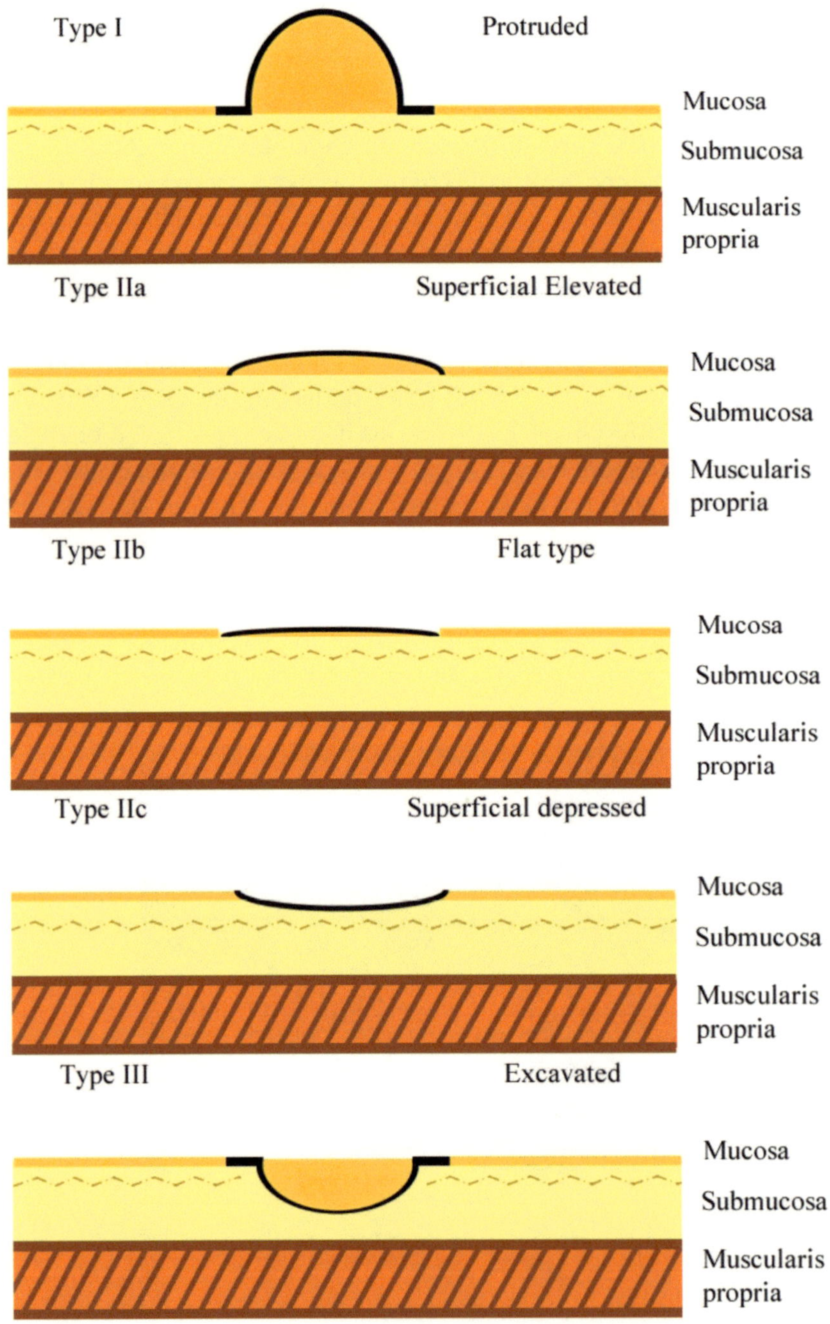

Figure 4. Japanese macroscopic classification of early gastric cancer

http://dx.doi.org/10.5772/54617

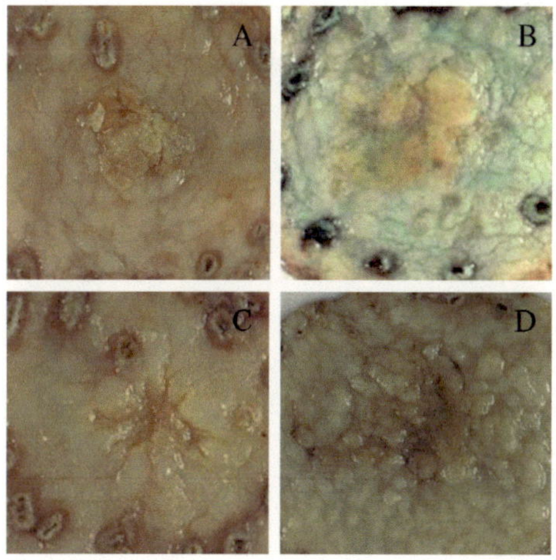

Figure 5. Early gastric cancer. A: EGC type I. The tumor shows a protruding lesion more than 2.5 mm in height. B: EGC type IIa. The tumor shows a slightly elevated, plaque-like lesion. C: EGC type IIc. A slightly depressed lesion with an irregular ulcer base mimicking a benign ulcer is seen. D: EGE type IIb+IIc. A combined flat and depressed lesion is accompanied with surrounding nodular gastric mucosa.

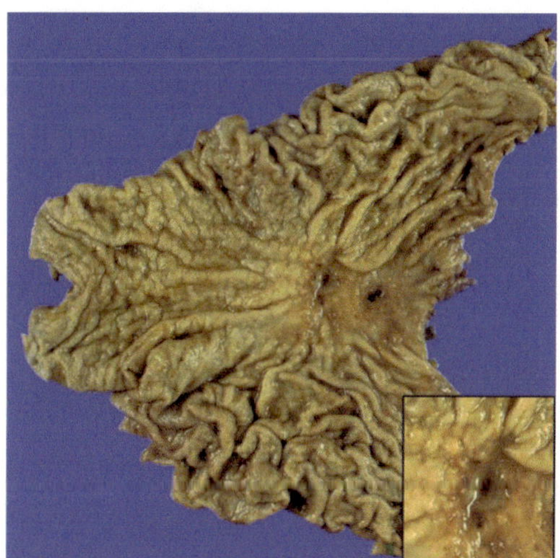

Figure 6. EGC type III. An ulcer-like excavated lesion with a prominent depression is present in the body of the lesser curvature.

3.4. Microscopic features

Histologically, the majority of EGCs are well differentiated, tubular adenocarcinomas. Most of the lesions are intestinal types with predominantly tubular (93%) and papillary (1%) histology (Fig.7) [73]. Mucinous carcinomas account for 1% of all EGCs. Signet ring cell carcinomas and poorly differentiated adenocarcinomas represent 5% and 30% of the cases, and are usually depressed or ulcerated types (types IIc or III) [73, 75] (Fig 8). Severe atrophic gastritis with diffuse intestinal metaplasia and pre-existing adenoma are frequently seen in the background of adenocarcinoma. It has been estimated that 10% of individuals with chronic atrophic gastritis would develop gastric carcinoma in a 15-year follow-up period [76].

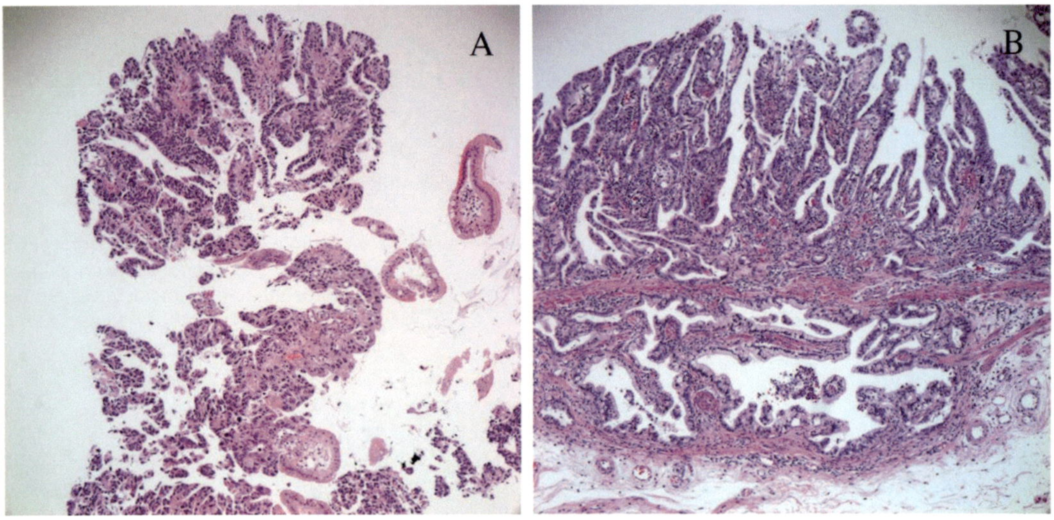

Figure 7. A. The biopsy shows well- differentiated papillary adenocarcinoma with invasion into the lamina propria. B. The endoscopic submucosal dissection specimen shows that the tumor invades into submucosa.

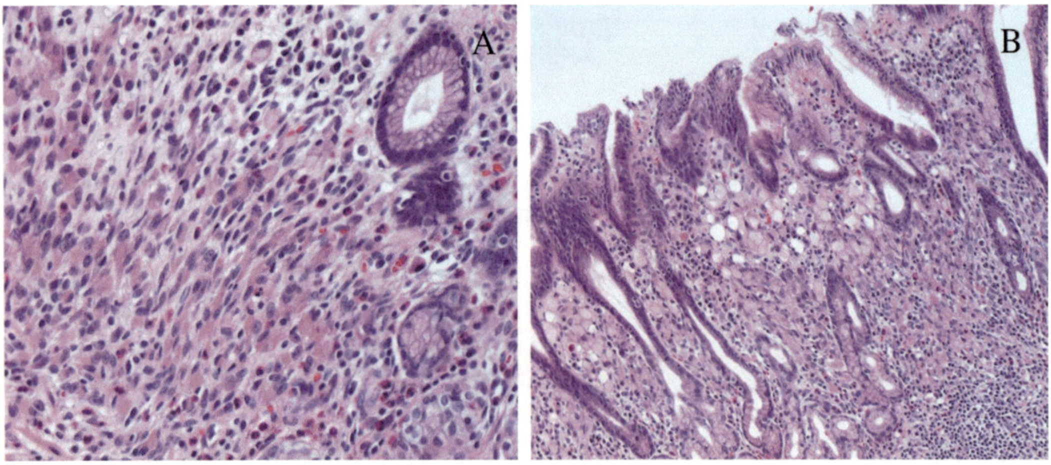

Figure 8. A. Intramucosal signet ring cell carcinoma with eosinophilic cytoplasm. B. Goblet cells mimicking signet ring cell carcinoma are found in the same gastrectomy specimen.

There has been a disagreement between Western and Japanese pathologists in distinguishing between high grade dysplasia and intramucosal invasive adenocarcinoma of the stomach. In the United States and Western countries, intramucosal invasive adenocarcinoma of the stomach has been defined as a lesion that shows clear invasion of the lamina propria in the form of single cells or small clusters of cells and a diagnosis of high grade dysplasia is rendered when the lesion shows only cytologic atypia and architectural abnormalities without clear invasion [77]. However, for Japanese pathologists, a diagnosis of intramucosal invasive adenocarcinoma has also been made with cytologic atypia and architectural abnormalities as parts of diagnostic criteria for intramucosal invasive adenocarcinoma in addition to intramucosal invasion by tumor [78]. This discrepancy of diagnostic criteria between Japanese and Western pathologists had developed a new Vienna classification for gastric epithelial neoplasia; however, this classification has not been adopted widely.

3.5. Indications for endoscopic resection

In a meta-analysis of 5,265 patients with EGC who underwent gastrectomy with lymph node dissection, nodal metastasis was observed in only 2.7% of adenocarcinomas with invasion limited to the mucosa and in 18.6% of EGCs with invasion extending into submucosa [79]. This seminal paper induced the widespread application of EMR as a first-line therapy for EGCs meeting several criteria, as underscored by the Japanese Gastric Cancer Association. The current indication of EMR for the treatment of EGCs includes well or moderately differentiated adenocarcinoma histology. The lesions must be (1) confined to the mucosa; (2) smaller than or equal to 2 cm for superficially elevated type lesions; (3) smaller than or equal to 1 cm for the flat and depressed type lesions; (4) no ulcer or ulcer scar; (5) no venous or lymphatic involvement [80, 81]. However, EMR has a limitation to resect a lesion greater than 2 cm in size and a relatively high risk of local recurrence up to 35% when resected tissues are fragmented or margins are not clear [82]. Thus, a new technique of endoscopic submucosal dissection (ESD) was recently developed to dissect directly along the deep submucosal layer, facilitating one-piece resection. After the introduction of ESD, some institutions in Japan and Korea have tried to adopt the expanded criteria for ESD. The expanded criteria for ESD include intramucosal EGS without size limitation for resection (elevated type), tumor with differentiated type as well as undifferentiated type (≤ 2 cm), and an ulcerative lesion (≤ 3 cm) [83]. The classic and expanded criteria for EMR and ESD are listed in table 1. Recently, Hirasawa et al investigated 3,843 patients of solitary undifferentiated type EGC with status post gastrectomy and lymph node dissection to find clinicopathologic factors related with lymph node metastasis [84]. They found that none of 310 intramucosal invasive EGCs with 2.0 cm or less in size without lymphovascular invasion and ulcer was associated with lymph node metastasis, which supports the expanded criteria for the endoscopic resection. In addition, in large series by Ahn et al, patients with EGC underwent an ESD with the extended criteria have shown acceptable clinical outcomes with a relatively high complete resection (88.4%) and a low local recurrence rate (1.1%) [85]. Careful clinical and radiographic evaluation using endoscopy and EUS for an accurate local staging and an appropriate selection of patients are strongly recommended before the application of the expanded criteria for ESD.

	Intramucosal Carcinoma				Submucosal Carcinoma	
	Ulcer (-)		Ulcer (+)		Sm1 (≤500μm)	Sm2 (>500μm)
Size (mm)	≤ 20 mm	> 20 mm	≤ 30 mm	> 30 mm	≤ 30 mm	Any size
Differentiated carcinoma	EMR	ESD	ESD	Surgery	ESD	Surgery
Undifferentiated carcinoma	ESD or Surgery considered	Surgery	Surgery	Surgery	Surgery	Surgery

EMR indicates endoscopic mucosal resection; **ESD**, endoscopic submucosal dissection.

Table 1. Endoscopic indication for early gastric carcinoma

3.6. Histologic evaluation of EMR/ESD specimens

Proper handling EMR or ESD specimens is important to get an accurate histopathologic diagnosis. EMR or ESD specimens are evaluated carefully in slices at interval of 2 mm according to the recommendation by Japanese Classification of Gastric Carcinoma [70]. The risk stratification of lymph node metastasis in EMR or ESD requires careful and precise pathologic examination of the resected tissue. The location, size, gross appearance, histology, degree of differentiation, microscopic depth of tumor invasion, presence of ulceration, neoplastic involvement of the lateral and vertical margins, and involvement of the lymphatics and/or blood vessels in the submucosa must be reported in detail [82]. Invasion to the lateral margin of EMR or ESD specimens is classified into the following three groups based on endoscopic and histopathologic evidence: (1) Complete resection; when the lateral margin is clear endoscopically and pathologically (minimal probability of local recurrence); (2) Incomplete resection: when the tumor has definitely invaded the lateral margin endoscopically and pathologically (high probability of local recurrence); (3) Not evaluable: when the tumor has been removed endoscopically, but its lateral margin was not pathologically evaluable because of a burn effect (burned by diathermic treatment), or mechanical damage, or when reconstruction was difficult because of piecemeal resection [86]. The presence of submucosal invasion, positive vertical (deep) margin, and lymphovascular invasion (LVI) in the EMR or ESD specimens are indications for additional surgical intervention if any of these three histologic factors are present [87]. If only the lateral mucosal margin is positive as mapped out by the pathologists, a repeated ESD or ablative therapy of the involved area, may be attempted [88]. To date, large tumor size (> 3 cm), the presence of LVI, and deep submucosal invasion (>500 μm) are regarded as the most convincing indicators for a higher risk of lymph node metastasis in EGCs [89-91]. The recurrence rate of EGCs after EMR is highly variable, ranging from 2% to 35% in different studies, depending on the accomplishment of complete resection or not [92-95]. Every study agrees that EMR is associated with a higher risk of local recurrence compared to ESD due to the piecemeal resection of large lesions. Despite ESD has shown a higher frequency of enbloc and complete resections than EMR, the local recurrence rate of EGC after ESD still ranges from 1 to 5% [96-98]. Therefore, surveillance biopsy from post- EMR sites is an important step in the follow up of patients to evaluate the residual or recurrent tumors. Mitsuhashi et al described pathologic features of the post-EMR biopsies which included, (1) architectural changes such as foveolar hyperplasia, villiform configuration, and lobular glandular proliferation; (2) cytologic changes such as increased mitoses (>2 mitoses/foveola), epithelial cytologic atypia, anisonucleosis with or without microcystic configuration and flattened epithelia, clear cell degeneration, signet ring cell change, and mucin depletion; (3) stromal changes such as edema of the lamina propria, fibrinopurulent exudates and granulation tissue related to mucosal ulceration, acute and chronic inflammation, ecstatic blood vessels, ischemia, and hemorrhage [99]. Although most of mucosal changes seen in post-EMR biopsies seem to be benign, reactive and non-specific, among them, three pathologic features including lacy architectural change, clear cell differentiation, and signet ring cell-like change can create a diagnostic pitfall to pathologists, which should be distinguished from residual or recurrent adenocarcinoma based on the prior history of EMR and absence of nuclear atypia

4. Advanced gastric carcinoma

4.1. Clinical manifestation

Men are more frequently affected than women (male: female ratio; 2:1) and the median age at diagnosis is 70 years of age [3]. No specific physical signs or symptoms for gastric carcinoma exist. The common presenting symptoms and signs in advanced gastric cancer (AGC), however, include dysphagia, early satiety, epigastric pain, weight loss, anemia, anorexia, nausea, vomiting and melena. Dysphagia is frequently associated with proximal tumors, and early satiety can be caused by distal tumors or tumors with linitis plastica appearance due to gastric outlet obstruction or loss of stomach distensibility [100]. The symptom duration is less than 3 months in nearly 40% of patients and longer than 1 year in only 20% [101]. Presenting symptoms and signs in patients with distant metastasis of AGCs may be different from those with AGCs without distant metastasis. These patients may show enlarged abdominal mass or abdominal swelling due to tumor metastasis to the liver or malignant peritoneal effusion. Occasionally, the non-regional lymph node metastasis to the supraclavicular area can be superficial and palpable (Virchow's lymph node). Peritoneal metastatic spread may be evident as a palpable ovary on pelvic examination (Krukenberg tumor) or metastasis to the pouch of Douglas on rectal examination (Blumer's shelf sign) can be detected. Vaginal bleeding due to metastasis to the endometrium has been reported in premenopausal women with AGCs [102]. Patients with AGC may present with paraneoplastic syndromes such as diffuse seborrheic keratosis, acanthosis nigricans, microangiopathic hemolytic anemia, and Trousseau's syndrome [103]. The overall prognosis of AGCs is poor, with 5-year survival rate of 20% [104, 105]. Median survival for metastatic or unresectable disease is approximately 8 to 10 months [106].

4.2. Methods for evaluation and staging

An upper gastrointestinal tract radiography and endoscopy with biopsy have been used as gold standard tests for the detection of gastric cancer. Advantages of double-contrast upper gastrointestinal series are cost-effective, with a low risk of side effects and a high sensitivity ranging from 85% to 95% for the diagnosis of gastric carcinoma [107]. However, in some cases, the differentiation between a benign ulcer from a malignant one or gastric lymphoma can be challenging for radiologists in regard to subtle radiologic findings. Therefore, endoscopy with histologic confirmation has been a choice of procedure for evaluation of gastric cancer. The diagnostic accuracy rate of endoscopy with biopsy for upper gastrointestinal cancers is more than 95% [104, 108]. The diagnostic accuracy of the biopsies usually increases with the increased numbers of sample taken. Many endoscopists generally take eight to ten biopsies and a minimum of six biopsies from any lesions is highly recommended with one from each quadrant and two from the center of the lesion [103]. Biopsy should be taken from the edge of an ulcerative lesion not from the base because when the biopsy is taken from the base of the ulcer, only necrotic tissue may be obtained. Gastric forcep biopsy may have limitation for the proper diagnosis and determination of degree of differentiation in some cases. Takao et al investigated the discrepancy rates of diagnoses between biopsy samples and resection specimens and found 1.4 % of adenocarcinoma cases on resection specimens were under- diagnosed as either non-neoplastic lesions or adenomas in biopsies [109]. In regard to the discrepancy of the degree of differentiation, 97% of differentiated adenocarcinomas and 83% of undifferentiated adenocarcinoma in biopsies have concordant histology on resection specimens with a higher discordant rate in undifferentiated carcinoma cases in which undifferentiated component in biopsies may not represent the degree of differentiation in whole lesions. Therefore, they suggested endoscopic features should be considered together with the biopsy diagnosis to determine an appropriate treatment strategy for the lesions. Although a great effort has been made in search of specific markers that would enable for early detection of gastric carcinoma including CEA, CA19.9, CA72.4, CA50, and pepsinogen in the serum, and CEA, CA19.9, and fetal sulfoglycoprotein in the gastric juice [103, 110, 111], no specific biologic markers have been verified for specific gastric cancer markers. Once a diagnosis of gastric carcinoma has been made, endoscopic ultrasonography and computed tomography (CT) scan are usually employed for tumor staging. EUS is particularly useful to estimate the depth of tumor invasion for local staging. Accuracy of EUS for T staging in gastric carcinoma is approximately 82%, with a sensitivity and specificity of 70% to 100% and 87% to 100%, respectively [112-114]. However, differentiating T2 and T3 gastric carcinoma may be difficult in some cases due to associated fibrosis in T2 mimicking T3 lesions. Accuracy for T staging of gastric carcinoma by spiral CT is approximately 64%, lower than that of EUS [115]. Detection of lymph node involvement by spiral CT scan is not reliable with sensitivity rates ranging from 24% to 43% [116], because lymph node size is not a good parameter for determining nodal metastasis. CT scan has been used for identifying distant metastasis to lung, liver, bone, etc. Magnetic Resonance Imaging (MRI) has been known to be almost comparable to CT scan for staging of AGC and useful to confirm a liver metastasis in equivocal cases [117, 118]. However, currently, MRI is limitedly used when the patients have an allergy to iodine contrast or renal failure due to motion induced artifacts, longer scanning times and a higher cost than CT scan.

http://dx.doi.org/10.5772/54617

4.3. Gross features

Approximately 50% of AGCs arise in the distal stomach (the pyloric part of the stomach), frequently involving the lesser curvature and 16% of AGCs occur in the proximal stomach (cardia, the upper third of the body and fundus) [17]. AGCs may show various gross appearances with different growth patterns. For standardization of the common morphologic features of AGCs, several classification systems have been proposed. The most widely used classification for macroscopic appearance of AGC is Bormann classification, dividing AGCs into four types [119]:

Type 1 Polypoid: Well circumscribed polypoid tumors (Fig. 9).

Type 2 Fungating: Fungating tumors with marked central infiltration (Fig. 10).

Type 3 Ulcerated: Ulcerated tumors with infiltrative margins (Fig. 11).

Type 4 Infiltrating: Diffusely infiltrated tumors (Fig. 12).

In one large series, the percentage of each subtype was type 1 in 7%; type 2 in 36%; type 3 in 25%; and type 4 in 26% [120]. The most common macroscopic type is a type 2 fungating tumor, which are frequently located in the lesser curvature of antrum. In contrast, polypoid (type 1) and ulcerated (type 3) types are commonly found in the greater curvature of corpus. On cut surface, AGC presents as a gray-white to yellow-white solid mass with a firm to hard consistency and contains areas of hemorrhage and necrosis.

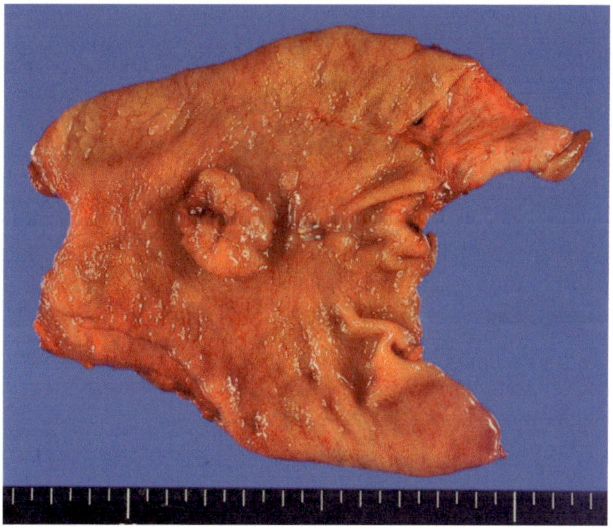

Figure 9. Bormann type 1. Polypoid carcinoma of the stomach is located in the antrum of the lesser curvature. This elevating solid mass shows focal superficial hemorrhage.

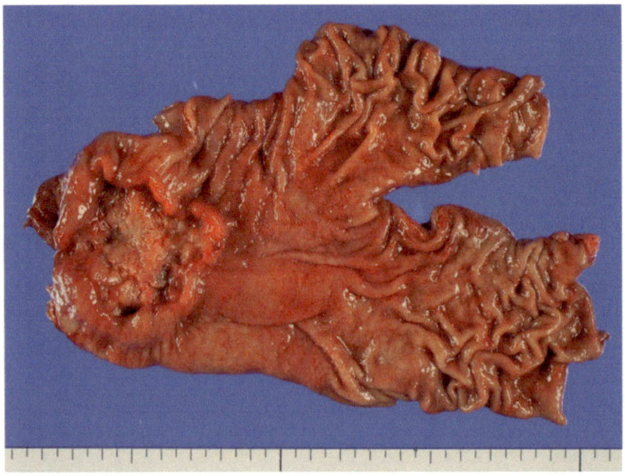

Figure 10. Bormann type 2. Fungating carcinoma of the stomach with extensive central ulceration involves the antrum.

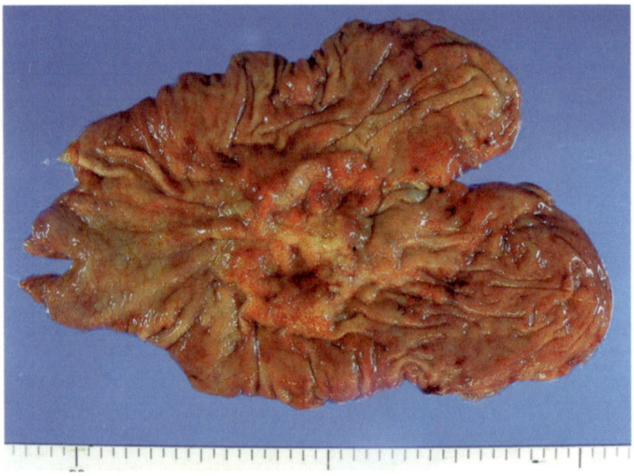

Figure 11. Bormann type 3. Ulcerated carcinoma of the stomach with infiltrative and heaped-up margins is present in the lower body of the lesser curvature.

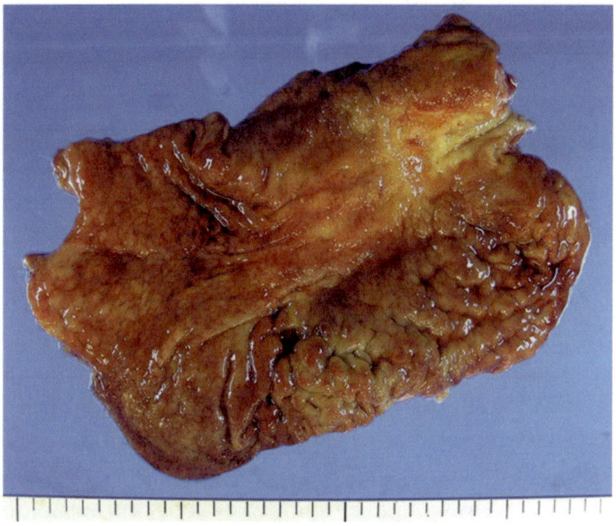

Figure 12. Bormann type 4. Linitis plastica, diffusely infiltrating carcinoma of the stomach with thickening of gastric rugae involves the whole stomach.

4.4. Microscopic features and morphologic classifications

Adenocarcinoma accounts for approximately 95% of all malignant gastric neoplasms. Because of heterogeneity and complexity in the morphologic characteristics of gastric carcinoma, many histologic classification systems have been proposed. The primary histopathologic classification used for gastric carcinoma was first described in 1965 by Lauren [121]. This system provided a general understanding of histogenesis and biology of this disease. This classification simply divides gastric carcinomas morphologically into two types: diffuse and intestinal types, which have shown different genetic alterations and biologic behaviors. This classification has been applied to determine a clinical indication of endoscopic procedure or surgery and has supported unified epidemiologic data of gastric cancers by researchers.

Intestinal type adenocarcinoma usually arises in the older population with an increased incidence in men and is frequently associated with chronic atrophic gastritis, intestinal metaplasia and Helicobacter pylori infection in neighboring mucosa [122]. They constitute approximately 60% of gastric carcinoma in high-risk population and occur frequently in the antrum as exophytic bulky lesions [123]. These tumors have a tendency to spread hematogeneously and often result in liver metastasis. Helicobacter pylori infection, high-salt diet and smoking have been recognized as risk factors of intestinal type adenocarcinoma [6]. In regard to the carcinogenesis of intestinal type gastric carcinoma, Correa et al proposed a multistep progression from Helicobacter pylori infection and gastritis to intestinal type gastric carcinoma [124]. The sequence of changes in the stomach has been proposed that Helicobacter pylori infection or autoimmune gastritis causes atrophic gastritis with intestinal metaplasia, and transforms to dysplasia (adenoma) and further progress to adenocarcinoma.

Multiple genetic alterations or mutations occur and accumulate in each step of carcinogenesis and result in malignant transformation. However, this hypothetical model only can apply to intestinal type adenocarcinoma but not to diffuse type. Microscopically, intestinal type adenocarcinomas show well developed glandular structures, either with papillary or tubular component, surrounded by a variable degree of desmoplastic stroma and a mixed inflammatory infiltration (Fig.13).

In contrast, diffuse type adenocarcinoma frequently occurs in younger patients, with equal distribution among men and women [122]. It tends to spread by direct tumor extension, resulting in peritoneal metastasis. Diffuse type adenocarcinoma has been believed to derive de novo from the peripheral stem cells of gastric gland neck proliferation zone without a recognizable precursor lesion [125, 126]. Grossly, this tumor frequently shows ulcerations and occasionally combines with rigid, thickened, leather-bottle appearance of the gastric wall, called linitis plastica. Microscopically, diffuse type adenocarcinoma is composed of individual tumor cells with or without signet ring cell configuration or small clusters of discohesive pleomorphic cells with little or no gland formation, which commonly deeply invade the full thickness layers of the gastric wall with desmoplastic reaction. Different clinicopathologic features of intestinal and diffuse type gastric carcinomas are listed in table 2.

Diffuse gastric cancer rarely can be hereditary with an autosomal dominant disorder which accounts for less than 1% of all cases of gastric carcinoma [6]. This disease is caused by germline mutation of CDH1 gene that encodes the cell adhesion protein E-cadherin, which plays an essential role in maintenance of the epithelial glandular structure [127]. Diffuse gastric carcinoma is the main cause of cancer mortality in patients with CDH1 gene mutation [128].

	Intestinal adenocarcinoma	**Diffuse adenocarcinoma**
Age	Old age	Young age
Sex	M > F	M = F
Risk factors	Helicobacter pylori infection, high salt diet, and smoking	CDH1 gene mutation
Precursors	Adenoma or dysplasia	Tubule-neck dysplasia or signet ring cell carcinoma in situ
Surrounding gastric mucosa	Atrophic gastritis with intestinal metaplasia	Non-atrophic gastritis or nonmetaplastic mucosa
Common location	Antrum and angulus	Corpus and whole stomach
Gross feature	Exophytic lesion	Ulcerative lesion and linitis plastic
Microscopy	Well - developed tubular architecture	Discohesive cells or signet ring cells
Routes of cancer dissemination	Hematogenous spread	Direct invasion into the surrounding organs

Table 2. Clinicopathologic features of intestinal and diffuse types of gastric adenocarcinomas

Some AGCs may not fit into one of two types clearly, and thus fall into mixed or unclassified categories. Mixed type gastric carcinoma accounts for approximately 14% of all gastric carcinoma [121, 129, 130]. However, there have been only a few studies investigating the clinicopathologic features of mixed type AGCs. In recent series by Zheng et al, mixed type adenocarcinomas exhibit larger size, deeper invasion, more frequent local invasion, and lymph node metastasis compared to intestinal or diffuse type gastric carcinomas [131]. Kozuki et al also demonstrated a similar result; prominent lymphatic permeation and lymph node metastasis were more frequently observed in mixed type than the pure type of gastric carcinoma [132]. These findings suggest that mixed type adenocarcinoma of the stomach may have more aggressive behavior than two pure types and could be separated as a distinct entity.

In 1977, Ming proposed another classification system of gastric carcinoma based on the pattern of tumor growth and invasiveness as an indicator of biological behavior, expanding vs. infiltrative type [133]. The expanding type adenocarcinomas grow predominantly by expansion with a sharply delineated periphery, resulting in a nodular growth of tumor. In contrast, the infiltrative type tumors show diffuse infiltration of tumor cells into the layers of gastric wall, without forming masses or nodules. There are some overlapping features between Lauren and Ming classifications. In most of cases, expanding types of AGC by Ming's classification are classified as intestinal types and infiltrative adenocarcinomas are diffuse types. However, Ming's classification was made based on the predominant tumor growth pattern, which limits its value to gastrectomy specimen and cannot be applied to biopsy specimens [134].

In 1992, Goseki et al proposed a classification system of AGC based on the degree of tubular differentiation and the amount of intracellular mucin production [135]. This system divides AGCs into four groups based on tubular differentiation and mucin production by tumor cells. Four grades of tumor were proposed: group I: well differentiated tubules, intracellular mucin poor; group II: well differentiated tubules, intracellular mucin rich; group III: poorly differentiated tubules, intracellular mucin poor; group IV: poorly differentiated tubules, intracellular mucin rich. The prognostic value of Goseki's classification has been investigated in only a few studies in patients with AGCs and its prognostic value remains controversial [136-140].

Although the Lauren and other classifications provide a simplified categorization of usual gastric carcinomas and better understanding of their biology and behavior in large epidemiologic studies, they are less useful to apply to a variety of histologic subtypes of gastric carcinoma for predicting their clinical outcome. World Health Organization (WHO) proposed a classification to meet this need based on traditional histopathologic features and the degree of differentiation of gastric carcinoma [141]. Gastric adenocarcinomas are graded like other glandular neoplasms based on the degree of glandular differentiation into well, moderately, and poorly differentiated subtypes. Well differentiated carcinoma consists predominantly of recognizable, well-formed glands with greater than 95% of glandular component in a tumor. Poorly differentiated tumors have a little gland formation consisting of pleomorphic tumor cells arranged in solid sheets or clusters with less than 50% of gland formation in a tumor. Moderately differentiated tumors are intermediate with 50-95% of gland formation in a tumor. The degree of differentiation is considered as an important prognostic factor that is highly associated with the depth of tumor invasion and a risk of lymph node metastasis [142-144]. WHO classification has been also used for determining the therapeutic options of patients with gastric carcinoma. The degree of differentiation is one of the important criteria for performing endoscopic resection.

In WHO classification, gastric carcinomas are divided into five categories based on histopathologic features including adenocarcinoma, adenosquamous carcinoma, squamous cell carcinoma, undifferentiated carcinoma, and unclassified carcinoma [145]. Adenocarcinomas are subdivided into papillary, tubular, mucinous and signet ring cell types. Generally, papillary and tubular variant are classified into intestinal, expanding, or differentiated type, whereas, mucinous and signet ring cell variants are categorized into diffuse, infiltrative, or undifferentiated type [146].

Tubular adenocarcinoma consists of tubular-shaped branching glands lined by pseudostratified columnar or cuboidal epithelium with elongated hyperchromatic nuclei having coarse chromatin and occasional mitotic figures (Fig. 14). Acinar structure may be present. The degree of cytologic atypia varies from low grade to high grade tumors. If tubular adenocarcinoma combines with papillary adenocarcinoma component, it is termed as a tubulopapillary variant.

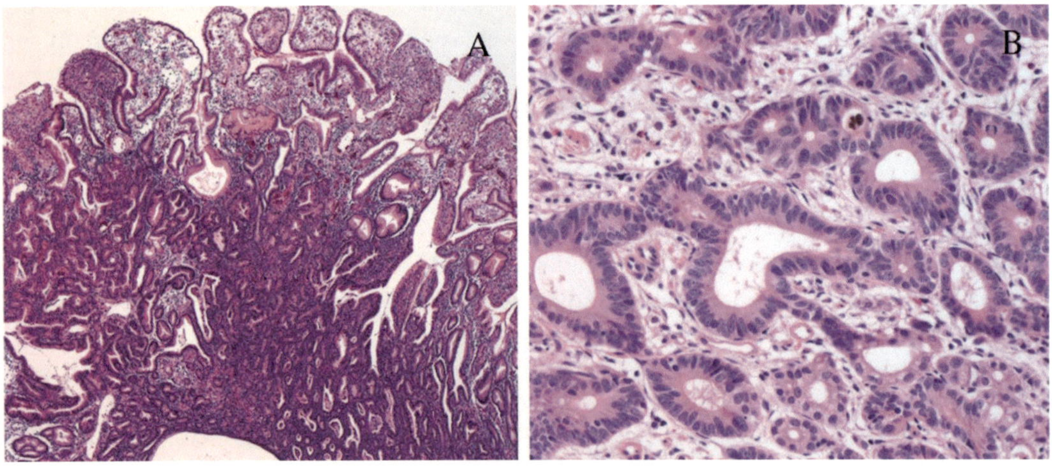

Figure 13. A. Gastric biopsy shows a well differentiated tubular adenocarcinoma. Adjacent to the carcinoma, regenerative foveolar epitheliums are admixed. B. In high power examination, the anastomosing glands are composed of atypical cells with vesicular nuclei and prominent nucleoli.

http://dx.doi.org/10.5772/54617

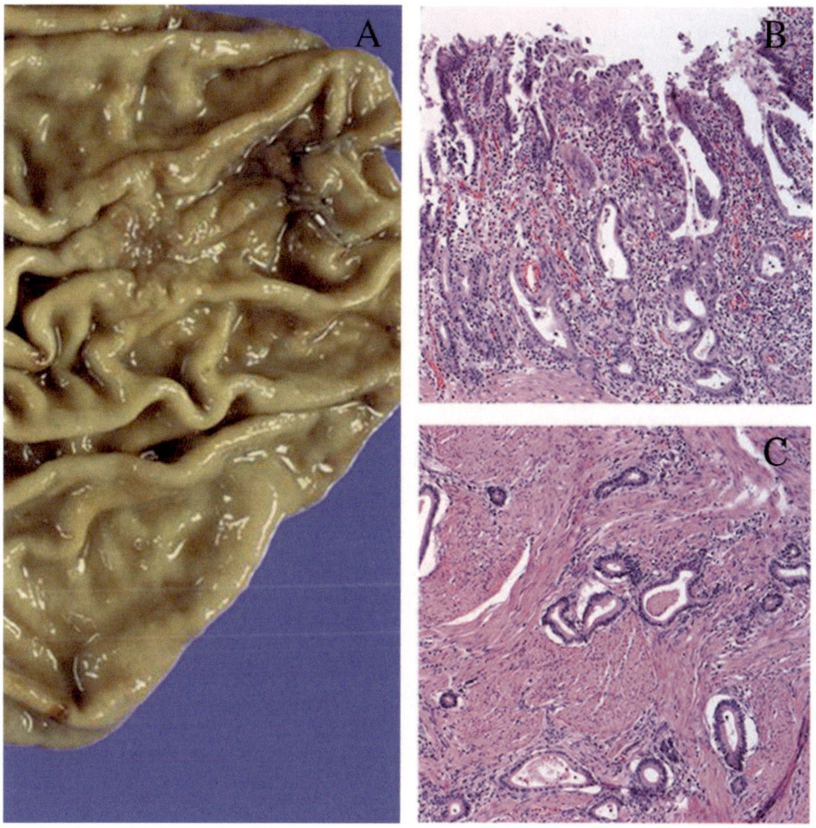

Figure 14. Tubular adenocarcinoma, well differentiated, in the resected stomach. A. Grossly, the tumor in the high body of greater curvature is advanced gastric carcinoma mimicking EGC type IIb. B. In the superficial area, the carcinoma mimics regenerative changes due to its bland morphology. C. However, the carcinoma infiltrates into subserosa.

Papillary adenocarcinoma is characterized by elongated finger-like processes that have a fibrovascular connective tissue core in the center and lined by cylindrical or cuboidal cells. The nuclear cytologic atypia varies from low to high grade. This tumor represents 6% to 11% of all gastric carcinomas [68, 147]. Papillary adenocarcinomas have distinct clinicopathologic features such as a higher frequency in aged patients, proximal location, and elevated macroscopic type [147]. Although papillary adenocarcinoma has been categorized into differentiated-type adenocarcinoma with low grade malignancy, some studies have shown that papillary adenocarcinomas of the stomach have a higher frequency of lymph node metastasis, liver metastasis and poorer surgical outcome compared to other types of gastric carcinoma [147-149]. Nakashima et al proposed a nuclear grading score for papillary adenocarcinoma of the stomach based on the extent of nuclear pleomorphism and nuclear polarity

[150]. They also reported that papillary adenocarcinoma with a high nuclear grade is usually accompanied by more advanced mural invasion, a higher risk of lymph node metastasis, higher chances of HER2 overexpression, and poorer prognosis. This study suggested that papillary adenocarcinomas with high nuclear grade of the stomach may be a good therapeutic candidate for anti-HER2 (trastuzumab) therapy.

Mucinous adenocarcinomas are also referred to as colloid, mucous, and muconodular carcinoma. This tumor accounts for 2 % to 6 % of all gastric carcinomas [151]. Mucinous adenocarcinoma is defined as a gastric adenocarcinoma with a substantial amount of extracellular mucin (≥ 50% of tumor volume) within tumors [145]. They may present in one of two forms; tubular glands with mucus-secreting epithelium surrounding collections of extracellular mucin and signet ring cells floating in the mucinous lake [152]. Sometimes, the tumor is predominantly composed of large acellular mucin pools with a few scattered tubular glands or signet ring cells (Fig. 15). The clinical outcome and prognosis of mucinous adenocarcinoma compared to non-mucinous adenocarcinoma is controversial. Some authors reported that the prognosis of patients with mucinous adenocarcinoma is poorer than that of patients with non-mucinous adenocarcinoma [153]. However, others demonstrated that the 5-year survival rates of mucinous and non-mucinous adenocarcinomas are not different when the tumors are compared stage by stage [152]. A recent study from South Korea reported that in mucinous gastric carcinomas, tumor size predicted prognosis more accurately than conventional pT stage (depth of invasion in a study with large number of cases) [154].

Signet ring cell adenocarcinoma of the stomach is characterized by diffuse infiltration of signet-ring type of tumor cells into the gastric wall. It accounts for 18% of total gastric carcinomas and 13.9% of all AGCs [155]. Histologically, signet ring cell carcinoma is defined as an adenocarcinoma in which the predominant component (more than 50% of the tumor) consists of isolated or small groups of malignant cells containing intracytoplasmic mucin with eccentric nuclei (Fig. 16) [145]. Most signet ring cell carcinomas accompany with marked desmoplasia within tumor. Signet ring cell carcinomas diffusely infiltrate through the muscular propria and subserosa with sparing the mucosa and present as firm and non-distensible texture, forming leather bottle appearance of stomach (linitis plastica). In these cases, because a few scattered tumor cells are embedded in the desmoplastic stroma, it is easy to overlook the presence of malignant cells. Therefore, a careful pathologic examination is strongly recommended for delineating free margins and depth of tumor invasion during evaluation for frozen sections as well as permanent sections of gastrectomy specimens. In problem cases, mucin stains (periodic acid-Schiff, Alcian blue, mucicarmine) and immunohistochemical staining for cytokeratin would be greatly helpful to demonstrate tumor cells. Li et al reported that the mean tumor size and depth of invasion of signet ring cell carcinoma is slightly larger and deeper than those of non-signet ring cell carcinoma [155]. This tumor is frequently discovered at an advanced stage such as, stage IIIb and IV, and shows a higher rate of lymph node metastasis and peritoneal dissemination [155, 156], and is associated with the poorer prognosis than other types of adenocarcinoma.

http://dx.doi.org/10.5772/54617

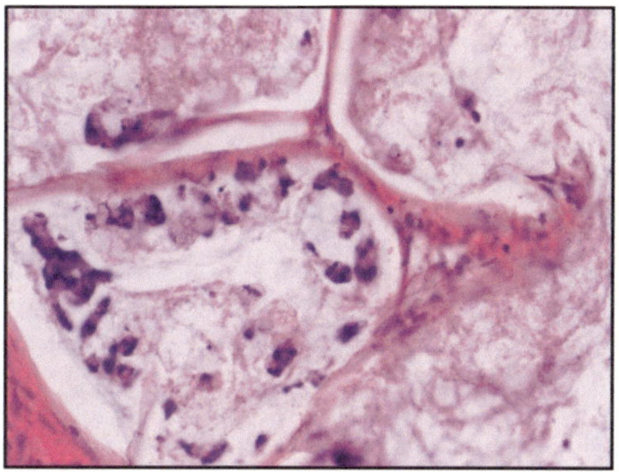

Figure 15. Mucinous carcinoma. Small clusters or strands of pleomorphic tumor cells containing mucin are present within mucin pool.

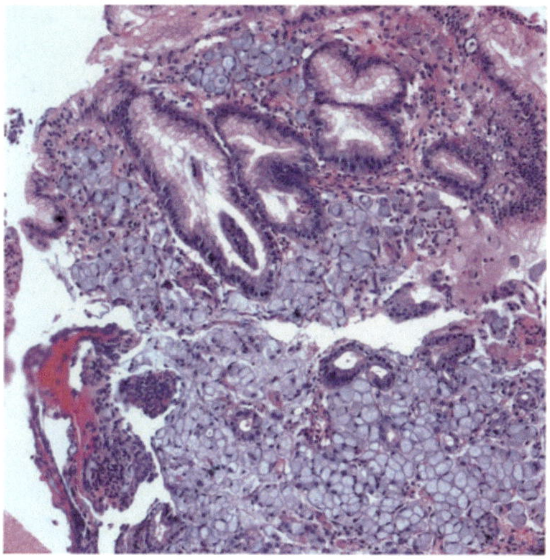

Figure 16. Signet ring cell carcinoma. Signet ring cells showing foamy or pale basophilic abundant cytoplasm and an eccentrically located nucleus infiltrate the lamina propria.

4.5. Immunohistochemistry

Gastric carcinomas have various amounts of differentiated tumor cells that may express heterogeneous phenotypes of mucin. Mucins are high molecular weight glycoproteins with complexity and diversity that constitute the major component of the mucus layer within the gastric epithelium. Up to date, twelve core proteins of human mucin have been described. It has known that normal human stomach can express MUC1, MUC5AC, and MUC6. MUC1 and MUC5AC are expressed in the superficial foveolar epithelium and mucous neck cells of both the antrum and corpus, whereas MUC6 is expressed in the pyloric glands of antrum and the mucous cells of the neck zone of the corpus [157-160]. In contrast, MUC2 is found in the Golgi region of foveolar cells in the antrum and predominantly express in the areas of intestinal metaplasia with vacuolar staining in goblet cells [161, 162]. MUC5B is expressed only during a brief period of fetal life [163]. Previous studies have shown that MUC5AC expression in gastric carcinoma is associated with diffuse type gastric carcinoma and EGC [164, 165]. The expression of MUC2 is closely correlated with mucinous carcinoma and cardia adenocarcinoma [164]. In additional studies by Pinto-de-Sousa et al, MUC5B was aberrantly expressed in 22% of gastric carcinomas and is associated with differentiation and co-expression of MUC5AC [166]. Expression of MUC1 is less frequent in adenoma compared to associated carcinoma [167]. In contrast, MUC2, an intestinal type mucin, was highly expressed in the adenomas, but either persisted or decreased after malignant transformation to adenocarcinomas. These findings suggest that MUC2 expression would be an early event, while MUC1 expression would be a late event in the carcinogenesis of the stomach [159]. The pattern of mucin expression may help to understand the differentiation pathway of gastric carcinoma and to predict its biologic behavior. However, it is still controversial whether expressions of mucin in gastric carcinoma have a prognostic significance or not.

Immunohistochemical staining of cytokeratin 7 and cytokeratin 20 show various expression in the stomach. Cytokeratin 20 is usually positive for antral epithelium, while cytokeratin 7 highlights the columnar cells of the cardia. It has known that adenocarcinomas of GEJ are more likely expressed CK7 and distal gastric adenocarcinoma are likely express CK20 [168].

5. Molecular pathology of gastric cancer

Although the carcinogenesis of gastric carcinoma is not clear, a rapid progress in the molecular biology of cancer helps us to understand a complex process of malignant transformation of the gastric epithelium caused by the accumulation of aberrant genetic mutations. Gastric cancer is a heterogeneous disease with multiple environmental etiologies and alternative pathways of carcinogenesis. Beyond mutations in TP53, alterations in other genes or pathways account for only small subsets of the disease [169]. Recent studies using next-generation sequencing (NGS) have revealed an extensive repertoire of potential cancer-deriving genes in several cancer types. In stomach, recent exome sequencing data with 22 AGCs showed that genes involved in chromatin modification to be commonly mutated. A downstream validation study confirmed frequent inactivating mutations or protein deficiency of ARID1A, which encodes a member of the SWI-SNF chromatin remodeling family, in 83% of gastric cancers with microsatellite instability (MSI), 73% of those with Epstein-Barr virus (EBV) infection and 11% of those that were not infected with EBV and microsatellite stable (MSS). Subsequent exome sequencing data with 15 AGCs showed similar genetic alterations; frequently mutated genes in the adenocarcinomas included TP53 (73%), PIK3CA (20%), and ARID1A (20%), and suggested that FAT4 and ARID1A may thus be key tumorigenetic events in subset of gastric cancers [170]. In a search for COSMIC (Catalogue Of Somatic Mutations in Cancer) data, TP53 mutations is the most frequent mutation followed by CDH1, ARID1A, MSH6, PIK2CA, CDK2A, APC, FBXW7, KRAS, CTNNB1, PTEN,EGFR, ERBB2, HRAS and BRAF (Fig.17). Recent high throughput mutation profiling showed similar results [171, 172]. Lee et al first described that mutations of CTNNB1 were significantly more frequent in EBV-associated gastric carcinoma [171].

Molecular targeted therapies have significantly emerged as an effective treatment and improved clinical outcomes of many common malignancies, including breast, colorectal, and lung cancers. Although studies for targeting agents of gastric cancer did not show promising results in the past decades, recently, trastuzumab has been approved by US Food and Drug Administration (FDA) and European Medicine Agency as a first-line therapy in Human epidermal growth factor receptor (HER) 2 positive metastatic gastric cancers and GEJ cancers based on the result of a landmark clinical trial, so called ToGA (Trastuzumab for Gastric Cancer) study. Currently, many other molecular targeted agents for AGCs are undergoing clinical trials, including vascular epithelial growth factor (VEGF) inhibitor, other HER family targeted agents, and etc. In this chapter, we focus on two main targeting agents, HER2 and VEGF inhibitors, and discuss about their biologic pathways and the results of clinical trials.

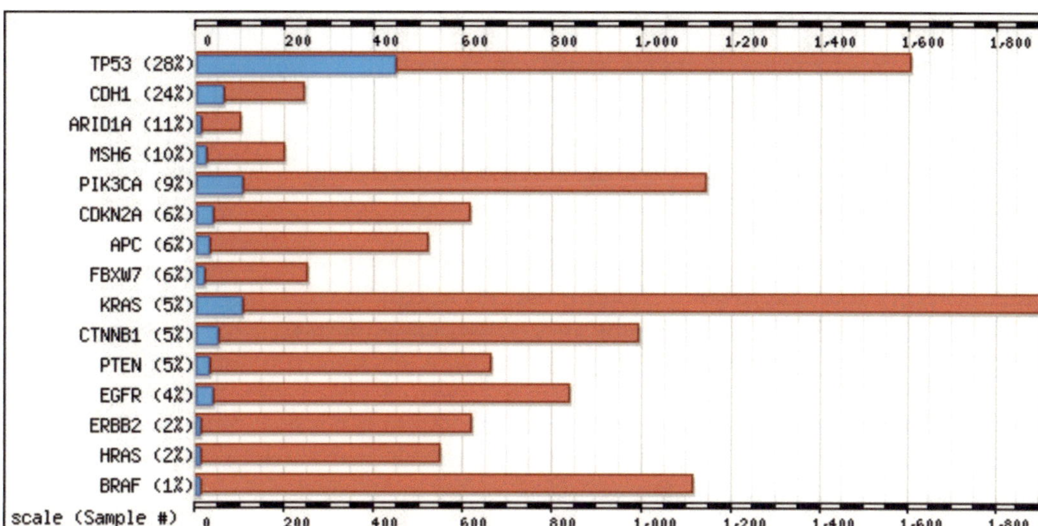

Figure 17. The graph highlights the most significantly mutated genes of gastric cancer from the Cancer Gene Census. *Source*: COSMIC: a open information showing somatic mutation related with human cancer, Sanger Institute. http://www.sanger.ac.uk/genetics/CGP/cosmic/

5.1. Next-generation sequencing of gastric cancer

Recent genome-wide sequencing studies demonstrated that mutations of AT-rich interactive domain 1A gene (ARIDI1A) were identified in 8-11 % of gastric cancer and frequently in EBV-positive gastric cancer and MSI-high gastric cancers [170, 173, 174]. ARIDI1A is one of the subunits of the Switch/Sucrase Non-fermentable (SWI/SNF) chromatin remodeling complex and involves the regulation of gene expression by binding to AT-rich DNA sequences [175]. ARIDI1A seems to act like a tumor suppressor gene that involves DNA repair, differentiation, development, and has a regulatory role in proliferation [175, 176]. ARIDI1A gene mutation has been reported in ovarian cancer, predominantly clear and endometrioid subtypes, and its rearrangement or deletion were identified in breast and lung cancer cell lines [176-178]. Recently, Wang et al demonstrated that gastric cancers with ARIDI1A mutation and loss are a distinct molecular subtype affecting predominantly EBV-positive and MSI-high gastric cancers, with a better prognosis and different carcinogenesis compared to the conventional gastric adenocarcinoma. They also demonstrated that ARIDI1A mutations are reversely associated with mutations of TP53 but concur with PIK3CA mutations. In large retrospective series by Abe et al, loss of ARIDI1A correlates with larger tumor size, advanced invasion depth, lymph node metastasis, and poor prognosis in EBV negative and MSS gastric cancers [174]. They also suggested that loss of ARIDI1A in EBV-positive gastric cancer is an early event in carcinogenesis and may precede EBV infection in gastric epithelial cells.

5.2. Activation of oncogenes

The MET proto-oncogene encodes a tyrosine kinase receptor for the hepatocyte growth factor and stimulates mitogenesis, motogenesis, vasculogenesis, and morphogenesis of the cells [179]. Its overexpression was found in 20% of diffuse and 40% of intestinal type gastric carcinomas. [180-182]. In series of MET gene activation, tumors with c-met protein tended to display increased invasiveness and poorly differentiated histology with poor prognosis on multivariate analysis [183, 184].

Fibroblast growth factor receptors (FGFRs) consist of four different variants and their overexpressions are associated with a poorer prognosis in patients with gastric carcinoma [185, 186]. FGFR type II encoding a receptor for keratinocyte growth factor is overexpressed in 33% of diffuse type of AGCs but not in intestinal type carcinomas [186, 187].

Another proto-oncogene, epidermal growth factor receptor genes including HER2 is overexpressed in 20% of intestinal type AGCs but not in diffuse type carcinomas [188]. More detailed description of ERBB2 is in the next section.

5.3. Inactivation of tumor suppressor genes

The TP53 gene located at 17p13.1 encodes a nuclear protein, which involves cell cycle control, DNA repair, cell differentiation and programmed cell death [181]. Mutation or loss of heterozygosity(LOH) of the TP53 gene has frequently been demonstrated in gastric adenocarcinoma. LOH occurs in 64 % and mutations in approximately 30-50% of gastric carcinomas [189]. Most alterations of the TP53 gene occur in AGCs. In intestinal type gastric carcinomas, although p53 gene mutations have been identified in 50% of EGCs and seem to be an early event, there was no proven relationship with tumor stage or progression [190, 191]. However, in diffuse type gastric carcinomas, TP53 gene mutations are significantly increased in advance stage, indicating the importance of TP53 mutations for tumor stage progression.

Deletions or mutations of the adenomatous polyposis coli (APC) gene located on chromosome 5q21 have been detected in up to one third of gastric carcinoma cases [192]. LOH of the APC gene occur in approximately 20% of intestinal type gastric carcinomas but not in diffuse type [193]. However, the frequency of APC gene mutations by histological types has been controversial and the role of APC gene in the carcinogenesis of gastric carcinoma is not clear yet compared to colorectal counterpart.

RUNX3 is a recently discovered tumor suppressor gene that is involved in gastric carcinogenesis. RUNX3 plays an important role for the suppression of cell proliferation in the gastric epithelium by inducing p21 expression in cooperation with TGF-β activated SMAD [194]. Loss of RUNX3 by hypermethylation of the promoter CpG island is observed in 45-65% of gastric carcinomas [195, 196].

Phosphatase and tensin homologue (PTEN) is located on chromosome 10q23.3 and acts as a plasma membrane lipid phosphatase. PTEN dephosphorylates the second messenger phosphatidylinositol-3,4,5-triphosphate, the product of phosphatidylinositol-3-kinase [197]. PTEN opposes the downstream signaling of phosphatidylinositol-3-kinase/ATP dependent tyrosine kinase pathway (PI3K) which involves the regulation of apoptosis, cell proliferation, migration, angiogenesis, and glucose metabolism [198]. Mina et al reported that PTEN deletion was found in 8 of 180 gastric cancer cases (4.4%) by fluorescence in-situ hybridization (FISH) and correlated with a higher rate of lymph node metastasis and distant metastasis indicating an aggressive behavior, which is similar to previous studies [199-201]. Interestingly, Esteva et al reported that PTEN loss in patients with HER2 positive metastatic breast cancer was significantly associated with a poor response to trastuzumab therapy and a shorter survival time, suggesting its pivotal role in trastuzumab resistance [202].

5.4. Cell-adhesion molecules and metastasis-related gene

The Wnt signaling pathway plays an essential role in embryonic development and a variety of processes including cell cycle regulation in differentiated cells. The Wnt signaling pathway also includes the regulation of β-catenin, which has multiple cellular functions, from cell surface signaling involving E-cadherin to nuclear translocation [106]. Mutations in the genes encoding Wnt pathway components are associated with various malignancies including tumors of gastrointestinal tract, in particular gastric cancer. E-cadherin, one of the members of the cadherins, acts as an adhesive molecule and plays an important role in growth development and carcinogenesis. E-cadherin gene located at chromosome 16q22 can be inactivated by mutation, LOH, and hypermethylation [181]. Because E-cadherin is a components of adhering junctions, the mutations of E-cadherin and related genes result in the dyscohesiveness of tumor cells in the morphology of diffuse type adenocarcinoma. Decreased expression of E-cadherin is predominantly found in undifferentiated, diffuse type gastric carcinomas, particularly in signet ring cell carcinoma and associated with invasiveness and a higher metastatic potential of gastric carcinomas resulting in a poorer prognosis [203, 204]. Hereditary diffuse gastric cancer is caused by germline mutations of E-cadherin (CDH1) [205]. Hypermethylation of E-cadherin promoter is another alternative pathway to inactivate E-cadherin gene and found in 83% of cases with sporadic diffuse type gastric carcinoma [206]. The Wnt signaling pathway would be less implicated for malignant transformation of intestinal type adenocarcinoma than diffuse type. APC gene mutations and mutations in the exon 3 of β-catenin lead to decreased phosphorylation of β-catenin and reduced proteolytic degradation of this protein in the Wnt pathway, which result in cytosolic accumulation of β-catenin, its nuclear translocation, and following malignant transformation of the gastric epithelium into intestinal type gastric carcinoma [207, 208].

5.5. Epigenetic alteration

Aberrant methylation of promoters may lead to the transcriptional silencing of various genes including E-cadherin, p16, p15, MGMT, CDKN2A, RUNX3 and MLH1. It has been reported that 40% of gastric carcinomas have CpG island methylation with frequent methylation in p16 and MLH1 genes [209]. CpG islands are DNA segments that are at least 0.5 kb in size, rich in G:C and CpG content, and found in approximately 70% of human gene promoters as an unmethylated status [210]. Promotor CpG island hypermethylation is found in almost all cancers and involves in carcinogenesis and aging process by affecting on the tumor related genes and the inactivation of tumor suppressor genes. Kang et al suggested that promotor CpG island hypermethylation occurs in an early step of the gastric carcinogenesis and accumulate during malignant transformation [211].

MSI is a DNA mismatch repair deficiency that is one of the pathways of gastric carcinogenesis. MSI has been found in 13%-44% of sporadic gastric carcinomas [212-214]. In gastric carcinomas, MSI is mainly caused by promoter CpG island hypermethylation of MLH1 gene [215, 216]. MSI due to epigenetic inactivation of MLH1 is found in 15%-39% of sporadic intestinal type carcinomas, 70% of which are associated with loss of MLH1 by hypermethylation of the promoter [215, 217]. Gastric carcinomas can be classified as MSI-low and MSI-high depending on the degree of genomic instability. MSI-high gastric carcinomas have some distinct clinicopathologic characteristic such as an association with intestinal type, distal stomach (antrum), and more favorable prognosis compared to MSS and MSI-low carcinomas [218]. In addition, some studies have shown that MSI-high gastric carcinomas have a lower risk of lymph node metastasis, near-diploid DNA content and tumoral lymphoid infiltration [219-221]. It is controversial that MSI involves in the early or late stage of gastric carcinogenesis due to contrary data. Particularly, EBV-positive gastric carcinoma is well known for global and nonrandom CpG island methylation of the promoter regions of cancer-related genes. Previous studies demonstrated that EBV-positive gastric carcinomas were strongly associated with CpG-island methylator phenotype and having multiple methylation of cancer related genes including genes of DNA repair and protection (MLH1, MGMT, and GSTP1), cell cycle regulation (p14,15,16, and cox2), cell adherence and metastasis (E-cadherin, bcl-2, and p73)[222-225]. However, the relationship between EBV-positive gastric cancer and MSI is not clear because some studies reported that EBV-positive gastric carcinomas presented with MSI-high but others showed no MSI in EBV-positive gastric carcinomas [212, 226-228]. Recently, Park et al reported that in multiple gastric carcinomas, EBV infection allows the gastric mucosa to escape from aberrant methylation of MLH1 and induces a malignant pathway independent of MSI [229].

Human telomerase reverse transcriptase (hTERT) is an important determinant of telomerase activity, the enzyme that catalyses the telomere DNA synthesis [230]. It has been reported that the majority of intestinal type gastric carcinomas have shortened telomere length, high levels of telomerase activity and a significant expression of hTERT [231, 232].

5.6. Molecular targeted therapies and related molecular changes

Therapeutic response and prognosis may be highly variable in patients with AGC within the same stage and chemotherapy regimens. Considering cancer is a product of accumulated genetic aberrations, elucidation of complex biological mechanism of cancer results in developing new molecular markers that would be specific for only tumor cells. Molecules that are closely associated with cell proliferation, invasion, and metastasis have been studied as potential candidates for targeted therapy. In gastric and GEJ carcinomas, some candidate molecules for targeted therapy such as epidermal growth factor (EGFR), vascular endothelial growth factor (VEGF), and P13K/AKT/mTOR pathway, as well as insulin-like growth factor receptor (IGFR), MET pathways, and FGFR have been actively investigated [179]. Two molecular target agents approached to phase III clinical trial are EGFR and VEGF inhibitors.

HER2 (c-erbB2) protooncogene is located on chromosome 17q11.2-12 and encodes a tyrosine kinase receptor that is overexpressed in several types of cancer, including gastric and breast cancers [233]. The HER family proteins regulate cell growth, survival, adhesion, migration, and differentiation, which can be amplified or weakened in tumor cells. It has been reported that HER2 gene amplification and/or protein overexpression in 13% to 23% of gastric and GEJ carcinoma [234-237]. HER2 overexpression is strongly associated with poor clinical outcome and disease aggressiveness [238-241]. Recently, the ToGA trial which compared trastuzumab plus chemotherapy vs. chemotherapy alone in patients with HER2-positive AGCs, mostly AGCs and GEJ cancers, [234] demonstrated that adding trastuzumab to the conventional chemotherapy is therapeutically superior in patients with HER2- positive AGCs than chemotherapy alone group.

Lapatinib is another HER2 targeted agent which is a dual tyrosine kinase inhibitor of EGFR and HER2. It has been actively investigated as a candidate agent for patients with trastuzumab-resistant gastric and GEJ cancers [242].

VEGF is a signal protein produced by cells that plays a key role in angiogenesis within a tumor and increases microvascular permeability [243]. It has been well known that tumors cannot grow beyond a certain limited size if it does not have an adequate blood supply. Tumors produce and secret VEGF and related receptors to enhance neovascularization. Increased expression of VEGF has been found in approximately 43% of gastric cancers and is associated with advanced stage, a higher risk of recurrence, and poor prognosis [244]. Karayiannakis et al reported that the serum VEGF concentration is strongly associated with metastasis and poor prognosis in patients of gastric and GEJ carcinomas [245]. These data have shown that VEGF would be a good molecular marker which can be detected not only from tumor tissue but also from serum. The recently introduced and evaluated anti-VEGF therapy are composed of the monoclonal antibody, bevacizumab, and multitargeted tyrosine kinase inhibitors, sunitinib and sorafenib [242]. Bevacizumab is a combinant humanized monoclonal antibody that targets VEGF. Previous studies have shown that a combination therapy with bevacizumab and chemotherapy significantly enhances the efficacy of chemotherapy in colorectal, lung, and renal cell carcinoma as well as recurrent glioblastoma [246-249]. The first phase III study of bevacizumab (generic name, avastin), the Avastin in Gastric Cancer (AVAGAST) trial, was to evaluate the therapeutic efficacy of bevacizumab combined with chemotherapy (capecitabine plus cisplatin) vs. chemotherapy alone as a first line therapy in patients with unresectable AGCs [250]. Although AVAGAST trial did not get a satisfying result with no significant difference in overall survival, however, both progression-free survival and overall response rate were improved in some patients treated with bevacizumab compared to the placebo control group. Although this strategy has demonstrated delayed tumor progression in some patients, the results are more modest than predicted. Several mechanisms of resistance have been recently proposed and emerging evidence indicates that, under certain experimental conditions, antiangiogenic agents increase intratumoral hypoxia by promoting vessel pruning and inhibiting neoangiogenesis [251].

In near future, the collection and dissemination of molecular targeted therapy research in gastric cancer will provide insight into the molecular understanding of gastric carcinogenesis and interconnectedness of biological processes and allow rapid correlation with clinical data, accelerating the impact on gastric cancer diagnosis, prognostication and treatment.

Author details

Sun-Mi Lee[1], Kyoung-Mee Kim[2] and Jae Y. Ro[3*]

*Address all correspondence to: jaero@tmhs.org

1 Departments of Pathology, University of Texas Health Science Center at San Antonio, San Antonio, TX, USA

2 SamSung Medical Center, SungKunkwan University School of Medicine, Seoul, Korea

3 The Methodist Hospital, Weill Medical College of Cornell University, Houston, TX, USA

References

[1] Kamangar, F., G.M. Dores, and W.F. Anderson, Patterns of cancer incidence, mortality, and prevalence across five continents: defining priorities to reduce cancer dispari-

ties in different geographic regions of the world. J Clin Oncol, 2006. 24(14): p. 2137-50.

[2] Siegel, R., D. Naishadham, and A. Jemal, Cancer statistics, 2012. CA Cancer J Clin, 2012. 62(1): p. 10-29.

[3] NCI. SEER Cancer Statistics Review,1975-2009. http://seer.cancer.gov/csr/1975_2009_pops09/ 2012.

[4] Yamaoka, Y., M. Kato, and M. Asaka, Geographic differences in gastric cancer incidence can be explained by differences between Helicobacter pylori strains. Intern Med, 2008. 47(12): p. 1077-83.

[5] Ferlay, J., et al., GLOBOCAN 2002 cancer incidence, mortality and prevalence worldwide. version 2.0 ed. IARC cancer base no.5. 2004, Lyon: IARC Press.

[6] Piazuelo, M.B., M. Epplein, and P. Correa, Gastric cancer: an infectious disease. Infect Dis Clin North Am, 2010. 24(4): p. 853-69, vii.

[7] Hisamichi, S., Screening for gastric cancer. World J Surg, 1989. 13(1): p. 31-7.

[8] Sue-Ling, H.M., et al., Early gastric cancer: 46 cases treated in one surgical department. Gut, 1992. 33(10): p. 1318-22.

[9] Devesa, S.S., W.J. Blot, and J.F. Fraumeni, Jr., Changing patterns in the incidence of esophageal and gastric carcinoma in the United States. Cancer, 1998. 83(10): p. 2049-53.

[10] Wijetunge, S., et al., Association of adenocarcinomas of the distal esophagus, "gastroesophageal junction," and "gastric cardia" with gastric pathology. Am J Surg Pathol, 2010. 34(10): p. 1521-7.

[11] Edge SB, Byrd DR, and Compton CC, AJCC Cancer Staging Manual. 7th ed. 2009, New York: Springer-Verlag. 103-115.

[12] Tokunaga, M., et al., Impact of esophageal invasion on clinicopathological characteristics and long-term outcome of adenocarcinoma of the subcardia. J Surg Oncol, 2012.

[13] Steup, W.H., et al., Tumors of the esophagogastric junction. Long-term survival in relation to the pattern of lymph node metastasis and a critical analysis of the accuracy or inaccuracy of pTNM classification. J Thorac Cardiovasc Surg, 1996. 111(1): p. 85-94; discussion 94-5.

[14] Crew, K.D. and A.I. Neugut, Epidemiology of upper gastrointestinal malignancies. Semin Oncol, 2004. 31(4): p. 450-64.

[15] Devesa, S.S. and J.F. Fraumeni, Jr., The rising incidence of gastric cardia cancer. J Natl Cancer Inst, 1999. 91(9): p. 747-9.

[16] Blot, W.J., et al., Rising incidence of adenocarcinoma of the esophagus and gastric cardia. JAMA, 1991. 265(10): p. 1287-9.

[17] Liu, Y., S. Kaneko, and T. Sobue, Trends in reported incidences of gastric cancer by tumour location, from 1975 to 1989 in Japan. Int J Epidemiol, 2004. 33(4): p. 808-15.

[18] Cunningham, D., et al., Perioperative chemotherapy versus surgery alone for resectable gastroesophageal cancer. N Engl J Med, 2006. 355(1): p. 11-20.

[19] DeMeester, S.R., Adenocarcinoma of the esophagus and cardia: a review of the disease and its treatment. Ann Surg Oncol, 2006. 13(1): p. 12-30.

[20] Kattan, M.W., et al., Postoperative nomogram for disease-specific survival after an R0 resection for gastric carcinoma. J Clin Oncol, 2003. 21(19): p. 3647-50.

[21] Maeda, H., et al., Clinicopathologic features of adenocarcinoma at the gastric cardia: is it different from distal cancer of the stomach? J Am Coll Surg, 2008. 206(2): p. 306-10.

[22] MacDonald, W.C. and J.B. MacDonald, Adenocarcinoma of the esophagus and/or gastric cardia. Cancer, 1987. 60(5): p. 1094-8.

[23] Gray, J.R., A.J. Coldman, and W.C. MacDonald, Cigarette and alcohol use in patients with adenocarcinoma of the gastric cardia or lower esophagus. Cancer, 1992. 69(9): p. 2227-31.

[24] Husemann, B., Cardia carcinoma considered as a distinct clinical entity. Br J Surg, 1989. 76(2): p. 136-9.

[25] Kajiyama, Y., et al., Prognostic factors in adenocarcinoma of the gastric cardia: pathologic stage analysis and multivariate regression analysis. J Clin Oncol, 1997. 15(5): p. 2015-21.

[26] Ohno, S., et al., Clinicopathologic characteristics and outcome of adenocarcinoma of the human gastric cardia in comparison with carcinoma of other regions of the stomach. J Am Coll Surg, 1995. 180(5): p. 577-82.

[27] Lagergren, J., et al., Symptomatic gastroesophageal reflux as a risk factor for esophageal adenocarcinoma. N Engl J Med, 1999. 340(11): p. 825-31.

[28] Inomata, Y., et al., Preservation of gastric acid secretion may be important for the development of gastroesophageal junction adenocarcinoma in Japanese people, irrespective of the H. pylori infection status. Am J Gastroenterol, 2006. 101(5): p. 926-33.

[29] Kamada, T., et al., Relationship between Gastroesophageal Junction Adenocarcinoma and Helicobacter pylori Infection in Japan. Digestion, 2012. 85: p. 256-60.

[30] Siewert, J.R. and H.J. Stein, Classification of adenocarcinoma of the oesophagogastric junction. Br J Surg, 1998. 85(11): p. 1457-9.

[31] International Classification of Disease. 9th Revision. Clinical Modification (ICD-9-CM). 6th ed. 2008, Maryland: National Center for Health Statistics.

[32] Leers, J.M., et al., Clinical characteristics, biologic behavior, and survival after esophagectomy are similar for adenocarcinoma of the gastroesophageal junction and the distal esophagus. J Thorac Cardiovasc Surg, 2009. 138(3): p. 594-602; discussion 601-2.

[33] Gertler, R., et al., How to classify adenocarcinomas of the esophagogastric junction: as esophageal or gastric cancer? Am J Surg Pathol, 2011. 35(10): p. 1512-22.

[34] Hirota, T., S. Ming, and M. Itabashi, Pathology of early gastric carcinoma, 1993, Tokyo: Springer-Verlag. 66-86.

[35] Fujita, S., Biology of early gastric carcinoma. Pathol Res Pract, 1978. 163(4): p. 297-309.

[36] Shimizu, S., M. Tada, and K. Kawai, Early gastric cancer: its surveillance and natural course. Endoscopy, 1995. 27(1): p. 27-31.

[37] Holscher, A.H., et al., Early gastric cancer: lymph node metastasis starts with deep mucosal infiltration. Ann Surg, 2009. 250(5): p. 791-7.

[38] Lawrence, M. and M.H. Shiu, Early gastric cancer. Twenty-eight-year experience. Ann Surg, 1991. 213(4): p. 327-34.

[39] Fielding, J.W., et al., Natural history of "early" gastric cancer: results of a 10-year regional survey. Br Med J, 1980. 281(6246): p. 965-7.

[40] Oliveira, F.J., et al., Early gastric cancer: Report of 58 cases. Gastric Cancer, 1998. 1(1): p. 51-56.

[41] Traynor, O.J., et al., Diagnostic and prognostic problems in early gastric cancer. Am J Surg, 1987. 154(5): p. 516-9.

[42] Axon, A., Symptoms and diagnosis of gastric cancer at early curable stage. Best Pract Res Clin Gastroenterol, 2006. 20(4): p. 697-708.

[43] Taylor, R.H., et al., Misleading response of malignant gastric ulcers to cimetidine. Lancet, 1978. 1(8066): p. 686-8.

[44] Wayman, J., N. Hayes, and S.M. Griffin, The response of early gastric cancer to proton-pump inhibitors. N Engl J Med, 1998. 338(26): p. 1924-5.

[45] Sakita, T., et al., Observations on the healing of ulcerations in early gastric cancer. The life cycle of the malignant ulcer. Gastroenterology, 1971. 60(5): p. 835-9 passim.

[46] Tsukuma, H., et al., Natural history of early gastric cancer: a non-concurrent, long term, follow up study. Gut, 2000. 47(5): p. 618-21.

[47] Kohli, Y., K. Kawai, and S. Fujita, Analytical studies on growth of human gastric cancer. J Clin Gastroenterol, 1981. 3(2): p. 129-33.

[48] Kikuchi, S., et al., Survival after surgical treatment of early gastric cancer: surgical techniques and long-term survival. Langenbecks Arch Surg, 2004. 389(2): p. 69-74.

[49] Onodera, H., et al., Surgical outcome of 483 patients with early gastric cancer: prognosis, postoperative morbidity and mortality, and gastric remnant cancer. Hepatogastroenterology, 2004. 51(55): p. 82-5.

[50] Moreaux, J. and J. Bougaran, Early gastric cancer. A 25-year surgical experience. Ann Surg, 1993. 217(4): p. 347-55.

[51] Sano, T., et al., Recurrence of early gastric cancer. Follow-up of 1475 patients and review of the Japanese literature. Cancer, 1993. 72(11): p. 3174-8.

[52] Kurihara, M., et al., Diagnosis of small early gastric cancer by X-ray, endoscopy, and biopsy. Cancer Detect Prev, 1981. 4(1-4): p. 377-83.

[53] Ito, Y., et al., The endoscopic diagnosis of early gastric cancer. Gastrointest Endosc, 1979. 25(3): p. 96-101.

[54] Maehara, Y., et al., Predictors of lymph node metastasis in early gastric cancer. Br J Surg, 1992. 79(3): p. 245-7.

[55] Yasuda, K., et al., Rate of detection of lymph node metastasis is correlated with the depth of submucosal invasion in early stage gastric carcinoma. Cancer, 1999. 85(10): p. 2119-23.

[56] Choi, J., et al., Endoscopic prediction of tumor invasion depth in early gastric cancer. Gastrointest Endosc, 2011. 73(5): p. 917-27.

[57] Ono, H. and S. Yohida, Endoscopic diagnosis of the depth of cancer invasion for gastric cancer. Stomach Intestine, 2001. 36: p. 6.

[58] Yanai, H., et al., Endoscopic ultrasonography and endoscopy for staging depth of invasion in early gastric cancer: a pilot study. Gastrointest Endosc, 1997. 46(3): p. 212-6.

[59] Kim, J.H., et al., Clinicopathologic factors influence accurate endosonographic assessment for early gastric cancer. Gastrointest Endosc, 2007. 66(5): p. 901-8.

[60] Lewin, K.J. and H.D. Appleman, Tumors of the esophagus and stomach, ed. J. Rosai. 1996, Washington D.C.: Armed Forces Institute of Pathology.

[61] Biasco, G., et al., Early gastric cancer in Italy. Clinical and pathological observations on 80 cases. Dig Dis Sci, 1987. 32(2): p. 113-20.

[62] Nakamura, K. and H. Sugano, Microcarcinoma of the stomach measuring less than 5 mm in the largest diameter and its histogenesis. Prog Clin Biol Res, 1983. 132D: p. 107-16.

[63] Shiroshita, H., et al., Re-evaluation of mucin phenotypes of gastric minute well-differentiated-type adenocarcinomas using a series of HGM, MUC5AC, MUC6, M-GGMC, MUC2 and CD10 stains. Pathol Int, 2004. 54(5): p. 311-21.

[64] Mori, M., M. Enjoji, and K. Sugimachi, Histopathologic features of minute and small human gastric adenocarcinomas. Arch Pathol Lab Med, 1989. 113(8): p. 926-31.

[65] Otsuji, E., et al., Clinicopathologic characteristics and prognosis of synchronous multifocal gastric carcinomas. Am J Surg, 2005. 189(1): p. 116-9.

[66] Choi, J., et al., Lymph node metastasis in multiple synchronous early gastric cancer. Gastrointest Endosc, 2011. 74(2): p. 276-84.

[67] Oohara, T., et al., Clinical diagnosis of minute gastric cancer less than 5 mm in diameter. Cancer, 1984. 53(1): p. 162-5.

[68] Hirota, T., et al., Clinicopathologic study of minute and small early gastric cancer. Histogenesis of gastric cancer. Pathol Annu, 1980. 15(Pt 2): p. 1-19.

[69] Ishida, M., et al., Metachronous liver metastasis from early gastric cancer. J Gastrointest Surg, 2012. 16(4): p. 837-41.

[70] Japanese classification of gastric carcinoma: 3rd English edition. Gastric Cancer, 2011. 14(2): p. 101-12.

[71] Update on the Paris classification of superficial neoplastic lesions in the digestive tract. Endoscopy, 2005. 37(6): p. 570-8.

[72] Tan, Y.K. and J.W. Fielding, Early diagnosis of early gastric cancer. Eur J Gastroenterol Hepatol, 2006. 18(8): p. 821-9.

[73] Xuan, Z.X., et al., Time trends of early gastric carcinoma. A clinicopathologic analysis of 2846 cases. Cancer, 1993. 72(10): p. 2889-94.

[74] Craanen, M.E., et al., Early gastric cancer: a clinicopathologic study. J Clin Gastroenterol, 1991. 13(3): p. 274-83.

[75] Everett, S.M. and A.T. Axon, Early gastric cancer: disease or pseudo-disease? Lancet, 1998. 351(9112): p. 1350-2.

[76] Sung, J., Early gastric cancer: diagnosis, treatment and prevention. Eur J Gastroenterol Hepatol, 2006. 18(8): p. 817-9.

[77] Srivastava, A. and G.Y. Lauwers, Gastric epithelial dysplasia: the Western perspective. Dig Liver Dis, 2008. 40(8): p. 641-9.

[78] Schlemper, R.J., et al., The Vienna classification of gastrointestinal epithelial neoplasia. Gut, 2000. 47(2): p. 251-5.

[79] Gotoda, T., et al., Incidence of lymph node metastasis from early gastric cancer: estimation with a large number of cases at two large centers. Gastric Cancer, 2000. 3(4): p. 219-225.

[80] Tsujitani, S., et al., Less invasive surgery for early gastric cancer based on the low probability of lymph node metastasis. Surgery, 1999. 125(2): p. 148-54.

[81] Kim, S.G., Endoscopic treatment for early gastric cancer. J Gastric Cancer, 2011. 11(3): p. 146-54.

[82] Soetikno, R., et al., Endoscopic mucosal resection for early cancers of the upper gastrointestinal tract. J Clin Oncol, 2005. 23(20): p. 4490-8.

[83] Sugano, K., Gastric cancer: pathogenesis, screening, and treatment. Gastrointest Endosc Clin N Am, 2008. 18(3): p. 513-22, ix.

[84] Hirasawa, T., et al., Incidence of lymph node metastasis and the feasibility of endoscopic resection for undifferentiated-type early gastric cancer. Gastric Cancer, 2009. 12(3): p. 148-52.

[85] Ahn, J.Y., et al., Endoscopic and oncologic outcomes after endoscopic resection for early gastric cancer: 1370 cases of absolute and extended indications. Gastrointest Endosc, 2011. 74(3): p. 485-93.

[86] Ono, H., Early gastric cancer: diagnosis, pathology, treatment techniques and treatment outcomes. Eur J Gastroenterol Hepatol, 2006. 18(8): p. 863-6.

[87] Rembacken, B.J., et al., Endoscopic mucosal resection. Endoscopy, 2001. 33(8): p. 709-18.

[88] Alfaro, E.E. and G.Y. Lauwers, Early gastric neoplasia: diagnosis and implications. Adv Anat Pathol, 2011. 18(4): p. 268-80.

[89] Amano, Y., et al., An assessment of local curability of endoscopic surgery in early gastric cancer without satisfaction of current therapeutic indications. Endoscopy, 1998. 30(6): p. 548-52.

[90] Habu, H., et al., Lymph node metastasis in early gastric cancer. Int Surg, 1986. 71(4): p. 244-7.

[91] Ishigami, S., et al., Carcinomatous lymphatic invasion in early gastric cancer invading into the submucosa. Ann Surg Oncol, 1999. 6(3): p. 286-9.

[92] Ono, H., et al., Endoscopic mucosal resection for treatment of early gastric cancer. Gut, 2001. 48(2): p. 225-9.

[93] Oka, S., et al., Advantage of endoscopic submucosal dissection compared with EMR for early gastric cancer. Gastrointest Endosc, 2006. 64(6): p. 877-83.

[94] Tanabe, S., et al., Clinical outcome of endoscopic aspiration mucosectomy for early stage gastric cancer. Gastrointest Endosc, 2002. 56(5): p. 708-13.

[95] Manner, H., et al., Long-term results of endoscopic resection in early gastric cancer: the Western experience. Am J Gastroenterol, 2009. 104(3): p. 566-73.

[96] Watanabe, K., et al., Clinical outcomes of EMR for gastric tumors: historical pilot evaluation between endoscopic submucosal dissection and conventional mucosal resection. Gastrointest Endosc, 2006. 63(6): p. 776-82.

[97] Isomoto, H., et al., Endoscopic submucosal dissection for early gastric cancer: a large-scale feasibility study. Gut, 2009. 58(3): p. 331-6.

[98] Goto, O., et al., Outcomes of endoscopic submucosal dissection for early gastric cancer with special reference to validation for curability criteria. Endoscopy, 2009. 41(2): p. 118-22.

[99] Mitsuhashi, T., et al., Post-gastric endoscopic mucosal resection surveillance biopsies: evaluation of mucosal changes and recognition of potential mimics of residual adenocarcinoma. Am J Surg Pathol, 2006. 30(5): p. 650-6.

[100] Clark, C.J., et al., Current problems in surgery: gastric cancer. Curr Probl Surg, 2006. 43(8-9): p. 566-670.

[101] Abeloff, M.D., et al., Abeloff's Clinical Oncology, ed. M.D. Abeloff. 2008, Philadelphia: Churchill Livingstone.

[102] Stemmermann, G.N., Extrapelvic carcinoma metastatic to the uterus. Am J Obstet Gynecol, 1961. 82: p. 1261-6.

[103] Catalano, V., et al., Gastric cancer. Crit Rev Oncol Hematol, 2009. 71(2): p. 127-64.

[104] Kurtz, R.C. and P. Sherlock, The diagnosis of gastric cancer. Semin Oncol, 1985. 12(1): p. 11-8.

[105] Wanebo, H.J., et al., Cancer of the stomach. A patient care study by the American College of Surgeons. Ann Surg, 1993. 218(5): p. 583-92.

[106] Shah, M.A., Gastric cancer: an update. Curr Oncol Rep, 2006. 8(3): p. 183-91.

[107] Low, V.H., et al., Diagnosis of gastric carcinoma: sensitivity of double-contrast barium studies. AJR Am J Roentgenol, 1994. 162(2): p. 329-34.

[108] Halvorsen, R.A., Jr., J. Yee, and V.D. McCormick, Diagnosis and staging of gastric cancer. Semin Oncol, 1996. 23(3): p. 325-35.

[109] Takao, M., et al., Discrepancies in histologic diagnoses of early gastric cancer between biopsy and endoscopic mucosal resection specimens. Gastric Cancer, 2012. 15(1): p. 91-6.

[110] Hakama, M., et al., Tumour markers and screening for gastrointestinal cancer: a follow up study in Finland. J Med Screen, 1994. 1(1): p. 60-4.

[111] Pectasides, D., et al., CEA, CA 19-9, and CA-50 in monitoring gastric carcinoma. Am J Clin Oncol, 1997. 20(4): p. 348-53.

[112] Willis, S., et al., Endoscopic ultrasonography in the preoperative staging of gastric cancer: accuracy and impact on surgical therapy. Surg Endosc, 2000. 14(10): p. 951-4.

[113] Kelly, S., et al., A systematic review of the staging performance of endoscopic ultrasound in gastro-oesophageal carcinoma. Gut, 2001. 49(4): p. 534-9.

[114] Bhandari, S., et al., Usefulness of three-dimensional, multidetector row CT (virtual gastroscopy and multiplanar reconstruction) in the evaluation of gastric cancer: a

comparison with conventional endoscopy, EUS, and histopathology. Gastrointest Endosc, 2004. 59(6): p. 619-26.

[115] Paramo, J.C. and G. Gomez, Dynamic CT in the preoperative evaluation of patients with gastric cancer: correlation with surgical findings and pathology. Ann Surg Oncol, 1999. 6(4): p. 379-84.

[116] Davies, J., et al., Spiral computed tomography and operative staging of gastric carcinoma: a comparison with histopathological staging. Gut, 1997. 41(3): p. 314-9.

[117] Sohn, K.M., et al., Comparing MR imaging and CT in the staging of gastric carcinoma. AJR Am J Roentgenol, 2000. 174(6): p. 1551-7.

[118] Kim, A.Y., et al., MRI in staging advanced gastric cancer: is it useful compared with spiral CT? J Comput Assist Tomogr, 2000. 24(3): p. 389-94.

[119] Borrmann, R., Handbuch der Speziellen Patho-logischen Anatomie und Histologie. Geshwulste des Magens und Duodenums, 1926: p. 865.

[120] Ming, S., Classification of gastric carcinoma. Gastric Carcinoma, ed. M. Filipe and J. Jass. 1986, Edinburgh: Carleston-Livingston. 3.

[121] Lauren, P., The Two Histological Main Types of Gastric Carcinoma: Diffuse and So-Called Intestinal-Type Carcinoma. An Attempt at a Histo-Clinical Classification. Acta Pathol Microbiol Scand, 1965. 64: p. 31-49.

[122] Noda, S., K. Soejima, and K. Inokuchi, Clinicopathological analysis of the intestinal type and diffuse type of gastric carcinoma. Jpn J Surg, 1980. 10(4): p. 277-83.

[123] Vauhkonen, M., H. Vauhkonen, and P. Sipponen, Pathology and molecular biology of gastric cancer. Best Pract Res Clin Gastroenterol, 2006. 20(4): p. 651-74.

[124] Correa, P., Human gastric carcinogenesis: a multistep and multifactorial process--First American Cancer Society Award Lecture on Cancer Epidemiology and Prevention. Cancer Res, 1992. 52(24): p. 6735-40.

[125] Carneiro, F., et al., Model of the early development of diffuse gastric cancer in E-cadherin mutation carriers and its implications for patient screening. J Pathol, 2004. 203(2): p. 681-7.

[126] Houghton, J., et al., Gastric cancer originating from bone marrow-derived cells. Science, 2004. 306(5701): p. 1568-71.

[127] Guilford, P., B. Humar, and V. Blair, Hereditary diffuse gastric cancer: translation of CDH1 germline mutations into clinical practice. Gastric Cancer, 2010. 13(1): p. 1-10.

[128] Oliveira, C., et al., Genetic screening for familial gastric cancer. Hered Cancer Clin Pract, 2004. 2(2): p. 51-64.

[129] Borch, K., et al., Changing pattern of histological type, location, stage and outcome of surgical treatment of gastric carcinoma. Br J Surg, 2000. 87(5): p. 618-26.

[130] Stelzner, S. and P. Emmrich, The mixed type in Lauren's classification of gastric carcinoma. Histologic description and biologic behavior. Gen Diagn Pathol, 1997. 143(1): p. 39-48.

[131] Zheng, H.C., et al., Mixed-type gastric carcinomas exhibit more aggressive features and indicate the histogenesis of carcinomas. Virchows Arch, 2008. 452(5): p. 525-34.

[132] Kozuki, T., et al., Differences in p53 and cadherin-catenin complex expression between histological subtypes in diffusely infiltrating gastric carcinoma. Histopathology, 2002. 41(1): p. 56-64.

[133] Ming, S.C., Gastric carcinoma. A pathobiological classification. Cancer, 1977. 39(6): p. 2475-85.

[134] Davessar, K., et al., Gastric adenocarcinoma: prognostic significance of several pathologic parameters and histologic classifications. Hum Pathol, 1990. 21(3): p. 325-32.

[135] Goseki, N., T. Takizawa, and M. Koike, Differences in the mode of the extension of gastric cancer classified by histological type: new histological classification of gastric carcinoma. Gut, 1992. 33(5): p. 606-12.

[136] Songun, I., et al., Classification of gastric carcinoma using the Goseki system provides prognostic information additional to TNM staging. Cancer, 1999. 85(10): p. 2114-8.

[137] Dixon, M.F., et al., Goseki grading in gastric cancer: comparison with existing systems of grading and its reproducibility. Histopathology, 1994. 25(4): p. 309-16.

[138] Martin, I.G., et al., Goseki histological grading of gastric cancer is an important predictor of outcome. Gut, 1994. 35(6): p. 758-63.

[139] Roy, P., et al., Prognostic comparison of the pathological classifications of gastric cancer: a population-based study. Histopathology, 1998. 33(4): p. 304-10.

[140] Guglielmi, A., et al., [Prognostic value of histologic classifications of advanced stomach cancer: comparative study of Lauren's and Goseki's classifications]. Chir Ital, 1997. 49(3): p. 45-9.

[141] WHO, Tumors of the digestive system. World Health Organization classification of tumors, ed. S.R. Hamilton and L.A. Aaltonen. 2000, Lyon: IARC Press. 37-68.

[142] Adachi, Y., et al., Pathology and prognosis of gastric carcinoma: well versus poorly differentiated type. Cancer, 2000. 89(7): p. 1418-24.

[143] Kuroda, T., et al., Presence of poorly differentiated component correlated with submucosal invasion in the early diffuse-type gastric cancer. Hepatogastroenterology, 2008. 55(88): p. 2264-8.

[144] Wu, C.Y., et al., Lymph node metastasis in early gastric cancer: a clinicopathological analysis. Hepatogastroenterology, 2002. 49(47): p. 1465-8.

[145] Watanabe, H., J. Jass, and L. Sobin, Histological typing of oesophageal and gastric tumors. 2nd ed. WHO international histological classification of tumors. 1990, Berlin: Springer-Verlag.

[146] Carneiro, F., M. Seixas, and M. Sobrinho-Simoes, New elements for an updated classification of the carcinomas of the stomach. Pathol Res Pract, 1995. 191(6): p. 571-84.

[147] Yasuda, K., et al., Papillary adenocarcinoma of the stomach. Gastric Cancer, 2000. 3(1): p. 33-38.

[148] Hirota, T., A. Ochiai, and M. Itabashi, Significance of histological type of gastric carcinoma as a prognostic factor. Stomach Intestine, 1991. 26: p. 9.

[149] Ito, E., T. Takizawa, and N. Shiraishi, Differentiated adenocarcinoma of the gastric and intestinal phenotype-histological appearance and biological behavior. Stomach Intestine, 2003. 38: p. 6.

[150] Nakashima, Y., et al., Nuclear atypia grading score is a useful prognostic factor in papillary gastric adenocarcinoma. Histopathology, 2011. 59(5): p. 841-9.

[151] Kunisaki, C., et al., Clinicopathologic characteristics and surgical outcomes of mucinous gastric carcinoma. Ann Surg Oncol, 2006. 13(6): p. 836-42.

[152] Adachi, Y., et al., A clinicopathologic study of mucinous gastric carcinoma. Cancer, 1992. 69(4): p. 866-71.

[153] Wu, C.Y., et al., A clinicopathologic study of mucinous gastric carcinoma including multivariate analysis. Cancer, 1998. 83(7): p. 1312-8.

[154] Sung, C.O., et al., Tumor size predicts survival in mucinous gastric carcinoma. J Surg Oncol, 2012.

[155] Li, C., et al., Advanced gastric carcinoma with signet ring cell histology. Oncology, 2007. 72(1-2): p. 64-8.

[156] Hyung, W.J., et al., Early gastric carcinoma with signet ring cell histology. Cancer, 2002. 94(1): p. 78-83.

[157] Ho, S.B., et al., Mucin gene expression in normal, preneoplastic, and neoplastic human gastric epithelium. Cancer Res, 1995. 55(12): p. 2681-90.

[158] Ho, S.B., et al., Heterogeneity of mucin gene expression in normal and neoplastic tissues. Cancer Res, 1993. 53(3): p. 641-51.

[159] Reis, C.A., et al., Immunohistochemical study of MUC5AC expression in human gastric carcinomas using a novel monoclonal antibody. Int J Cancer, 1997. 74(1): p. 112-21.

[160] Reis, C.A., et al., Expression of fully and under-glycosylated forms of MUC1 mucin in gastric carcinoma. Int J Cancer, 1998. 79(4): p. 402-10.

[161] Sakamoto, H., et al., Mucin antigen expression in gastric carcinomas of young and old adults. Hum Pathol, 1997. 28(9): p. 1056-65.

[162] Reis, C.A., et al., Immunohistochemical study of the expression of MUC6 mucin and co-expression of other secreted mucins (MUC5AC and MUC2) in human gastric carcinomas. J Histochem Cytochem, 2000. 48(3): p. 377-88.

[163] Buisine, M.P., et al., Developmental mucin gene expression in the gastroduodenal tract and accessory digestive glands. I. Stomach. A relationship to gastric carcinoma. J Histochem Cytochem, 2000. 48(12): p. 1657-66.

[164] Pinto-de-Sousa, J., et al., Mucins MUC1, MUC2, MUC5AC and MUC6 expression in the evaluation of differentiation and clinico-biological behaviour of gastric carcinoma. Virchows Arch, 2002. 440(3): p. 304-10.

[165] Fiocca, R., et al., Characterization of four main cell types in gastric cancer: foveolar, mucopeptic, intestinal columnar and goblet cells. An histopathologic, histochemical and ultrastructural study of "early" and "advanced" tumours. Pathol Res Pract, 1987. 182(3): p. 308-25.

[166] Pinto-de-Sousa, J., et al., MUC5B expression in gastric carcinoma: relationship with clinico-pathological parameters and with expression of mucins MUC1, MUC2, MUC5AC and MUC6. Virchows Arch, 2004. 444(3): p. 224-30.

[167] Lee, H.S., et al., MUC1, MUC2, MUC5AC, and MUC6 expressions in gastric carcinomas: their roles as prognostic indicators. Cancer, 2001. 92(6): p. 1427-34.

[168] Taniere, P., et al., Cytokeratin expression in adenocarcinomas of the esophagogastric junction: a comparative study of adenocarcinomas of the distal esophagus and of the proximal stomach. Am J Surg Pathol, 2002. 26(9): p. 1213-21.

[169] Wang, K., et al., Exome sequencing identifies frequent mutation of ARID1A in molecular subtypes of gastric cancer. Nat Genet, 2011. 43(12): p. 1219-23.

[170] Zang, Z.J., et al., Exome sequencing of gastric adenocarcinoma identifies recurrent somatic mutations in cell adhesion and chromatin remodeling genes. Nat Genet, 2012. 44(5): p. 570-4.

[171] Lee, J., et al., High-throughput mutation profiling identifies frequent somatic mutations in advanced gastric adenocarcinoma. PLoS One, 2012. 7(6): p. e38892.

[172] MacConaill, L.E., et al., Profiling critical cancer gene mutations in clinical tumor samples. PLoS One, 2009. 4(11): p. e7887.

[173] Jones, S., et al., Somatic mutations in the chromatin remodeling gene ARID1A occur in several tumor types. Hum Mutat, 2012. 33(1): p. 100-3.

[174] Abe, H., et al., ARID1A expression loss in gastric cancer: pathway-dependent roles with and without Epstein-Barr virus infection and microsatellite instability. Virchows Arch, 2012.

[175] Reisman, D., S. Glaros, and E.A. Thompson, The SWI/SNF complex and cancer. Oncogene, 2009. 28(14): p. 1653-68.

[176] Huang, J., et al., Genomic and functional evidence for an ARID1A tumor suppressor role. Genes Chromosomes Cancer, 2007. 46(8): p. 745-50.

[177] Jones, S., et al., Frequent mutations of chromatin remodeling gene ARID1A in ovarian clear cell carcinoma. Science, 2010. 330(6001): p. 228-31.

[178] Wiegand, K.C., et al., ARID1A mutations in endometriosis-associated ovarian carcinomas. N Engl J Med, 2010. 363(16): p. 1532-43.

[179] Oshima, T. and M. Masuda, Molecular targeted agents for gastric and gastroesophageal junction cancer. Surg Today, 2012. 42(4): p. 313-27.

[180] Nakajima, M., et al., The prognostic significance of amplification and overexpression of c-met and c-erb B-2 in human gastric carcinomas. Cancer, 1999. 85(9): p. 1894-902.

[181] Panani, A.D., Cytogenetic and molecular aspects of gastric cancer: clinical implications. Cancer Lett, 2008. 266(2): p. 99-115.

[182] Kuniyasu, H., et al., Frequent amplification of the c-met gene in scirrhous type stomach cancer. Biochem Biophys Res Commun, 1992. 189(1): p. 227-32.

[183] Kuniyasu, H., et al., Aberrant expression of c-met mRNA in human gastric carcinomas. Int J Cancer, 1993. 55(1): p. 72-5.

[184] Huang, T.J., et al., Overexpression of the c-met protooncogene in human gastric carcinoma--correlation to clinical features. Acta Oncol, 2001. 40(5): p. 638-43.

[185] Smith, M.G., et al., Cellular and molecular aspects of gastric cancer. World J Gastroenterol, 2006. 12(19): p. 2979-90.

[186] Hattori, Y., et al., K-sam, an amplified gene in stomach cancer, is a member of the heparin-binding growth factor receptor genes. Proc Natl Acad Sci U S A, 1990. 87(15): p. 5983-7.

[187] Hara, T., et al., Amplification of c-myc, K-sam, and c-met in gastric cancers: detection by fluorescence in situ hybridization. Lab Invest, 1998. 78(9): p. 1143-53.

[188] Yokota, J., et al., Genetic alterations of the c-erbB-2 oncogene occur frequently in tubular adenocarcinoma of the stomach and are often accompanied by amplification of the v-erbA homologue. Oncogene, 1988. 2(3): p. 283-7.

[189] Rhyu, M.G., et al., Allelic deletions of MCC/APC and p53 are frequent late events in human gastric carcinogenesis. Gastroenterology, 1994. 106(6): p. 1584-8.

[190] Wu, M.S., et al., Genetic alterations in gastric cancer: relation to histological subtypes, tumor stage, and Helicobacter pylori infection. Gastroenterology, 1997. 112(5): p. 1457-65.

[191] Brito, M.J., et al., Expression of p53 in early (T1) gastric carcinoma and precancerous adjacent mucosa. Gut, 1994. 35(12): p. 1697-700.

[192] Horii, A., et al., The APC gene, responsible for familial adenomatous polyposis, is mutated in human gastric cancer. Cancer Res, 1992. 52(11): p. 3231-3.

[193] Hsieh, L.L. and Y.C. Huang, Loss of heterozygosity of APC/MCC gene in differentiated and undifferentiated gastric carcinomas in Taiwan. Cancer Lett, 1995. 96(2): p. 169-74.

[194] Chi, X.Z., et al., RUNX3 suppresses gastric epithelial cell growth by inducing p21(WAF1/Cip1) expression in cooperation with transforming growth factor {beta}-activated SMAD. Mol Cell Biol, 2005. 25(18): p. 8097-107.

[195] Kim, T.Y., et al., Methylation of RUNX3 in various types of human cancers and premalignant stages of gastric carcinoma. Lab Invest, 2004. 84(4): p. 479-84.

[196] Sakakura, C., et al., Frequent downregulation of the runt domain transcription factors RUNX1, RUNX3 and their cofactor CBFB in gastric cancer. Int J Cancer, 2005. 113(2): p. 221-8.

[197] Maehama, T. and J.E. Dixon, The tumor suppressor, PTEN/MMAC1, dephosphorylates the lipid second messenger, phosphatidylinositol 3,4,5-trisphosphate. J Biol Chem, 1998. 273(22): p. 13375-8.

[198] Blanco-Aparicio, C., et al., PTEN, more than the AKT pathway. Carcinogenesis, 2007. 28(7): p. 1379-86.

[199] Im, S.A., et al., Potential prognostic significance of p185(HER2) overexpression with loss of PTEN expression in gastric carcinomas. Tumori, 2005. 91(6): p. 513-21.

[200] Zhou, Y.J., et al., Inactivation of PTEN is associated with increased angiogenesis and VEGF overexpression in gastric cancer. World J Gastroenterol, 2004. 10(21): p. 3225-9.

[201] Zheng, H.C., et al., Role of PTEN and MMP-7 expression in growth, invasion, metastasis and angiogenesis of gastric carcinoma. Pathol Int, 2003. 53(10): p. 659-66.

[202] Esteva, F.J., et al., PTEN, PIK3CA, p-AKT, and p-p70S6K status: association with trastuzumab response and survival in patients with HER2-positive metastatic breast cancer. Am J Pathol, 2010. 177(4): p. 1647-56.

[203] Mayer, B., et al., E-cadherin expression in primary and metastatic gastric cancer: down-regulation correlates with cellular dedifferentiation and glandular disintegration. Cancer Res, 1993. 53(7): p. 1690-5.

[204] Ascano, J.J., et al., Inactivation of the E-cadherin gene in sporadic diffuse-type gastric cancer. Mod Pathol, 2001. 14(10): p. 942-9.

[205] Suriano, G., et al., The intracellular E-cadherin germline mutation V832 M lacks the ability to mediate cell-cell adhesion and to suppress invasion. Oncogene, 2003. 22(36): p. 5716-9.

[206] Tamura, G., et al., E-Cadherin gene promoter hypermethylation in primary human gastric carcinomas. J Natl Cancer Inst, 2000. 92(7): p. 569-73.

[207] Ebert, M.P., et al., Increased beta-catenin mRNA levels and mutational alterations of the APC and beta-catenin gene are present in intestinal-type gastric cancer. Carcinogenesis, 2002. 23(1): p. 87-91.

[208] Ebert, M.P., et al., Loss of beta-catenin expression in metastatic gastric cancer. J Clin Oncol, 2003. 21(9): p. 1708-14.

[209] Sakata, K., et al., Hypermethylation of the hMLH1 gene promoter in solitary and multiple gastric cancers with microsatellite instability. Br J Cancer, 2002. 86(4): p. 564-7.

[210] Cervantes, A., et al., Molecular biology of gastric cancer. Clin Transl Oncol, 2007. 9(4): p. 208-15.

[211] Kang, G.H., et al., Profile of aberrant CpG island methylation along the multistep pathway of gastric carcinogenesis. Lab Invest, 2003. 83(5): p. 635-41.

[212] Chong, J.M., et al., Microsatellite instability in the progression of gastric carcinoma. Cancer Res, 1994. 54(17): p. 4595-7.

[213] Semba, S., et al., Microsatellite instability in precancerous lesions and adenocarcinomas of the stomach. Cancer, 1996. 77(8 Suppl): p. 1620-7.

[214] Ottini, L., et al., Microsatellite instability in gastric cancer is associated with tumor location and family history in a high-risk population from Tuscany. Cancer Res, 1997. 57(20): p. 4523-9.

[215] Leung, S.Y., et al., hMLH1 promoter methylation and lack of hMLH1 expression in sporadic gastric carcinomas with high-frequency microsatellite instability. Cancer Res, 1999. 59(1): p. 159-64.

[216] Herman, J.G. and S.B. Baylin, Gene silencing in cancer in association with promoter hypermethylation. N Engl J Med, 2003. 349(21): p. 2042-54.

[217] Fleisher, A.S., et al., Hypermethylation of the hMLH1 gene promoter in human gastric cancers with microsatellite instability. Cancer Res, 1999. 59(5): p. 1090-5.

[218] Halling, K.C., et al., Origin of microsatellite instability in gastric cancer. Am J Pathol, 1999. 155(1): p. 205-11.

[219] dos Santos, N.R., et al., Microsatellite instability at multiple loci in gastric carcinoma: clinicopathologic implications and prognosis. Gastroenterology, 1996. 110(1): p. 38-44.

[220] Oliveira, C., et al., The clinicopathological features of gastric carcinomas with microsatellite instability may be mediated by mutations of different "target genes": a study of the TGFbeta RII, IGFII R, and BAX genes. Am J Pathol, 1998. 153(4): p. 1211-9.

[221] Wu, M.S., et al., Clinicopathological significance of altered loci of replication error and microsatellite instability-associated mutations in gastric cancer. Cancer Res, 1998. 58(7): p. 1494-7.

[222] Kusano, M., et al., Genetic, epigenetic, and clinicopathologic features of gastric carcinomas with the CpG island methylator phenotype and an association with Epstein-Barr virus. Cancer, 2006. 106(7): p. 1467-79.

[223] Chang, M.S., et al., CpG island methylation status in gastric carcinoma with and without infection of Epstein-Barr virus. Clin Cancer Res, 2006. 12(10): p. 2995-3002.

[224] Enomoto, S., et al., Lack of association between CpG island methylator phenotype in human gastric cancers and methylation in their background non-cancerous gastric mucosae. Cancer Sci, 2007. 98(12): p. 1853-61.

[225] Chong, J.M., et al., Global and non-random CpG-island methylation in gastric carcinoma associated with Epstein-Barr virus. Cancer Sci, 2003. 94(1): p. 76-80.

[226] Leung, S.Y., et al., Microsatellite instability, Epstein-Barr virus, mutation of type II transforming growth factor beta receptor and BAX in gastric carcinomas in Hong Kong Chinese. Br J Cancer, 1999. 79(3-4): p. 582-8.

[227] Chang, M.S., et al., Epstein-Barr virus and microsatellite instability in gastric carcinogenesis. J Pathol, 2003. 199(4): p. 447-52.

[228] Wu, M.S., et al., Epstein-Barr virus-associated gastric carcinomas: relation to H. pylori infection and genetic alterations. Gastroenterology, 2000. 118(6): p. 1031-8.

[229] Park, H.Y., et al., EBV infection and mismatch repair deficiency mediated by loss of hMLH1 expression contribute independently to the development of multiple synchronous gastric carcinomas. J Surg Oncol, 2012.

[230] Yasui, W., et al., Molecular diagnosis of gastric cancer: present and future. Gastric Cancer, 2001. 4(3): p. 113-21.

[231] Yasui, W., et al., Expression of telomerase catalytic component, telomerase reverse transcriptase, in human gastric carcinomas. Jpn J Cancer Res, 1998. 89(11): p. 1099-103.

[232] Yasui, W., et al., Immunohistochemical detection of human telomerase reverse transcriptase in normal mucosa and precancerous lesions of the stomach. Jpn J Cancer Res, 1999. 90(6): p. 589-95.

[233] Herbst, R.S., Review of epidermal growth factor receptor biology. Int J Radiat Oncol Biol Phys, 2004. 59(2 Suppl): p. 21-6.

[234] Bang, Y.J., et al., Trastuzumab in combination with chemotherapy versus chemotherapy alone for treatment of HER2-positive advanced gastric or gastro-oesophageal junction cancer (ToGA): a phase 3, open-label, randomised controlled trial. Lancet, 2010. 376(9742): p. 687-97.

[235] Yano, T., et al., Comparison of HER2 gene amplification assessed by fluorescence in situ hybridization and HER2 protein expression assessed by immunohistochemistry in gastric cancer. Oncol Rep, 2006. 15(1): p. 65-71.

[236] Lorenzen, S. and F. Lordick, How will human epidermal growth factor receptor 2-neu data impact clinical management of gastric cancer? Curr Opin Oncol, 2011. 23(4): p. 396-402.

[237] Park, D.I., et al., HER-2/neu amplification is an independent prognostic factor in gastric cancer. Dig Dis Sci, 2006. 51(8): p. 1371-9.

[238] Yonemura, Y., et al., Evaluation of immunoreactivity for erbB-2 protein as a marker of poor short term prognosis in gastric cancer. Cancer Res, 1991. 51(3): p. 1034-8.

[239] Uchino, S., et al., Overexpression of c-erbB-2 protein in gastric cancer. Its correlation with long-term survival of patients. Cancer, 1993. 72(11): p. 3179-84.

[240] Mizutani, T., et al., Relationship of C-erbB-2 protein expression and gene amplification to invasion and metastasis in human gastric cancer. Cancer, 1993. 72(7): p. 2083-8.

[241] Allgayer, H., et al., c-erbB-2 is of independent prognostic relevance in gastric cancer and is associated with the expression of tumor-associated protease systems. J Clin Oncol, 2000. 18(11): p. 2201-9.

[242] Liu, L., N. Wu, and J. Li, Novel targeted agents for gastric cancer. J Hematol Oncol, 2012. 5: p. 31.

[243] Ferrara, N., H.P. Gerber, and J. LeCouter, The biology of VEGF and its receptors. Nat Med, 2003. 9(6): p. 669-76.

[244] Maeda, K., et al., Prognostic value of vascular endothelial growth factor expression in gastric carcinoma. Cancer, 1996. 77(5): p. 858-63.

[245] Karayiannakis, A.J., et al., Circulating VEGF levels in the serum of gastric cancer patients: correlation with pathological variables, patient survival, and tumor surgery. Ann Surg, 2002. 236(1): p. 37-42.

[246] Hurwitz, H., et al., Bevacizumab plus irinotecan, fluorouracil, and leucovorin for metastatic colorectal cancer. N Engl J Med, 2004. 350(23): p. 2335-42.

[247] Sandler, A., et al., Paclitaxel-carboplatin alone or with bevacizumab for non-small-cell lung cancer. N Engl J Med, 2006. 355(24): p. 2542-50.

[248] Miller, K., et al., Paclitaxel plus bevacizumab versus paclitaxel alone for metastatic breast cancer. N Engl J Med, 2007. 357(26): p. 2666-76.

[249] Spasic, M., et al., Molecular characteristics and pathways of Avastin for the treatment of glioblastoma multiforme. Neurosurg Clin N Am, 2012. 23(3): p. 417-27.

[250] Ohtsu, A., et al., Bevacizumab in combination with chemotherapy as first-line therapy in advanced gastric cancer: a randomized, double-blind, placebo-controlled phase III study. J Clin Oncol, 2011. 29(30): p. 3968-76.

[251] Rapisarda, A. and G. Melillo, Overcoming disappointing results with antiangiogenic therapy by targeting hypoxia. Nat Rev Clin Oncol, 2012. 9(7): p. 378-90.

Chapter 8

Variants of Gastric Carcinoma: Morphologic and Theranostic Importance

Sun-Mi Lee, Kyoung-Mee Kim and Jae Y. Ro

Additional information is available at the end of the chapter

http://dx.doi.org/10.5772/54342

1. Introduction

Variants of gastric cancer account for approximately 5% of all carcinomas of the stomach. Some variant carcinomas, such as lymphoepithelioma-like carcinoma, hepatoid carcinoma with or without α-fetoprotein (AFP) production, small cell or neuroendocrine carcinoma, adenosquamous and squamous carcinoma, choriocarcinoma, sarcomatoid carcinoma, parietal cell or oncocytic carcinoma, micropapillary carcinoma, mucoepidermoid carcinoma, chief cell carcinoma, and Paneth cell carcinoma have been described, and recognition of the specific subtype is important due to not only their correlation with a distinct clinical course and prognosis but also differential diagnosis from metastasis from the outside of the stomach and different therapeutic modalities, particularly in the era of targeted treatment. Gastric lymphoepithelioma-like carcinoma and parietal cell or oncocytic carcinoma have been found to have a lower risk of lymph node metastasis and better prognosis. However, other variants such as hepatoid carcinoma, small cell or neuroendocrine carcinoma, adenosquamous and squamous carcinoma, choriocarcinoma, sarcomatoid carcinoma, and micropapillary carcinoma have shown to be associated with a poorer prognosis and a higher risk of metastasis to the lymph node and other organs, compared to conventional intestinal or diffuse type of gastric adenocarcinomas.

In recent years, early detection, endoscopic mucosal resection (EMR) for early gastric cancer, and neoadjuvant therapy have made a remarkable progress in the management and prognosis of gastric cancers. Thus, the prediction of aggressive behavior and accurate risk stratification in the variants of gastric cancer has become more important than ever. The World Health Organization (WHO) classification and the degree of differentiation have not been applied to some variants of gastric carcinoma. Considering that EMR and neoadjuvant therapy are selectively applied to patients with gastric carcinoma based on the tumor size, WHO classification, and degree of differentiation, further specific subclassification for each variant should be discussed to allow treatment to be directed to appropriate patient groups..

Recently, Giuffre et al analyzed the HER2 status in a cohort of rare histologic variants of advanced gastric adenocarcinoma such as hepatoid adenocarcinoma and oncocytic adenocarcinoma [1]. This series demonstrated that one of rare variants of gastric carcinoma, hepatoid adenocarcinoma, has shown an increased HER2 overexpression in up to 42.86% of cases compared to the intestinal (31.25%) and diffuse (3.45%) types of gastric adenocarcinoma. Trastuzumab has been known as an additional useful therapeutic standard option for patients with HER2-positive advanced gastric cancer. Therefore, this result and further studies may bring a significant progress in clinical course and prognosis in patients with aggressive variants of gastric carcinoma such as hepatoid adenocarcinoma. However, future studies are needed to evaluate overexpression of HER2 in other variants of gastric carcinoma. The variants of gastric carcinoma are listed in Table 1.

2. Epstein-Barr virus associated lymphoepithelioma-like carcinoma

Lymphoepithelioma-like carcinoma of the stomach (LELCS), also known as gastric carcinoma with lymphoid stroma, undifferentiated carcinoma with lymphoid stroma or medullary carcinoma, is a unique variant of gastric adenocarcinoma which is highly associated with Epstein-Barr virus (EBV) infection. This variant was described originally by Watanabe et al in 1976 and accounts for approximately 4% of all gastric carcinomas [2-4]. It has recently been emphasized that the role of EBV infection in the carcinogenesis of LELCS. The incidence of EBV-associated gastric adenocarcinoma varies from 1.3% to 20.1% in different areas, with an average of 10% worldwide [5, 6]. The prevalence of EBV infection has been found approximately 75 % of LELCS and 16% of conventional gastric adenocarcinoma in North America by EBV-encoded ribonucleic acids in situ hybridization (EBER-ISH) [7].

The clinicopathologic and molecular characteristics of EBV-associated LELCSs are quite different from those of conventional gastric carcinoma, such as a male predominance (male to female ratio: 2-3.4:1), predisposition to proximal stomach, frequent association with multiple and remnant gastric cancers, a lower frequency of lymph node metastasis, a relatively favorable prognosis, and aberrant concordant methylation of multiple genes [4, 8-10]. The mean age of diagnosis is 54.8 years, younger than conventional gastric carcinomas [11]. The clinical symptoms of LELCS are similar with conventional gastric adenocarcinoma, and patients with EBV-associated gastric carcinoma are known for elevated antibodies against EBV-related antigens. Levine et al reported that patients with EBV-associated gastric carcinoma have significantly high IgG and IgA antibody titer to EBV viral capsid antigen more than 5 years preceding their first diagnoses [12].

Watanabe and Yanai et al had reported the specific endoscopic findings of EBV-related LELCs in early and advanced lesions [4, 8]. In their series, approximately 80 % of LELCS appear to be a superficial depressed type, such as IIc, IIc+III, and IIa+IIc, frequently combined with ulcer in an early stage. Endoscopic ultrasonography of this variant demonstrates a hypoechoic

Histologic type	Incidence	Mean age	Sex	Clinical importance	Morphologic feature	Prognosis
EBV-associated lymphoepithelioma-like carcinoma	4%	54.8 yrs	M:F= 2-3.4:1	Possible good candidate for EMR and DNA methyltransferase inhibitor	Undifferentiated tumor cells embedded within a lymphoid stroma	Better prognosis compared to CoA (5-YSR: 71.4%)
Hepatoid adenocarcinoma	0.4-0.7%	64.5 yrs	M:F=3.5:1	Possible good candidate for anti-HER2 therapy (HER2 overexpression)	Tumor showing hepatoid differentiation with an immunoreactivity of AFP and glycan3	Worse prognosis compared to CoA (5-YSR: 9%)
Neuroendocrine cell carcinoma	0.1-0.6%	65 yrs	M:F=2.9:1	Response well to chemotherapy	Monotonous polygonal cells having fine granular chromatin and inconspicuous nucleoli with an immunoreactivity of neuroendocrine markers	Unfavorable prognosis (median survival: 1.7 years)
Squamous and adenosquamous carcinoma	0.04-0.9%	64 yrs	M:F=5:1	Differentiation from squamous or adenosquamous cell carcinoma arising from distal esophagus	Tumors with definite squamous differentiation including keratinization, squamous pearl formation, and intercellular bridges with or without a glandular component	Unfavorable prognosis (mean survival: 1.6 years)
Choriocarcinoma	0.08%	58.6 yrs	M:F=2.3:1	Elevated serum β-HCG Frequent cause of gastrointestinal bleeding and some hormone effects	Tumor with an admixture of cytotrophoblasts and syncytiotrophoblasts	Unfavorable prognosis (maximum survival: one year)
Sarcomatoid carcinoma	50 cases reported	45 yrs	M:F=2.3:1	Diagnosed at an advance stage with lymph node and liver metastasis	Tumor with a high grade sarcomatous component	Unfavorable prognosis (mean survival: 10 months)
Acinar cell carcinoma	10 cases reported	64.8 yrs	M:F=1:1	Tumor arising from pancreatic heterotopias or de novo acinar metaplasia	Tumor with acinar cell differentiation and pancreatic exocrine enzyme production confirmed by immunohistochemistry	Undetermined
Invasive micropapillary carcinoma	0.07%	66.2 yrs	M:F=2.5-3:1	High incidence of lymphovascular invasion and lymph node metastasis	Tumor with papillary clusters devoid of fibrovascular cores within lacunar spaces	Worse prognosis compared to CoA (5-YSR:30%)
Gastric adenocarcinoma of fundic gland type (chief cell predominant)	A few cases reported	65 yrs	M:F=1:1	Differentiation from a fundic gland polyp	Well differentiated adenocarcinoma admixed with predominantly chief cells and scattered parietal cells	Favorable prognosis expected but limited data
Parietal cell carcinoma and oncocytic carcinoma	Less than 30 cases reported	70.2 yrs	M:F=9:1	Occurs in an older population with a favorable prognosis	Tumors showing parietal cell differentiation with or without an immunoreactivity of H+/K+ ATPase	Favorable prognosis but limited data

M:F indicates male to female ratio; EMR: endoscopic mucosal resection; CA: conventional adenocarcinoma; AFP: Alpha-fetoprotein; 5-YSR: 5-year survival rate

Table 1. Variants of Gastric carcinoma

submucosal tumor-like protrusion with a large thickness compared to the length in an early lesion. Most LELCSs appear as a fungating mass (Bormann type II) accompanied by marked thickening of the gastric wall in an advanced stage (Fig. 1).

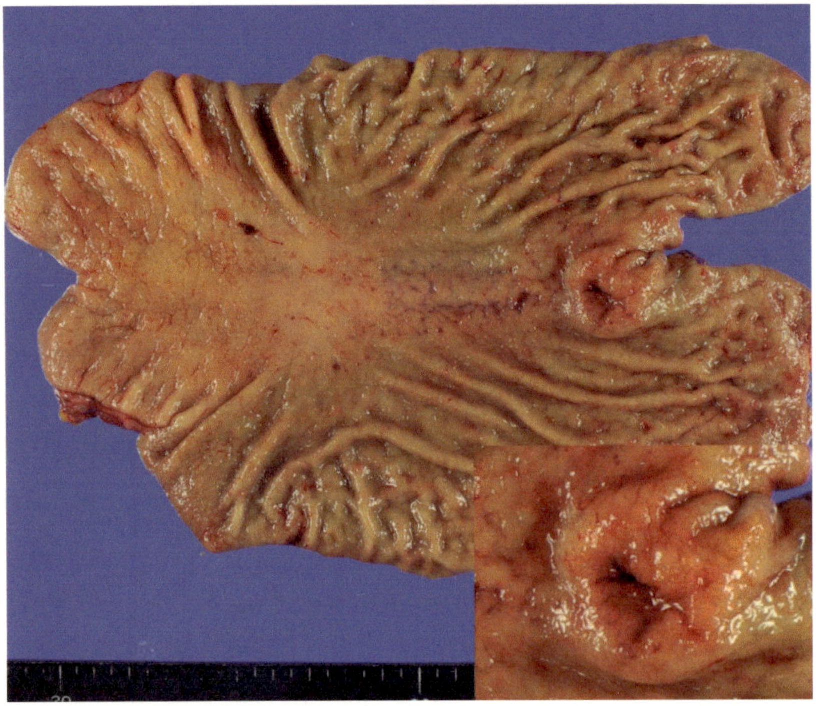

Figure 1. Gross photograph of EBV-associated lymphoepithelioma-like carcinoma in an advance stage. This tumor usually presents as a fungating mass (Bormann type II).

Histologically, LELCS has a well demarcated and pushing border and nests of poorly or undifferentiated tumor cells embedded within a lymphoid stroma. The tumor cells are arranged in syncytia, microalveolar, thin trabecular, or primitive tubular patterns. Also, they contain vesicular to clear nuclei, prominent nucleoli, and abundant eosinophilic polygonal cytoplasm with poorly defined cell borders (Fig 2). Generally, tumor cells grow in a diffuse manner intermixed with lymphocytes and plasma cells, mimicking malignant lymphoma (Schmincke type). However, a sharp demarcation between the tumor nests and lymphocyte stroma that is composed of variable amounts of lymphocytic infiltration, sometimes with lymphoid follicles, is noted (Regaud type) but no desmoplastic reaction is identified. Rarely, giant cells and epithelioid granulomas are observed within the lymphoid stroma [13, 14]. In the early lesion, LELCS shows a "lace pattern", which consists of columnar arrangement and intercolumnar fusion of neoplastic glands between dense lymphocytic infiltration at the intermediate zone of lamina propria [15]. This tumor is usually accompanied with severe atrophic gastritis in the background but not associated with intestinal metaplasia or Helicobacter pylori infection that are often observed in usual gastric adenocarcinoma [16].

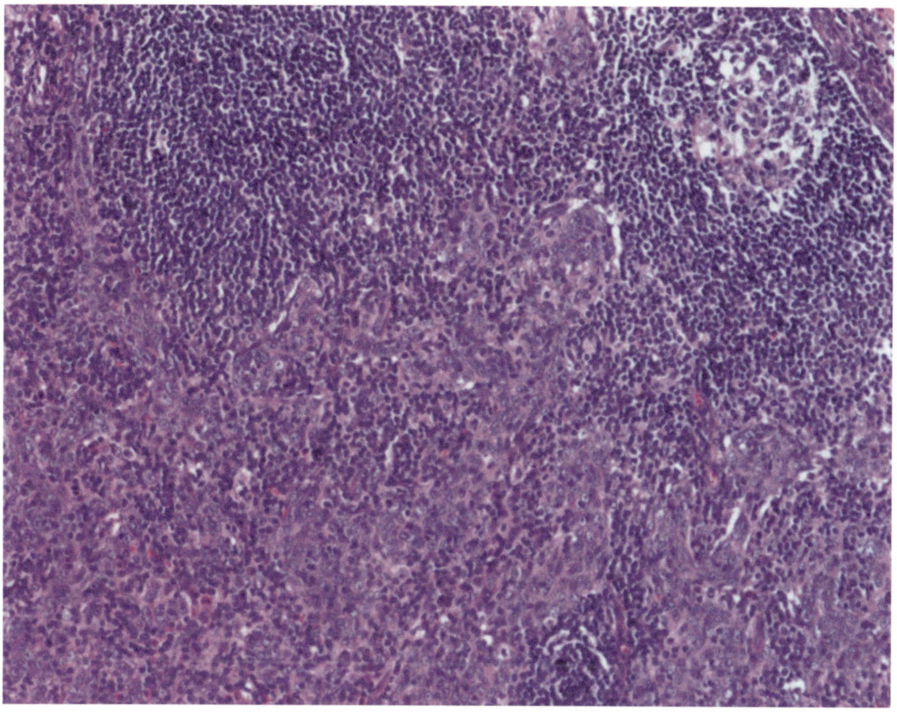

Figure 2. High magnification view of LELCS shows syncytial and solid nests of undifferentiated tumor cells with vesicular nuclei and prominent nucleoli surrounded by dense lymphocytic infiltration on H&E stain

The epithelial cell component of this variant is positive for keratins. Also HLA-DR expression of tumor cells associated with dense lymphocytic infiltrates can be detected in some cases of EBV-associated LELCS [17]. Increased dendritic cells within a lymphocyte stroma are also seen, which are positive for S100 and CD83. CD8+ T lymphocytes are the predominant cells infiltrating into tumor cell nests in EBV-associated LELCS, many of which express perforin and granzyme B [18]. Florid proliferation of CD8+ T lymphocytes within tumor cells seems to be associated with the host immune response to remove EBV antigen or cellular EBV-induced antigen [19].

EBV has specific latency expression patterns in different EBV-associated malignancies. EBV-associated LELCS can express viral latent genes and related products, not only EBV-encoded small ribonucleic acids (EBER) but also EBV-determined nuclear antigen type 1, BamHI A region rightward transcripts, and variable latent membrane protein 2A and 2B [20]. Polymerase chain reaction (PCR) to amplify EBV deoxyribonucleic acid fragments and EBER-ISH techniques could be used to detect EBV in tumor tissues; however, as a PCR test for amplifying EBV DNA is very sensitive and may cause a false positivity, and EBERs are always abundantly expressed in nearly 100% of tumor cell tissues (Fig.3), EBER-ISH technique is a gold standard test to detect EBV in paraffin-embedded tissues [21].

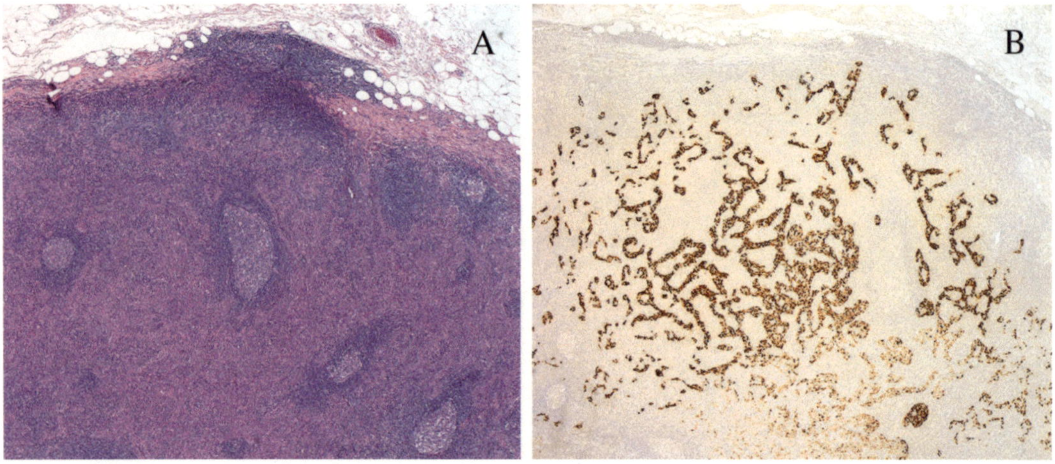

Figure 3. Microscope and EBER-ISH photographs of EBV-associated lymphoepithelioma-like carcinoma. **A.** A relatively well circumscribed mass with focal infiltration into subserosa. Reactive lymphoid follicles are scattered between tumor nests combined with dense lymphocytic infiltration. **B.** EBER-ISH highlights solid nests of EBV-infected tumor cells with cytoplasmic staining pattern in lymphoepithelioma-like carcinoma.

Previous studies of conventional gastric adenocarcinoma have been shown 34-60% of p53 overexpression. Some studies showed the frequency of p53 immunoreactivity, approximately 14%, was much lower in patients with EBV-associated LELCS compared to conventional gastric carcinoma [22]. However, other studies have almost same frequency of p53 expression with conventional gastric adenocarcinoma [23, 24]. The role of p53 mutation in the development of EBV-associated gastric carcinoma is still unclear.

If an accompanying lymphoid stroma contains multiple reactive follicles and intense lymphocytic infiltration in LELCS can be mistaken as a pseudolymphoma or lymphoma. It is important to examine the presence of malignant epithelial cell component carefully. Immunohistochemical markers for the cytokeratins, AE1/AE3 and CAM5.2, should be essential to detect in which only scarce undifferentiated malignant epithelial cells are present.

EBV is a ubiquitous γ-1 herpes virus usually acquired during childhood via salivary transmission, which establishes a life-long persistent infection of B cells in over 90% of adults [20]. EBV has been linked to the pathogenesis of several mesenchymal and epithelial neoplasms including nasopharyngeal carcinoma, B and T cell lymphomas, NK cell malignancies, and a subset of smooth muscle tumors [25]. The role of EBV in gastric carcinoma is considered to be directly oncogenic, but is still largely unknown. The infection of EBV is assumed to be occurred in the very early stage of carcinogenesis [23]. However, there is still a controversy over whether EBV infects gastric epithelial cells before or after the development of invasive gastric carcinoma [9].

Studies for genetic abnormality for EBV-associated gastric carcinoma are still limited and sparse. Several previous studies had failed to demonstrate any significant chromosomal loss or gain in comparative genome hybridization, changes of DNA copy number and microsatellite clearly. In contrast to inconsistent and negative results in genetic alteration, epigenetic alterations such as promoter hypermethylation, which bring in chromatin remodeling and silencing of tumor-related genes, plays a key role in the carcinogenesis of EBV-associated gastric carcinoma [26]. Kusano et al demonstrated that EBV-associated gastric carcinomas were strongly associated with high CpG-island methylation (CpG-island methylator phenotype- high, CIMP-H) by using methylation-specific polymerase chain method [27]. Other epigenetic series about EBV-associated gastric carcinoma have shown simultaneous methylation of multiple genes, including cell cycle regulation (p14, p15, p16, and cox2), DNA repair and protection (HMLH1, MGMT,GSTP1), cell adherence and metastasis (E-cadherin, TIMP3), angiogenesis (THBS1), apoptosis (DAP-kinase, bcl-2, p73), and signal transduction (APC, PTEN, RASSF1A) [28, 29]. Higher frequencies of hypermethylation of cancer-related genes found in EBV-associated gastric carcinoma suggest a close relationship between EBV infection and aberrant methylation of this variant during its carcinogenesis. Also, these findings suggest that DNA methyltransferase inhibitors such as 5-aza-2'-deoxycytidine (5-aza-CdR) or trichostatin A (TSA), which can induce the lytic phase of EBV infection in EBV positive gastric cancer cell lines, can be a promising therapeutic agent specially for EBV-associated gastric carcinoma [30].

Another interesting characteristic of EBV-associated gastric carcinoma is its higher occurrence among gastric remnant carcinomas, ranging from 27% to 42% [31-33]. Chen et al hypothesizes that the injuries of gastric mucosa and/or changes of the microenvironment within the remnant stomach may be involved in the development of EBV-associated gastric carcinoma [34].

EBV-associated LELCS has known to have a low risk of lymph node metastasis [35]. Interestingly, whether the presence of tumor metastasis within the regional lymph nodes or not, perigastric lymph nodes frequently show reactive hyperplasia that represents a host immune response against LELCS [4]. EBV-associated LELCS shows a very low rate of regional lymph node metastasis especially if the tumor involves in the mucosa and submucosa as an early gastric cancer [4]. The patients with this variant tumor can be good candidates for EMR in regard to a lower frequency of lymph node metastasis and a relative well circumscribed tumor margin that can be easily assessed endoscopically. Some clinical trials to remove EBV-associated LELCS in an early stage have been reported using an endoscopic resection such as EMR or submucosal dissection [36, 37]. The patients treated with endoscopic resection have shown a benign clinical course without recurrence or metastasis. The prognosis of EBV-associated gastric carcinoma has been considered better than conventional gastric carcinoma. Song et al reported that 5-year overall survival rate of EBV-associated gastric carcinoma was 71.4%, and disease-free survival rate was 67.5% compared to 56.1% and 55.2% of those usual gastric carcinoma and suggested the prognosis of EBV-associated gastric carcinoma depends on the patient's inflammatory response (tumor-infiltrating lymphocyte counts) [11].

3. Hepatoid adenocarcinoma

Hepatoid adenocarcinoma of the stomach (HACS) was first described by Ishikura et al in 1985 as a subtype of AFP producing gastric carcinoma, which has a histologic similarity with hepatocellular carcinoma and distinct clinicopathological properties [38]. The incidence of this variant ranges from 0.38% to 0.73% of all gastric cancer [39, 40]. The mean age of diagnosis is 64.5 years (range from 49 to 78 years), similar to that of conventional gastric carcinomas. The clinical symptoms are similar to those seen in patients with conventional gastric adenocarcinoma except marked elevated serum level of AFP in most patients. Characteristically, earlier studies demonstrated that HACS frequently combined with vascular invasion, liver metastasis, and a higher incidence of lymph node metastasis which result in a poorer prognosis than other common types of gastric adenocarcinoma [41, 42].

AFP is a serum protein produced by fetal liver, yolk sac cells, and some fetal gastrointestinal cells [43]. HACS is characterized by distinct hepatoid differentiation histologically and the production of liver specific proteins including AFP confirmed by immunohistochemistry. However, not all HACSs produce hepatic specific protein. Approximately 54 % of HACSs express AFP by immunohistochemistry and 63% of patients with HACS show an elevated serum AFP level [39, 44]. In addition, there are some histologic types of carcinoma other than HACS, tubular/papillary adenocarcinomas, poorly differentiated medullary carcinoma, and enteroblastic adenocarcinoma, also can produce and secrete AFP [38, 45-48].

The most commonly found macroscopic type of HACS is 0-IIc (superficial depressed type) in an early lesion [49]. This tumor can occur as a circumscribed mass, Bormann type II (fungating type) or III (ulceroinfiltrative type) as an advanced cancer in the antrum and lower body of the stomach (Fig.4) [44, 49]. Microscopically, this variant contains areas of hepatoid differentiation showing structural mimicry of liver tissue such as sheet-like or trabecular arrangement of tumor cells with sinusoid-like vasculature and bile canaliculus-like structure [50]. This tumor consists of cuboidal or polygonal cells with centrally located nuclei and abundant eosinophilic cytoplasm (Fig.5). However, there is no consensus for quantification of the proportion of hepatocellular differentiated component yet to accept as HACS. The proportion of hepatoid component ranges from 10 to 90% in reported cases of HACS [51]. The glandular component such as well-differentiated tubular or papillary adenocarcinoma frequently intermingles with the hepatoid component. The transition between glandular and hepatoid components of HACS can be gradual or abrupt. Occasionally, bile and periodic acid-Schiff-positive/diastase-resistant hyaline globules may be observed in intracellular and extracellular sites. In addition to the production of liver-specific proteins such as AFP as well as prealbumin, albumin, and transferrin, Proteins Induced by Vitamin K Absence - II (PIVKA-II) and Hep-par1 antigen can be detected in tumor cells [38, 52, 53]. Some HACSs exhibit extensive lymphovascular invasion, extending to veins with tumor emboli, which results in early metastasize to other organs, predominantly to the liver [39].

Immunohistochemically, the tumor cells are positive for CK8, CK18, CK19, CK20, but negative for CK7. Also this variant can express the canalicular pattern of polyclonal carcioembryonic antigen (CEA), α-1 antitrypsin, and α-1 antichymotrypsin [54]. The immunoreactivity of PIVKA-II and Hep-par1 are variably observed. Glypican-3 is a cell surface heparin sulfate proteoglycan considered to be an oncofetal protein because of its presence in fetal liver and liver tumors (hepatocellular cell carcinoma and hepatoblastoma) [55]. The immunohistochemical staining pattern of glypican-3 is strongly positive in membrane and cytoplasm of hepatoid

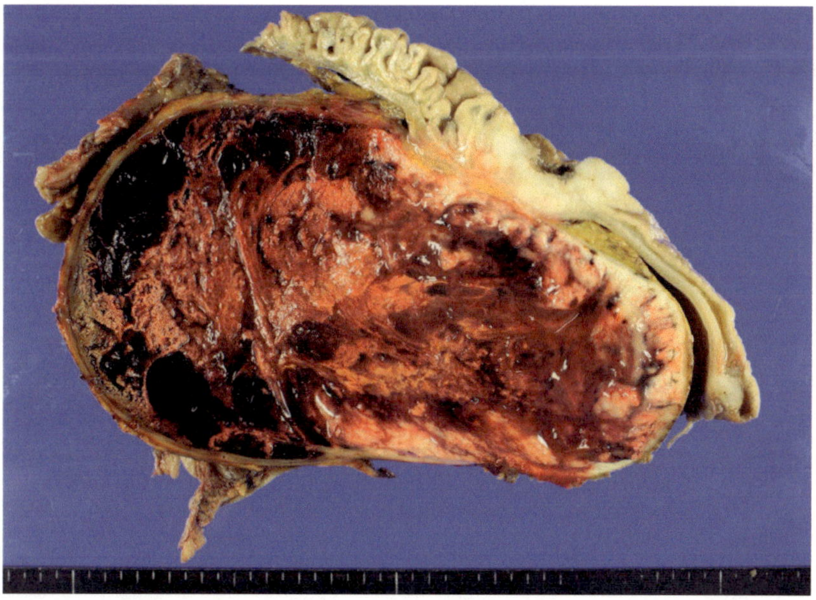

Figure 4. Gross photograph of hepatoid adenocarcinoma. The tumor presents as a fungating mass (Bormann type II) in the lower body of the stomach which projects exophytically into the abdominal cavity. The subserosal lesion shows extensive necrosis and hemorrhage on the cut surface.

tumor cells (Fig. 5). Hishinuma et al reported that glypican 3 is more sensitive (100% sensitivity) than either Hep-par1 or AFP but Hep-par1 is more specific as an immunohistochemical marker for HACS [51]. In a series by Kinjo et al showed that AFP has 81.1% of sensitivity and 46.1% of specificity and glypican-3 has 90.5% of sensitivity and 63.2% of specificity [49]. These studies support both AFP and glypican-3 could be useful markers to make a diagnosis of HACS.

Many cytogenetic and molecular studies had been undertaken to investigate pathogenesis and biological behavior of this variant. However, the histogenesis of HACS is still unclear. Kishimoto et al proposed that gastric carcinoma might acquire hepatic differentiation during the tumor progression, "HACS transdifferentiation"[56]. Akiyama et al demonstrated that the hepatoid component exhibited exactly same patterns of chromosome X inactivation, p53 gene mutation, the level of p53 expression, and loss of heterozygosity with conventional adenocarcinomatous component of HACS [57]. These findings suggest a monoclonal origin of both glandular and hepatoid elements of HACS and support "HACS transdifferentiation" as the most accepted histogenesis.

Differential diagnoses of HACS include other similar-appearing tumors (lung, pancreas, esophagus so on) and hepatocellular cell carcinoma. Particularly, the metastatic HACS to the liver may be almost indistinguishable from hepatocellular cell carcinoma due to overlapping clinicopathologic features such as elevated AFP level, hepatoid morphology, and immunoexpressions of AFP, polyclonal CEA, and alpha-1 antitrypsin. Moreover, the hepatoid component of HACS can be more prominent in metastatic lesions to perigastric lymph nodes or liver [45, 58]. The presence of underlying disease such as liver cirrhosis and the presence of primary

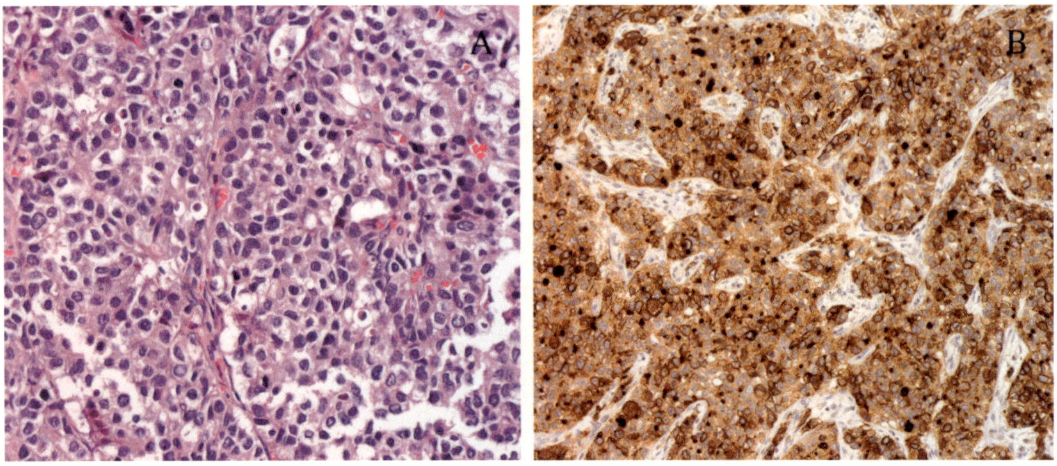

Figure 5. Microscopic photograph of hepatoadenocarcinoma and its immunostaining pattern of glycan-3. **A.** Solid nests of tumor cells are incompletely surrounded by sinusoid-like microvascular structure. This tumor is composed of polygonal cells with centrally located polymorphic nuclei and pale pinkish relatively abundant cytoplasm, resembling hepatocytes. **B.** The glycan-3 immunostain shows membranous and cytoplasmic staining pattern of tumor cells.

lesion detected by screening modalities such as endoscopy and abdominal computerized tomography scan would be useful to differentiate metastatic HACS and primary hepatocellular cell carcinoma. Although hepatocellular cell carcinoma arising in non-cirrhotic liver and without known risk factors is rare, this tumor has been reported to appear as a single nodule with pseudo-adenomatous or sclerosing pattern histologically [59, 60].

In recent clinical series by Baek et al, approximately 77% of patients with HACS at presentation were diagnosed as an advanced stage, stage III or IV [44]. Median overall survival and progression free survival of these patients after gastrectomy and/or palliative chemotherapy were 8.03 months (95% CI: 6.59-9.47) and 3.47 months (95% CI: 0.65-6.29), respectively. The incidence of liver metastasis of HACS is significantly higher than that of conventional gastric adenocarcinoma. Liu et al reported the overall incidence of liver metastasis was 75.6% including 8.9% synchronous and 73.2% metachronous liver metastasis in HACSs compared to 11.6 %, including 1.8% synchronous and 9.9% metachronous liver metastasis in conventional gastric adenocarcinoma [50]. The overall 5-year survival rate of HACS was 9% compared to 44% in conventional gastric adenocarcinoma [50]. Most of HACS cases clinically appear to chemoresistant and curative resections are limited due to advanced lesions at diagnosis. Kamata et al demonstrated multiple ATP-binding cassette transporters related with multidrug resistance of tumor such as multidrug resistant-associated proteins 1,2, and 6 were expressed frequently in HACS [61]. This finding suggested that ATP-binding cassette transporters participated in the mechanism of multidrug resistance in HACS.

HER2 gene amplification and protein overexpression have been introduced as the target therapy with anti-HER2 humanized monoclonal antibody (trastuzumab) in various cancers including gastric cancer in an advance stage. Although reported rates of HER2 overexpression have been variable, it accounts for approximately 20 % of all gastric carcinomas. Recently, Giuffre et al reported that a markedly increased HER2 amplification was more frequent in HACS (42.9%) than that seen in tubular gastric adenocarcinomas (31.3%) [1]. This finding shows trastuzumab can be a useful therapeutic standard option not only for patients with advanced gastric cancer but also in aggressive variants like HACS.

4. Neuroendocrine cell carcinoma

Primary small cell carcinoma of the stomach (PSCCS) is an exceedingly aggressive variant of gastric carcinoma with neuroendocrine differentiation. Since Matsusaka et al described this variant first in 1976, less than 230 cases have been reported in the literature [62]. This tumor also has been referred to "oat cell carcinoma" and "atypical carcinoid" and accounts for 0.1 - 0.6% of total gastric cancers [63, 64]. The mean age of presentation is 65 years (range, 42 to 84 years) and it commonly affects males [65]. The clinical presentation is similar to those seen in patients with conventional gastric adenocarcinoma in an advanced stage. PSCCS may rarely secrete hormones such as vasoactive intestinal peptide, neuron-specific enolase, pro-gastrin-releasing peptide, antidiuretic hormone, and adrenocorticotropic hormone [66-68]. A few cases of PSCCS have been reported in association with paraneoplastic syndromes including paraneoplastic neurological syndrome and Cushing syndrome by ectopic production of ACTH [69, 70].

PSCCS tends to metastasize early to regional lymph nodes and liver and extends to surrounding organs including liver, transverse colon, pancreas, and diaphragm at the presentation [71-74]. In the largest retrospective series, Chiba et al demonstrated that PSCCSs have a higher incidence rate of lymphatic invasion (88.9% vs. 56.6%), vascular invasion (75.6% vs. 31.6%), and lymph node metastasis (82.1% vs. 58.8%) compared to those of conventional gastric carcinoma [75].

Neuroendocrine cell carcinomas of the gastrointestinal tract are usually responded well to the chemotherapy. Although there has been no established chemotherapy regimen for PSCCS due to its rarity, generally it has been recognized that surgical resection alone may not be sufficient treatment and emphasize the importance of adjuvant chemotherapy, especially for advanced disease. Fukuda et al insisted that intensive chemotherapy with or without surgical resection should be recommended for this tumor at any stage [76]. Recently, some studies have reported good response of some chemoregimens routinely used for lung SCC such as etoposide/cisplatin, irinotecan/cisplatin, and S1/cisplatin [65, 68, 77, 78]. The 5-year survival rate of patients with gastric neuroendocrine carcinoma has been reported to be 22.1%- 43.8% and the median survival time is 19 month [68, 79, 80]. However, long-term survival up to 3 years was reported in a patient with aggressive adjuvant chemotherapy [68].

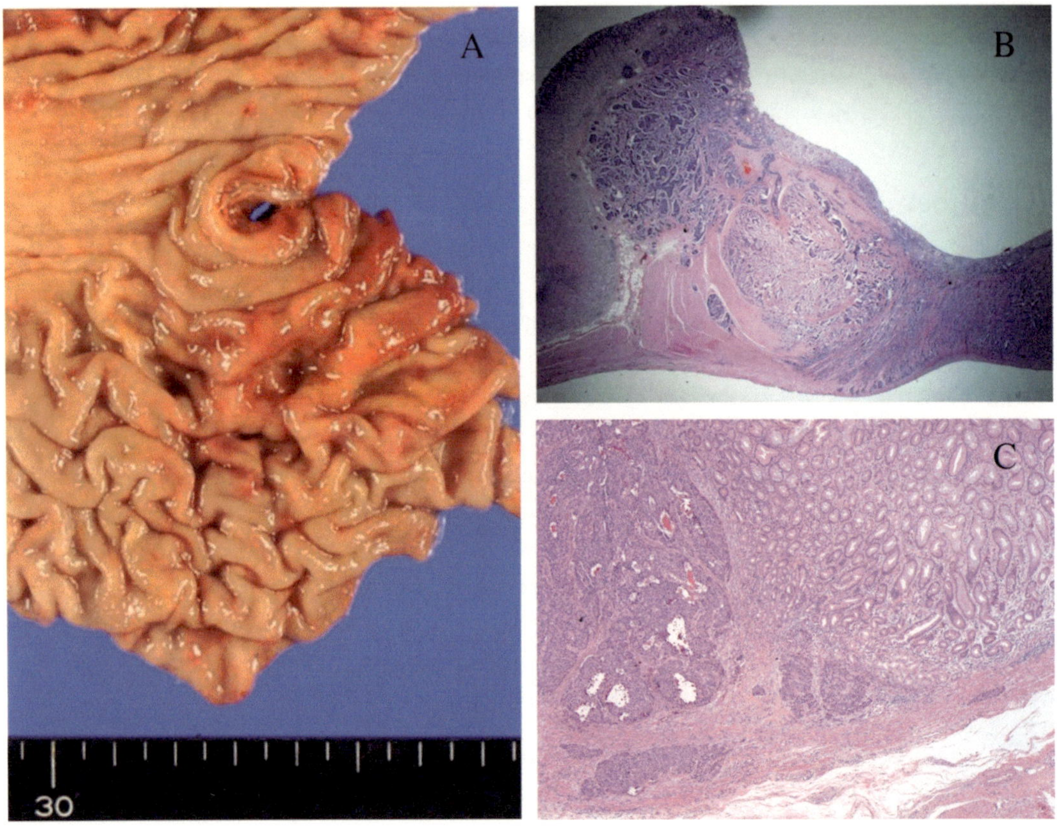

Figure 6. Gross and microscopic photographs of neuroendocrine carcinoma in the stomach. **A.** It forms an ulceroinfiltrative solid mass (Bormann type III) in the upper body of the stomach. **B.** At lower magnification, this solid tumor invades into the subserosa. **C.** Dark purple solid nests of poorly differentiated neuroendocrine carcinoma invades into the muscularis mucosa accompanied by desmoplastic reaction in the surrounding tissue.

Macroscopically, the average size of the tumor is approximately 6.3 cm [65]. This tumor is an ulcerative or protruding mass (70% of cases) with frequent invasion to subserosa (Fig.6) [65, 81]. PSCCS can be classified as pure (Fig.7) or mixed (composite) SCC (Fig.8) depending on the proportion of neuroendocrine cell component. However, regardless of the proportion of neuroendocrine carcinoma in total volume of gastric carcinoma, its presence has been correlated with a poor prognosis. Approximately 60% of PSCCS cases are associated with conventional gastric adenocarcinoma, and rare cases with sarcomatoid carcinoma, adenosquamous, and squamous carcinoma variants have been reported [82-85]. Histologically, diagnostic criteria for PSCCS are identical with those for pulmonary neuroendocrine tumors by the WHO/ International association for the Study of Lung Cancer [86]. First of all, the SCC histology is defined as having a markedly high nuclear/cytoplasmic ratio and hyperchromatic small nuclei (less than 3 resting lymphocytes) with finely granular chromatin and inconspicuous or rarely conspicuous nucleoli. Frequent nuclear molding might be present. Focal or extensive necrosis can be seen. The typical organoid architecture pattern of low grade neuroendocrine neoplasm (eg. carcinoid) is rarely present in PSCCS. As a high grade tumor, their proliferative rate is high, and all exhibit more than 10 mitoses per 10 high power fields, with a mean of 40 to 50 mitoses [87]. Intestinal metaplasia may be seen in the background of gastric mucosa. In cases with classic histologic features of neuroendocrine tumors, positive staining for neuroendocrine markers is not a requirement for a diagnosis [87].

The pathogenesis of neuroendocrine carcinoma of the stomach is unknown. The most commonly accepted hypothesis is the presence of a "pluripotent stem cell" that has a potential to grow and differentiate into other cell types producing mucin or keratin [88]. This hypothesis has been supported by some cases of composite neuroendocrine carcinomas with other glandular or squamous cell components [89, 90]. Other suggested theory is that neuroendocrine carcinoma of the stomach arises from neuroendocrine precursor cells in gastric adenocarcinoma during its genetic progression [91].

Since PSCCS could be occasionally misdiagnosed as poorly differentiated adenocarcinoma or malignant lymphoma due to accompanying crush artifact in small biopsies, Grimelius stain and immunohistochemistry would be useful to differentiate morphologic mimickers. Immunohistochemical staining for neuroendocrine markers, including chromogranin, synaptophysin, and CD56, is usually positive (Fig.9) [81, 92, 93]. Its intensity and distribution can vary, with most examples showing patchy and moderately intense immunoreactivity. Also, most PSCCSs show an immunoreactivity for keratin AE1/AE3 and CEA but not for high molecular cytokeratin CK34βE [87]. Recently, Li et al demonstrated the low molecular weight cytokeratin, CK8 (CAM 5.2), is more commonly expressed in SCC in gastrointestinal tract including PSCCS than is the expression of AE1/AE3 or epithelial membrane antigen, suggesting CK8 as a sensitive marker for SCCs of the gastrointestinal tract [94]. The proliferation index for Ki-67 is high, usually more than 25 % positive nuclei. Rindi et al have reported that angioinvasion, tumor size, clinicopathological type, mitotic count, and Ki-67 proliferation index are predictors of tumor malignancy and patient outcome in neuroendocrine tumors of the stomach [79].

At the current time, neuroendocrine carcinomas in the gastrointestinal tract are classified into neuroendocrine carcinoma (small and large cell subtypes) and mixed adenoneuroendocrine carcinoma by World Health Organization (WHO) [95]. Large cell neuroendocrine carcinoma of the stomach (LCNECS) is defined as a high grade or poorly differentiated malignant neuroendocrine tumor of non-small cell type. In the largest series by Jiang et al, LCNECSs account for at least 1.5% of all gastric cancer [96]. In this series, the mean age of the patients with LCNECS is 62.7 years (range, 47 to 79 years) and it mostly affects males.

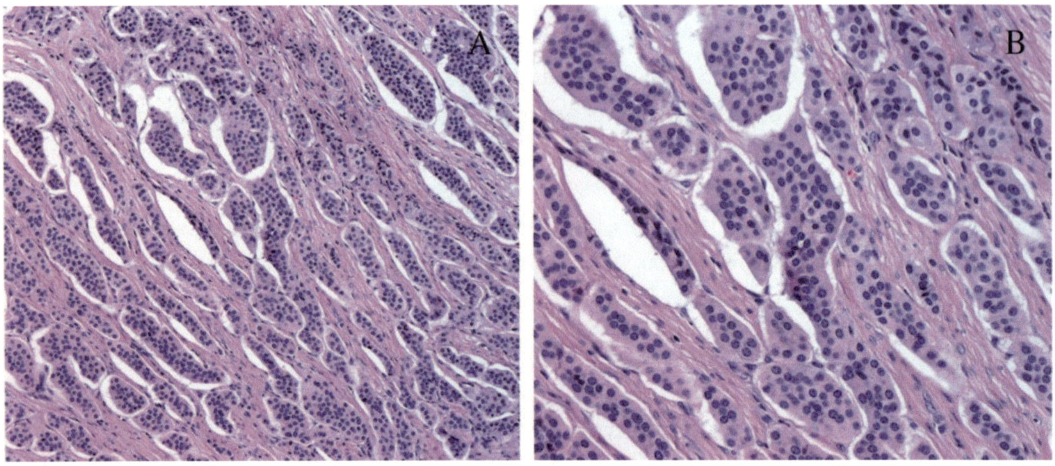

Figure 7. Pure well differentiated neuroendocrine carcinoma of the stomach. **A.** Well differentiated neuroendocrine carcinoma shows a typical organoid or solid nest growth pattern. **B.** At higher magnification, the tumor cells display characteristic cytologic features of neuroendocrine cells including hyperchromatic small nuclei with finely granular chromatin ("salt and pepper" nuclei) and inconspicuous nucleoli.

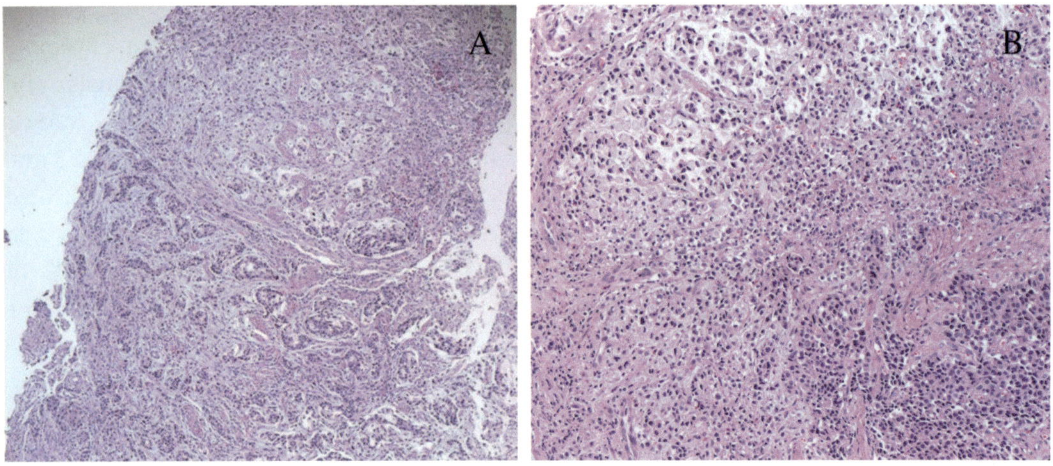

Figure 8. Mixed small cell carcinoma reveals an admixture of poorly differentiated adenocarcinoma with signet ring cell features and small cell carcinoma. **A.** In a small biopsy, neuroendocrine carcinoma component can be misled as a part of poorly differentiated adenocarcinoma. **B.** At high magnification, the upper part of this picture shows rounded aggregates of signet ring cell carcinoma with mucin. Adjacent to signet ring cell carcinoma, solid nests of poorly differentiated neuroendocrine tumor cells with a high nuclear to cytoplasmic ratio are present in the lower part of this picture.

Grossly, the mean size of the tumor is 6.4 cm (range 1.1 to 13.0 cm) and 66% of cases are Bormann type II or III in an advanced stage [96]. The diagnostic criteria for LCNECS is defined as having the following features: a diffuse growth pattern or "neuroendocrine architecture" (organoid, nesting, palisading, rosettes, or trabeculae), monotonous polygonal or round to oval cells with moderate amounts of slightly eosinophilic cytoplasm and ill defined cell border, granular or vesicular nuclei with evenly distributed granular chromatin, and with or without visible nucleoli [97]. Focal lumen formation or focal intracytoplasmic mucin might be seen, and are not feature for exclusion. LCNECSs usually combine with other common adenocarcinoma components. Immunohistochemical evidence of neuroendocrine differentiation is defined as positive staining for one of three neuroendocrine markers, chromogranin, synaptophysin, and CD56, in > 20% of the tumor cells [97]. In a relatively large study to compare LCNECS and PSCCS by Matsui et al, they demonstrated LCNECSs reveal a higher mitotic count, larger polygonal cells, a lower nuclear-cytoplasmic ratio, coarser nuclear chromatin, and more frequent conspicuous nucleoli than PSCCSs [81].

The main difficulty with the diagnosis of gastric neuroendocrine carcinoma is to distinguish them from poorly differentiated adenocarcinoma with solid growth pattern and malignant lymphoma. Preoperative diagnosis of neuroendocrine carcinoma from gastric endoscopic biopsy specimens would be challenging for the pathologists due to its histologic heterogeneity as well as the propensity of neuroendocrine tumor that mainly proliferates under the mucosal layer [65, 71]. Also, neuroendocrine carcinoma of the stomach cannot be easily recognizable due to less prominent neuroendocrine histologic features in high grade tumor cells. These factors can result in limited and demanding biopsy specimens for making a diagnosis of PSCCS preoperatively. However, careful evaluation for hidden or faint neuroendocrine architecture, cytologic features of neuroendocrine cells, and comparable immunohistochemical profiles would be useful to differentiate two disease entities. Sometimes ultrastructural study can help to demonstrate accumulation of electron-dense core neurosecretory granules measuring 200 nm in diameter in these tumors [98].

Primary gastric malignant lymphoma can be distinguished by immunoreactivity of CD45 and lack of cytokeratins. SCC of the lung metastatic to the stomach should always be considered in the differential diagnosis of PSCCS. With limited data, staining for the lung marker, thyroid transcription factor-1 (TTF1), seems to be almost always negative in neuroendocrine tumors of the gastrointestinal tract [99]. So TTF1 can be helpful to differentiate a metastatic lesion from SCC of the lung.

Another subtype of neuroendocrine carcinoma is a mixed neuroendocrine carcinoma. Although localized endocrine cell differentiation in benign or malignant glandular neoplasm of the gastrointestinal tract is relatively common, truly mixed glandular-endocrine neoplasms (adenoneuroendocrine carcinoma) are rare. These tumors are composed of both glandular component like conventional adenocarcinoma and recognizable neuroendocrine component of small or large cell type that comprises substantial proportions of the tumor volume with each component at least 30% of the lesion [100]. Most of mixed glandular-neuroendocrine neoplasms of the stomach are malignant tumors arising in the background of atrophic gastritis.

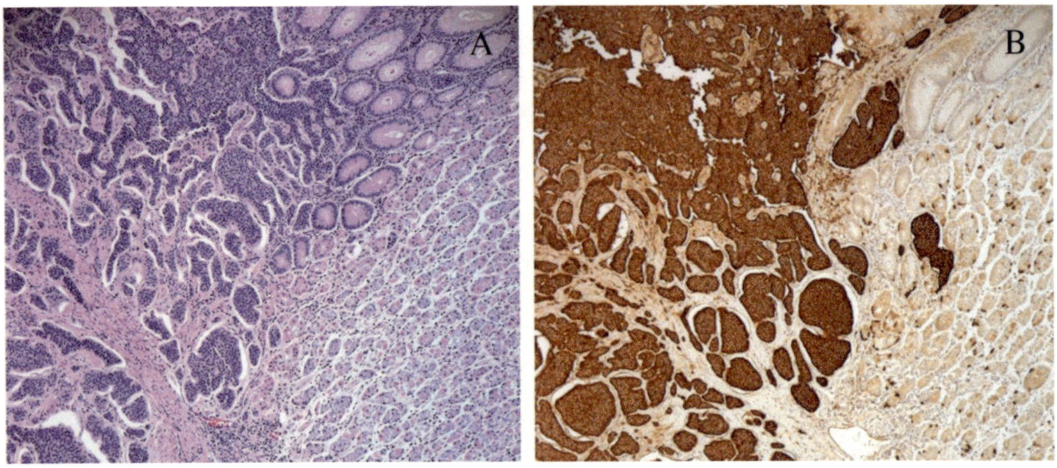

Figure 9. A. Small cell carcinoma of stomach forms solid nests or sheets of tumor cells that invades into the gastric mucosa. **B.** This variant shows a strong positivity for one of neuroendocrine markers, chromogranin.

5. Squamous and adenosquamous carcinoma

Primary squamous and adenosquamous carcinoma of the stomach is an extremely rare and aggressive variant of the stomach cancer that accounts for 0.04 to 0.9 % of all gastric carcinoma [101, 102]. Although clinical manifestation of the patients with primary squamous and adenosquamous carcinoma of the stomach is similar with patients with conventional gastric adenocarcinoma, it has been reported a mildly elevated serum level of squamous cell carcinoma antigen and a long history of smoking and alcohol abuse in some patients [103-105]. The mean age of presentation is 64 years (range, 17 to 89 years) and men are affected about five times as often as women [104]. Patients with primary squamous or adenosquamous carcinoma of the stomach frequently present with advanced stage disease (pT3 or T4) with or without metastases or involvement of other organs (stage III or IV) [106]. It has known that these variants do not response well to the routine chemoregimen for conventional gastric carcinoma. There is no established standard adjuvant chemoradiation therapy for patients with primary squamous and adenosquamous carcinoma in the stomach. However, one isolated case suggested that low-dose 5-fluorouracil plus cisplatin would be an effective preoperative chemoregimen to shrink the size of tumors and lower postoperative complications [106].

Although there is no specific macroscopic feature for primary squamous carcinoma of the stomach, recently Oono et al demonstrated a well demarcated, white superficial depressed area of primary squamous carcinoma as an early lesion which is not stained by 3.0% lugol solution on chromoendoscopy [107]. Main differential diagnosis of primary squamous carcinoma of the stomach is primary squamous carcinoma of the esophagus that involves the proximal stomach. Parks et al have proposed the diagnostic criteria for primary squamous carcinoma of the stomach based on not only histologically definite squamous features but also in regard to clinical findings as follows: (1) the tumor must not be located in the cardia; (2) the tumor must not extend into the esophagus; (3) there should be no evidence of squamous carcinoma in any other part of the body [108] (Fig.10). Another criteria for primary squamous carcinoma of the stomach by the Japanese Classification of Gastric Carcinoma are as follows: (1) the tumor must consist of only squamous carcinoma without any component of adenocarcinoma (pure squamous component only) (Fig.11) and (2) any tumor near esophagogastric junction must be excluded unless evidence for supporting the tumor originated from the stomach exists [109].

The origin of primary squamous carcinoma of the stomach is unclear, but four hypotheses concerning its development have been proposed, including (1) nests of ectopic squamous cells in gastric mucosa; (2) squamous metaplasia of the gastric mucosa before malignant transformation; (3) squamous differentiation in a preexisting adenocarcinoma; and (4) multipotential stem cells in the gastric mucosa [110-112].

Focal squamous differentiation in the intestinal-type adenocarcinoma is relatively common. Therefore, Straus et al established a diagnostic criteria for adenosquamous carcinoma of the stomach that the squamous component should be present in more than 25 percent of the resected tumor (Fig.12 and 13) [111]. Its biological behavior is usually determined by the adenocarcinoma component. Also the diagnostic criteria by Parks should be applied for the final diagnosis of primary gastric adenosquamous carcinoma to exclude primary esophageal cancer and metastatic lesion.

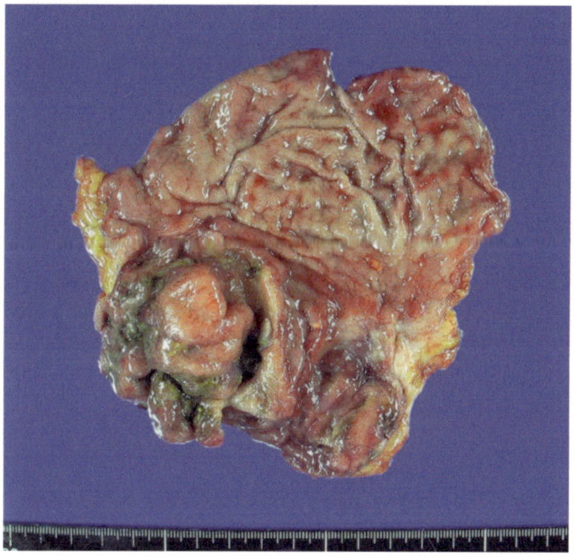

Figure 10. Gross photograph of pure squamous carcinoma. Gastrectomy specimen displays a large, fungating solid mass with surface ulceration and necrosis.

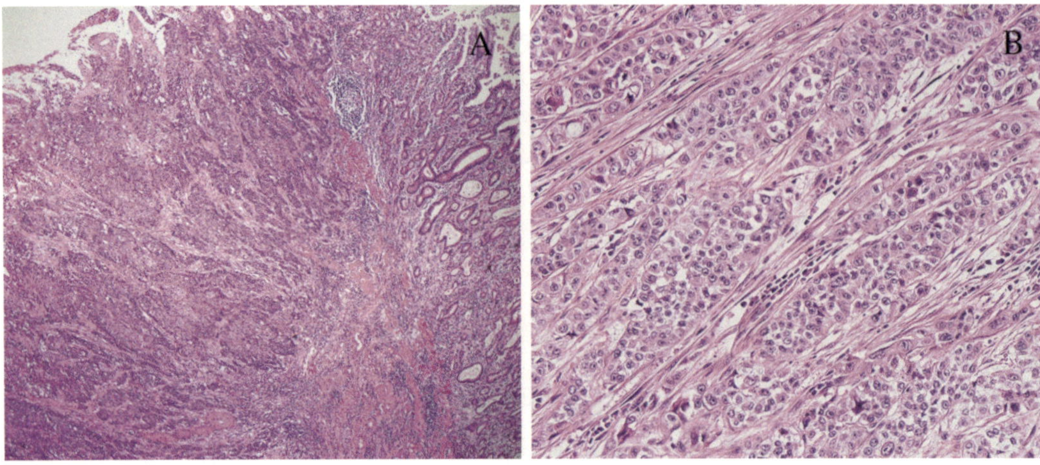

Figure 11. A. Dense solid sheets of squamous carcinoma invade into the submucosa. **B.** At high magnification, infiltrating solid nests of tumor cells show marked pleomorphism, intercellular bridges, and high mitotic counts.

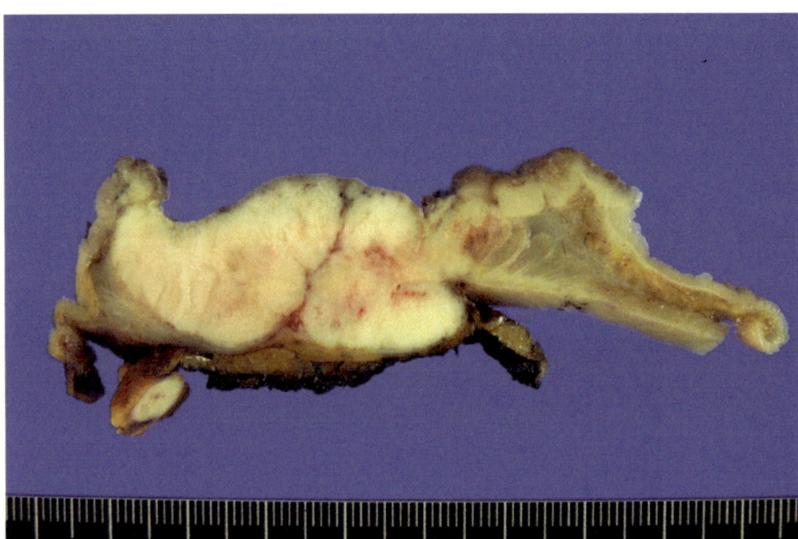

Figure 12. Gross photograph of adenosquamous carcinoma. Adenosquamous carcinoma with a pale yellow solid cut surface that involves all the gastric wall and an attached lymph node.

Differential diagnosis of primary squamous and adenosquamous carcinoma of the stomach include (1) gastric adenocarcinoma, intestinal type, with squamous differentiation; (2) chronic gastritis or ulcer with squamous metaplasia; (3) esophageal squamous carcinoma arising from the esophagogastric junction; (4) metastatic squamous carcinoma to the stomach. Most of reported cases of primary squamous and adenosquamous carcinoma of the stomach have demonstrated a poorer clinical course and prognosis than conventional gastric adenocarcinoma. The mean survival after surgery is less than 12 months (1-16 months) [113]. Radical surgical excision is the only option for localized disease. For advanced-stage disease, surgery plus adjuvant radio-and/or chemotherapy appears to achieve a better outcome than surgery alone in terms of longer survival, although experience is limited due to the rarity of this variant.

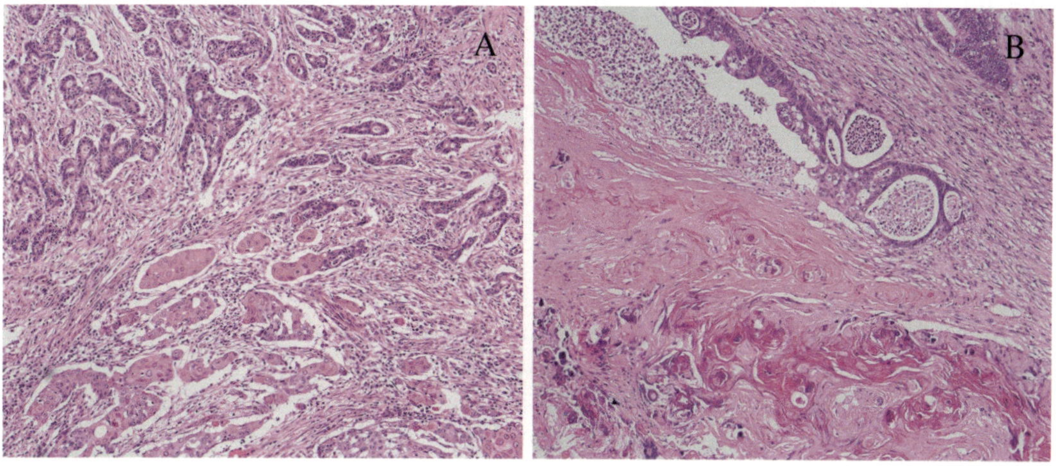

Figure 13. A. A mixed area of both glandular and squamous carcinoma. **B.** At high magnification, a mixed area of squamous carcinoma with prominent keratin formation and adjacent adenocarcinoma with intraluminal abscess is seen.

6. Choriocarcinoma

Primary choriocarcinoma of the stomach (PCCS) is a highly aggressive variant of gastric carcinoma that was described for the first time by Davidsohn in 1905 [114]. This variant represents approximately 0.08 % of all the gastric cancers [115]. Pure gastric choriocarcinomas are extremely rare and only less than twenty cases were reported [116-118]. Most of primary gastric choriocarcinomas have been reported as a composite or mixed tumor with a combination of predominant choriocarcinoma component and a variable degree of adenocarcinoma. Transitions between adenocarcinoma and choriocarcinoma component may be clear or not. Yolk sac tumor, small cell carcinoma, and hepatoid carcinoma components may be seen as well [119-122]. In the study by Kobayashi et al, the average age of the patients with PCCS is 62.4 years in men and 54.8 years in women with a male predominance (male: female ratio=2.3:1) [123]. The clinical presentation of this variant is similar to that of gastric adenocarcinoma, however, it is a frequent cause of gastrointestinal bleeding and may have some hormonal effects such as gynecomastia in men, precocious puberty, pregnancy mimicking symptoms including amenorrhea, nausea and vomiting in women [124, 125].

PCCS behaves more like gestational choriocarcinoma because it shows extensive hematogenous dissemination or metastasis by mixed or pure components of choriocarcinoma as opposed to the routine lymphatic spreading of gastric adenocarcinoma. Kobayashi et al analyzed previously reported 53 cases of PCCS and concluded that the most common cause of death in patients with PCCS is hepatic failure caused by liver metastasis followed by massive cancerous hemorrhage [123]. Untreated patients with PCCS have an average survival of several months [126]. Although no standard therapy has been established, complete surgical resection with neoadjuvant chemotherapy for non-gestational choriocarcinoma has been used in most of cases. Noguchi et al have reported a good response with the combination chemotherapy of 5-fluouracil and cisplatin after surgery [127]. However, radiotherapy did not show any improvement for clinical course and outcome [126]. Basically, accurate diagnosis by initial biopsy, curative resection, early and appropriate intervention by chemotherapy, and the absence of combined liver metastasis are favorable prognostic factors for patients with PCCS.

The significance of an elevated serum β-human chorionic gonadotropin (HCG) is controversial. Some studies suggested that it is associated with a shorten survival and poorer prognosis [128]. However, other insisted that it does not have any prognostic significance [129]. β-HCG can be detected in blood or tissue in about 10% of patients with conventional gastric carcinoma; however, many of these tumors do not show any histologic evidence of the presence of choriocarcinoma component [130-132]. Also, the elevation of serum β-HCG and HCG immunoreactivity on tissue in these patients were usually mild. Most of reported cases of PCCS have been accompanied by markedly elevated serum level of β-HCG level up to 53,000 IU/ml at the presentation preoperatively and it significantly declined to the low level or baseline several months after surgeries. So, monitoring serum β-HCG level may have a role in evaluating response to treatment and tumor recurrence.

Macroscopically, this tumor usually occurs as a large exophytic mass with extensive necrosis and hemorrhage. Radiographically, it is a heterogeneous mass with enhanced vascularity and hemorrhage, mimicking a vascular tumor such as cavernous hemangioma [133]. Microscopically, this variant consists of choriocarcinoma and conventional adenocarcinoma with a variable proportion. Choriocarcinoma exhibits a typical biphasic pattern of admixed cytotrophoblasts and syncytiotrophoblasts. Polygonal cytotrophoblasts are located with a central core and surrounded by a peripheral rim of multinucleated syncytiotrophoblasts. Cytotrophoblasts have large, round hyperchromatic nuclei, abnormal nuclear chromatin, irregular nuclear membranes, occasional prominent nucleoli, and dense eosinophilic to amphophilic cytoplasm. Pleomorphic and multinucleated large cells are syncytiotrophoblasts. The viable tumor cells are found mainly at the lesion's periphery while extensive hemorrhage and necrosis are often in the center of the tumor like gestational choriocarcinoma. Typical and atypical mitotic figures may be frequently found. This tumor can show vascular invasion with tumor thrombi and tumor cells lining vascular spaces occasionally. Adenocarcinoma components would be tubular or papillary type with varying degree of differentiation. This tumor has been frequently misdiagnosed as gastric adenocarcinoma at presentation due to the size of tumor, massive tumor necrosis, and combined adenocarcinoma element. The diagnosis may even more become difficult in a small gastric biopsy from the lesion because it may reveal only scant syncytiotrophoblasts intermixed with recognizable routine adenocarcinoma component. Only 8% of PCCS cases in a pooled analysis of 53 cases were correctly diagnosed as choriocarcinoma in an initial biopsy [123]. Therefore. an extensive and large tissue sampling would be required for a precise diagnosis of

PCCS prior to surgery. In addition, if the biopsy contain any suspicious elements that suggest syncytiotrophoblasts, immunohistochemical biomarkers for trophoblastic cells will help confirming the diagnosis. In most instances, choriocarcinomatous cells are strongly positive for cytokeratin, β-HCG, and weakly positive for human placental lactogen. However, PCCS may not express β-HCG in the tumor tissue by immunohistochemistry [134].

Regarding the pathogenesis of PCCS, several theories have been proposed. The dedifferentiation theory first proposed by Pick in 1926 has been the most accepted explanation for the pathogenesis of choriocarcinoma [135]. Liu et al reported the first interphase cytogenetic study of PCCS, the results of which support this theory that PCCS arises from an alternative differentiation pathway, a dedifferentiation, of primary gastric adenocarcinoma [135, 136]. In this study, PCCSs showed the gain of chromosome 12, which is frequently associated with choriocarcinoma, and other genomic imbalances (gains of function mutations in 2q, 7pq, 8pq, 13q, 17q, 18q, 20pq and deletions in 17p) that are common genomic mutations in conventional gastric adenocarcinoma.

The major differential diagnosis of PCCS is metastatic trophoblastic tumor from other sites, particularly a non-gestational gonadal or extragonadal germ cell tumor from men and intrauterine or extrauterine gestational trophoblastic tumor in reproductive aged women. Extensive radiologic and clinical evaluation is recommended to rule out metastatic trophoblastic tumor from genital tracts in the men and women to make an unequivocal PCCS diagnosis.

7. Sarcomatoid carcinoma

Since Queckenstedt described the existence of the sarcomatous component in the gastric adenocarcinoma in 1904, approximately 50 cases of gastric sarcomatoid carcinoma have been reported [137]. Sarcomatoid carcinoma of the stomach (SCS) - also referred to as carcinosarcoma, malignant mixed mesodermal tumor, spindle cell carcinoma, and pseudosarcoma- is an uncommon variant of gastric carcinoma which is a biphasic neoplasm composed of a mixture of malignant epithelial and mesenchymal components. The various terms in use represent the uncertain histogenesis of this tumor, whether sarcomatoid carcinomas represent a single or two separate entities (carcinoma with sarcomatoid differentiation versus collision tumor consisting of carcinoma and sarcoma) remains controversial; however, some stromal tumor cells of SCS showing epithelial features such as staining for cytokeratin favor a monoclonal origin with divergent transformation.

The mean age of presentation is 45 years (range, 27 to 74 years) and males are predominantly affected (2.3:1), with patients frequently having metastasis to regional lymph nodes and liver at the time of diagnosis [138, 139]. Due to this tumor detecting at advance stage and its rapid growth, most of SCSs are associated with a poor clinical outcome. Sato et al reported a mean survival of 10 months in patients with SCS [140]. The current standard therapy for SCS is partial or total gastrectomy with regional lymph node dissection. The effects of chemotherapy or radiotherapy have not been established [141]. SCS may present synchrononously with conventional adenocarcinoma. However, there is no case of SCS that develops secondarily in patients with prior chemotherapy, which is different from primary sarcomatoid carcinoma arising from other organs. SCS usually occurs in the antral or pyloric region and infiltrates the gastric wall frequently. Macroscopically, it is a polypoid, exophytic, or endophytic mass with ulceration (Fig.14) [139, 140, 142-146]. Histologically, SCS exhibits an adenocarcinoma component with variable differentiation and a high-grade sarcomatous component composed of spindle cells with high cellularity, frequent mitotic counts with atypical forms and pleomorphism (Fig.15). The spindle cells generally have plump, pleomorphic nuclei with a coarsely stippled chromatin pattern and small nucleoli with a haphazard arrangement. The transition between epithelial and sarcomatoid components can be abrupt but two components may intermix with each other. The epithelial component is predominantly composed of adenocarcinoma but rarely adenosquamous and neuroendocrine cell carcinoma can be accompanied [82, 83, 140]. Some cases represent atrophic gastritis and dysplasia in the background gastric epithelium [142, 145].

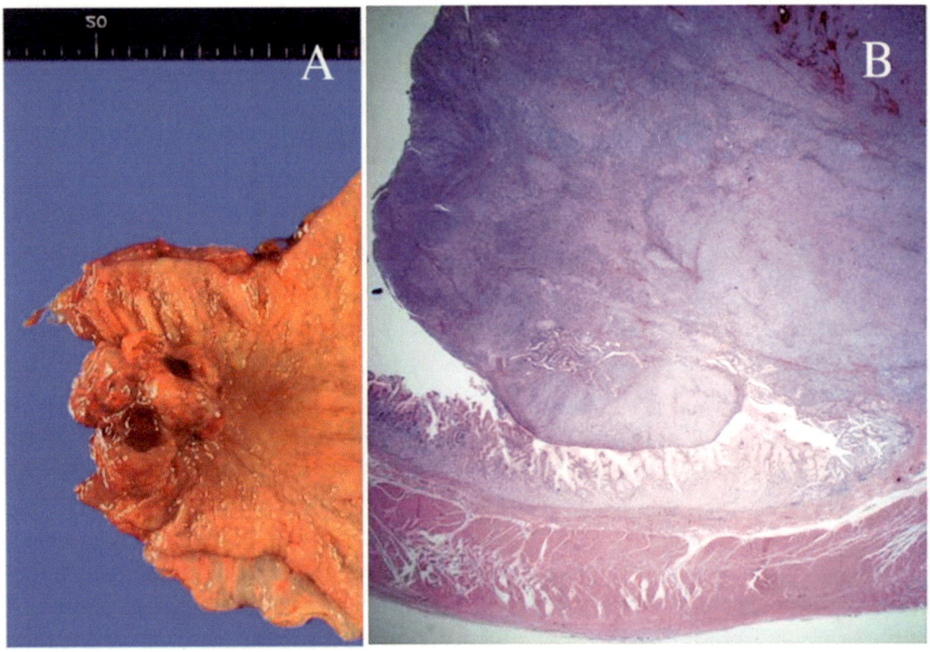

Figure 14. Gross and microscopic photographs of sarcomatoid carcinoma. **A.** This variant frequently appears as a polypoid or exophytic mass in the antrum. **B.** Low-magnification view shows a relatively well circumscribed dense mass.

The proportion of the sarcomatoid component is highly variable (5 % up to 80 %) [83, 139, 147]. In most instances, the pattern typically resembles that seen in high grade spindle sarcomas which lack specific immunohistochemical markers for identifying the line of differentiation [83, 84, 141, 148]. In some cases, the sarcomatous component can be heterologous, with osteosarcomatous, chondrosarcomatous, and rhabdomyosarcomatous or leiomyosarcomatous differentiation [82, 139, 146, 149, 150]. There have been three cases reported showing multidirectional differentiation including rhabdomyosarcoma, osteosarcoma, and chondrosarcoma [139, 147, 148].

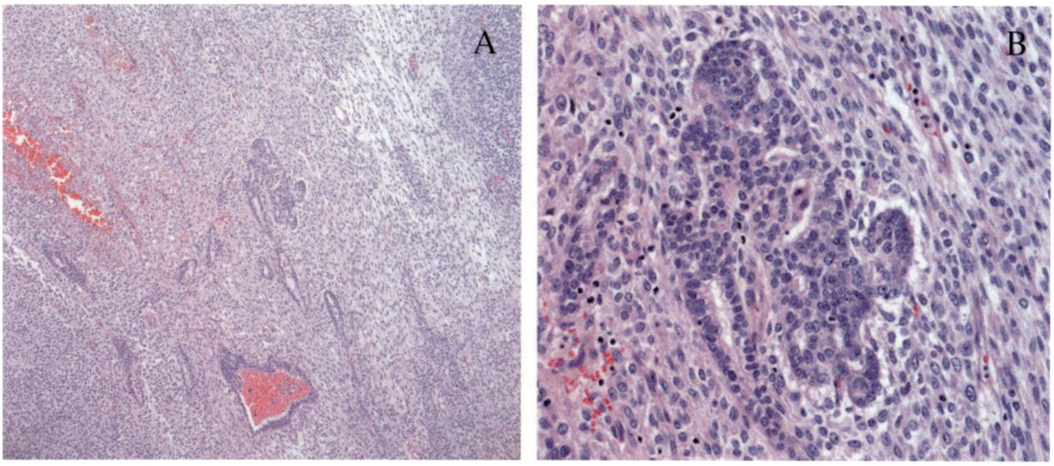

Figure 15. Microscopic photographs of sarcomatoid carcinoma. **A.** Adenocarcinoma component is entrapped by sarcomatoid cell component. **B.** At high magnification, the glandular component showing anastomosing or cribriform pattern is surrounded by dense spindle cells. The spindle cells show compact and hyperchromatic nuclei with marked pleomorphism. This biphasic pattern supports the diagnosis of this variant. The sarcomatous component may display heterologous differentiation toward skeletal and smooth muscle, bone, and cartilage.

The epithelial component is identified by CK, EMA, or Cam 5.2, whereas muscle markers like desmin, myogenin, or myoD1 may confirm rhabdomyoblastic differentiation and when chondrosarcoma or liposarcoma is suspected, S100 protein can be used to confirm the diagnosis. In rare cases such as the epithelial component containing neuroendocrine differentiation, neuroendocrine markers (synaptophysin, chromogranin, and CD56) would be useful.

Differential diagnoses of SCS include other primary gastric sarcomas. If primary gastric sarcoma is suspected based on radiologic and endoscopic findings, multiple and extensive sampling of the lesion should be performed to avoid missing an epithelial component. Another consideration is the extremely rare instance of osseous metaplasia arising in the conventional gastric adenocarcinoma. Unusual bone component in the stomach can be mistaken for a part of SCS element. However, the bone component is histologically benign [151, 152]. Similarly, differentiating SCS from benign, borderline, and malignant spindle cell tumors, such as inflammatory fibroid polyp, calcifying fibrous tumor, gastrointestinal stromal tumor, and plexiform angiomyxoid myofibroblastic tumor need to be considered.

8. Acinar cell carcinoma

Acinar cell carcinoma of the stomach (ACCS) defined to have immunohistochemical evidence of pancreatic exocrine enzyme production, is an uncommon variant of gastric adenocarcinoma that is morphologically resemble to primary pancreatic acinar cell carcinoma. Pure ACCS is extremely rare and only two cases had been reported [153, 154]. Most of reported ACCS are mixed tumors which combine with glandular and/or neuroendocrine carcinoma components.

Microscopically, this variant demonstrates acinar, solid, glandular/microglandular, and trabecular arrangement of cells forming large, densely cellular tumor nodules containing minimal stroma (Fig.16). Tumor cells forming acini are cuboidal or columnar cells similar to size of normal pancreatic acinar cells with basally located nuclei and apical eosinophilic granular cytoplasm (Fig 17). Nuclei are round to oval, with minimal to mild pleomorphism, indistinct nucleoli or occasional single nucleolus. Mitotic activity is variable. The cytoplasm is moderately abundant, eosinophilic, and granular. The non-neoplastic stomach shows chronic gastritis with intestinal metaplasia. ACCS can exhibit different morphologic features such as focal ductal differentiation and well-formed individual ductal elements with mucin production that are uncommon in primary acinar cell carcinoma of the pancreas [155]. Periodic acid-Schiff reaction after diastase digestion and Grimelius stains demonstrate characteristic positive granules within the cytoplasm of the tumor cells. By immunohistochemistry, the tumor cells express pancreatic exocrine enzymes, predominantly trypsin, and variably lipase, α-1 anti-trypsin, α-1 anti-chymotrypsin and chymotrypsin. Among many pancreatic enzymes, trypsin is one of the most common and useful markers for the diagnosis of ACCS. The frequency of trypsin expression in series varied from 71% to 100% (average, 97%), whereas chymotrypsin expression ranged from 39% to 100% (average, 66%) [156]. The antigens α-1 antitrypsin and α-1 chymotrypsin can be positive for some tumor cells but not specific for ACCS [153, 157]. Another important diagnostic feature of acinar cell carcinoma is the presence of zymogen granules, which are large (250 to 1000 μm) electron-dense, homogeneous granules on electron microscopy [155].

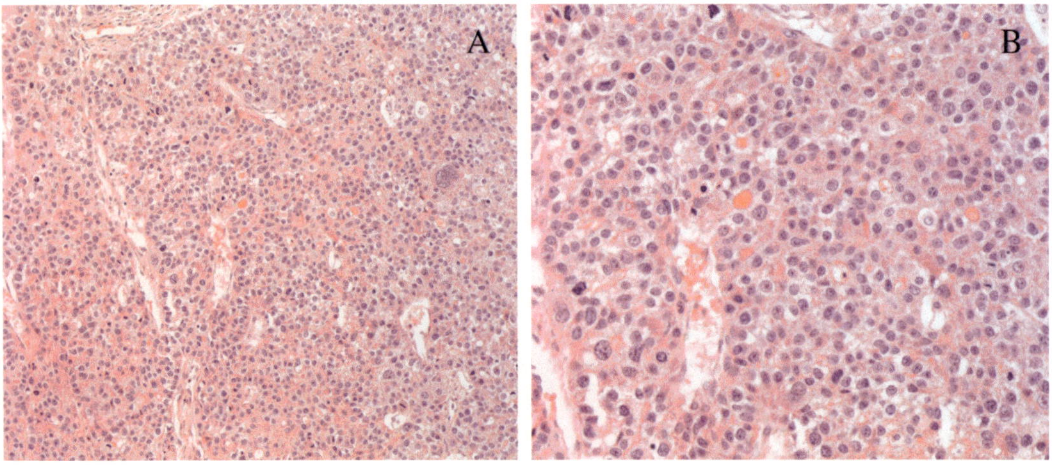

Figure 16. Microscopic photographs of acinar cell carcinoma. **A.** This variant shows trabecular and glandular arrangement of tumor cells. **B.** High magnification view demonstrates solid sheets of cuboidal cells with moderate pleomorphism and eosinophilic granular cytoplasm. Occasional mitoses and giant tumor cells are seen.

The histogenesis of ACCS is unclear. There are several hypotheses that may explain the origin of this variant. Because pancreatic heterotopia is relatively common in the stomach, origin in heterotopic pancreatic tissue was proposed first. Some ACCSs arising from heterotopic pancreas have been reported [158-163]. Acinar cell metaplasia is a relatively common finding in the gastric mucosa, either as a congenital abnormality, or in association with chronic gastritis [164-167]. ACCS may arise from this metaplastic process. Ambrosini-Spaltro et al reported an ACCS arising in association with pancreatic metaplasia in the gastric mucosa [168]. The possibility of the presence of "pluripotent stem cells" in the gastric mucosa, which have the potential to grow and differentiate to diverse cell types and neoplasms has been suggested by several studies of gastric composite tumors by morphology, ultrastructural examination, immunohistochemistry, and molecular genetics [157, 169, 170]. Fukunaga reported a gastric carcinoma resembling pancreatic mixed acinar-neuroendocrine carcinoma and proposed the possibility of a primitive multipotent cell with the capacity of divergent differentiation to explain acinar and neuroendocrine differentiation in the tumor [157].

The main differential diagnosis is metastatic lesion from pancreatic neoplasm. Since immunohistochemical expression of this tumor in the stomach and pancreas is exactly same, full clinical and radiographic evaluation would be essential to exclude the possibility of metastasis from pancreas.

The prognosis of primary ACCS is unknown due to the scarcity of reported cases. However, considering 50% of patients with primary pancreatic acinar cell carcinoma having metastases at presentation and a worse prognosis, the recognition of acinar cell component in gastric carcinoma may be important for the patients' treatment and prognosis.

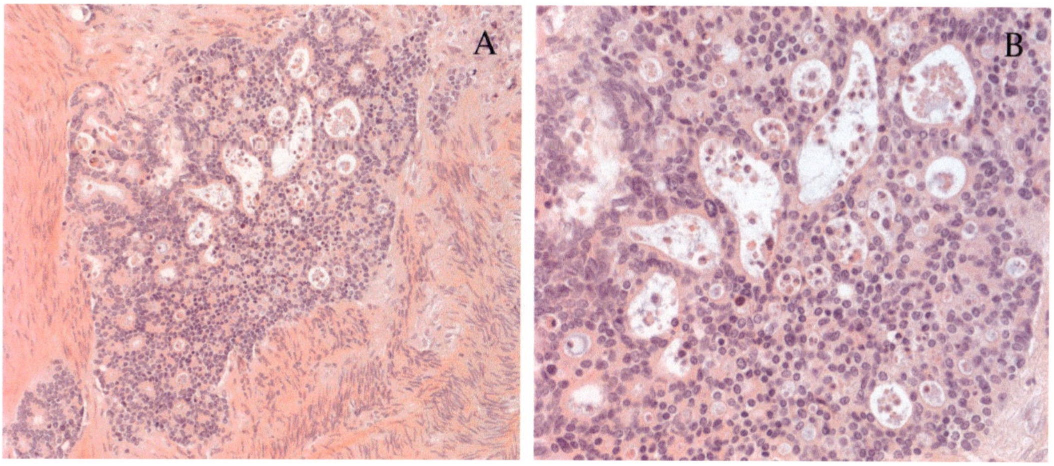

Figure 17. A and B. Microscopic photographs of acinar cell carcinoma. This tumor shows a prominent acinar growth pattern mimicking normal pancreatic acinar cells with prominent ductal elements with mucin.

9. Invasive micropapillary carcinoma

Recently, an unusual variant of gastric adenocarcinoma called " invasive micropapillary carcinoma of the stomach (IMPCS)" has been described by Shimoda et al in 2008 [171]. In a recent study by Roh et al, IMPCSs were present in up to 0.07% of 1,5254 total or subtotal gastrectomy specimens [172]. The mean age of this variant is 66.2 years (range 36-87 years) with a male predominance (male to female ratio: 2.5-3:1). This rare tumor demonstrates an aggressive behavior associated with a higher incidence of lymphovascular invasion and lymph node metastasis, resulting in a poor prognosis similar to invasive micropapillary carcinomas (IMPCs) of other organs including breast, urinary bladder, ureter, lung, parotid gland, and colon [173-179]. In the reported series to date, patients with IMPCS have an estimated 30% of 5- year overall survival rate compared to those with non-IMPCS having 67% of 5-year survival by Kaplan-Meir method [172].

Histologically, this variant consists of small tight cell clusters of papillary structure devoid of fibrovascular cores within lacunar spaces mimicking lymphatic or vascular channels (Fig.18). The lacunar spaces are artifactual tissue spaces and not lined by an endothelial cell. Several adjunct markers have been introduced to enhance the recognition of IMPCs. IMPCs in most organ systems are characterized by inverted polarity with MUC1 expression with membranous MUC1 staining facing the stroma [180]. Similarly, epithelial membrane antigen shows reverse polarity expression in IMPCs [181]. However, focal or heterogeneous staining pattern of IMPCs by MUC1 and EMA can be seen. Other immunohistochemical expressions of KL-6, CA125, and HER2/neu are frequently increased in IMPCs of the urinary tract but lack of specificity as an ancillary maker [181-184].

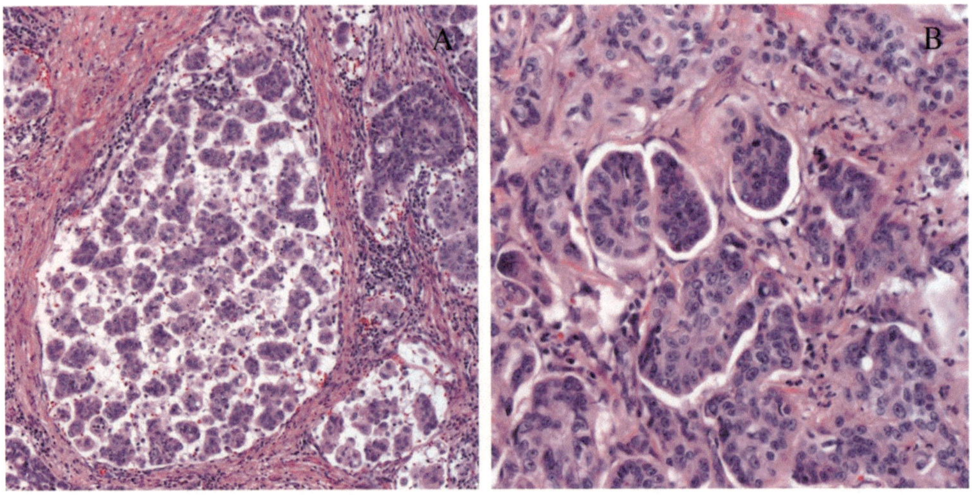

Figure 18. Invasive micropapillary carcinoma. **A.** Typical pathologic features of micropapillary carcinoma lined by clear spaces without lining cells nor mucin are seen. Papillary adenocarcinoma within lymphatic space is a lesion mimicking micropapillary carcinoma. **B.** In lymphatic spaces, the numbers of papillae are more than two unlike one in micropapillary carcinoma.

http://dx.doi.org/10.5772/54342

No" pure" form of IMPCS has been reported and all cases of IMPCS reported have been combined with conventional or papillary gastric adenocarcinoma. In the series of 72 IMPCS cases by Eom et al, most of the combined adenocarcinoma components were characterized as intestinal type (64/72 cases, 88.9%) and papillary adenocarcinoma (43/72 cases, 59.7%), and the remaining were classified as diffuse type (8/72 cases, 11.1%) and tubular adenocarcinoma (21/72 cases, 29.2%) [185].

Although IMPC has become increasingly well recognized as a distinct and aggressive variant in stomach as well as other organs from recent vigorous studies. Diagnostic criteria for a diagnosis of IMPCS remain imprecise. In a recent study about interobserver reproducibility in the diagnosis of IMPC of the urinary tract, this study recommended a combination of some histologic features included small tumor cell nests within stromal retraction spaces, back-to-back lacunae, multiple tumor nests within each single retraction space are useful to make a diagnosis for "classic" IMPC that may bring a better reproducibility. Additional associated histologic features to be considered including epithelial ring forms, intracytoplasmic vacuolization, elongated epithelial nests (i.e., micropapillae), and peripherally oriented nuclei. These diagnostic criteria of IMPC in the urinary tract based on a combination of several histologic features would be highly useful to make a diagnosis of IMPCs in other organs including stomach. In addition, the threshold for a diagnosis of IMPCs based on the percentage/volume of IMPC component is undetermined. There has been no validated clinicopathologic data that support the threshold of IMPC proportion in association with a clinical outcome in patients with IMPC. One study of IMPCs in the urinary tract showed a trend towards an association between the proportion of IMPC and survival with >50 % IMPC component imparting a relative mortality risk of 2.4, compared to with < 50% IMPC of those [186]. However, Kim et al suggested that the proportion of IMPC component with respect the whole tumor is not related with the prognosis of the patients with IMPC in the colorectum [187]. In the stomach, Roh et al failed to find any significant clinicopathologic differences between a group with ≤ 20% of IMPC component and another group with > 20% of IMPC component [172]. Some studies suggest an arbitrary cutoff of IMPCS as ≥ 5% of IMPC proportion in total tumor volume but ≥ 10% of IMPC proportion in other studies [172, 185]. Approximately 70% of reported cases in the stomach were found that the proportion of IMPC component to the entire tumor ranged from 10% to 70%. In previous published cases of IMPC of the colorectum, the proportion of IMPC component ranged from 5 % to 80 % but was usually less than 30 % of the entire lesion [178, 187, 188]. Comperat et al analyzed 72 cases of IMPC of the urinary bladder and the proportions of IMPC component are: 10% of cases with less than 10% of IMPC component, 47% of cases with 10%-50% of those, and 43% of cases with more than 50% of these [189]. Further studies are needed to have an established criteria for IMPCS showing a good reproducibility among inter-and intraobservers and to evaluate a diagnostic threshold of IMPC proportion in total volume of the tumor that correlate best with the clinical outcome.

The incidence of metastasis of IMPC from other organs to the stomach is uncommon. The possible metastatic lesions of IMPCs from other organs included urinary bladder, breast, lung, and ovary. Lotan et al investigated immunohistochemical markers to identify the primary site and differentiate metastatic lesions of IMPC [190]. They recommended that an immunohistochemical panel consisting of uroplakin, CK20, TTF-1, ER and WT-1, and/or PAX8, and mammaglobin is the best one for accurately classifying the likely primary site of IMPC. In their studies, urothelial IMPC were usually positive for uroplakin and CK20, whereas p63, high molecular weight cytokeratin, and thrombomodulin were less sensitive and specific. Lung IMPC was uniformly TTF-1 positive. Breast IMPC was ER positive, mammaglobin positive, and PAX8/WT-1 negative, while ovarian IMPC was ER positive, mammaglobin negative, and PAX/WT-1 positive. However, no specific marker has been introduced for verifying specifically IMPCS.

The main differential entity of IMPCS is papillary adenocarcinoma or conventional adenocarcinoma with multiple endolymphatic tumor emboli. Morphologically, when a distinction of IMPC within lacunar spaces from lymphovascular tumor emboli may be difficult, immunohistochemical studies including factor VIII, *Ulex europaeus*, CD31, CD34, and D2-40 as well as FLI1 and Erg nuclear stains would be useful to rule out lymphovascular tumor emboli from other types of adenocarcinoma (Fig.19) [191].

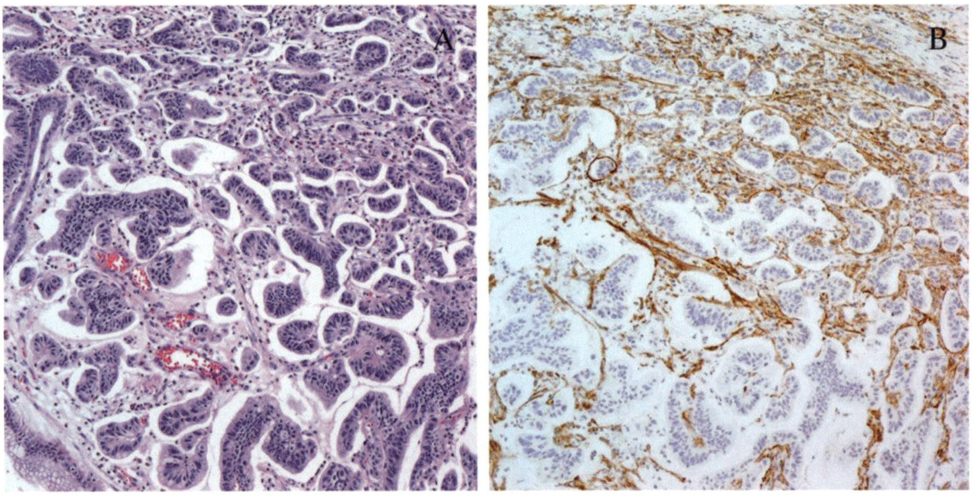

Figure 19. A. Invasive micropapillary variant showing tight small clusters of papillary structures within lacunar spaces. **B.** Immunohistochemical stain for D2-40 would be useful to rule out lymphatic tumor emboli.

10. Gastric adenocarcinoma of fundic gland type (chief cell predominant type)

Recently, Ueyama et al proposed gastric adenocarcinoma of fundic gland type for a new entity of gastric carcinoma [192]. Although gastric adenocarcinomas with foveolar and pyloric gland type differentiation are relatively common, only a few cases of gastric adenocarcinomas with fundic gland differentiation have been reported. This variant is a well differentiated adenocarcinoma composed of mixed chief and parietal cells mimicking fundic glands (Fig.20). In

http://dx.doi.org/10.5772/54342

addition to histologic similarity of chief and parietal cells, immunohistochemical staining with pepsinogen I (a marker for chief cells) and H+/K+ATPase (a marker for parietal cells) exhibit differentiation toward the chief and parietal cells in gastric adenocarcinoma. In the series by Ueyama et al and Singhi et al, the patients' age range from 42 to 79 years (average: 65 years) with a relatively equal sex distribution [192, 193].

Gastric adenocarcinoma of fundic gland type is a relatively small tumor, the maximum diameter of tumors range from 0.2 to 2 cm (average 0.6 cm) [192, 193]. Characteristically, gastric adenocarcinomas of fundic gland type are located in areas with oxyntic mucosa, in the upper third of the stomach, fundus and cardia [192, 193]. Macroscopic findings of this variant in early lesion are the superficial depressed type (type 0-IIc) or superficial elevated type (type 0-IIa) [192]. Histologically, this variant is a well-differentiated adenocarcinoma composed of columnar cells admixed with predominantly chief cells, with pale grey-blue, basophilic cytoplasm, and scattered parietal cells, with coarse granular eosinophilic cytoplasm. Both cells exhibit mildly enlarged and hyperchromatic nuclei with slight pleomorphism. Mitotic activity is absent or very low.

Differential diagnosis includes fundic gland polyps that are small benign mucosal polyps that occur in the gastric fundus. Histologically, they are composed of dilated glands lined by oxyntic mucosa without atypia.

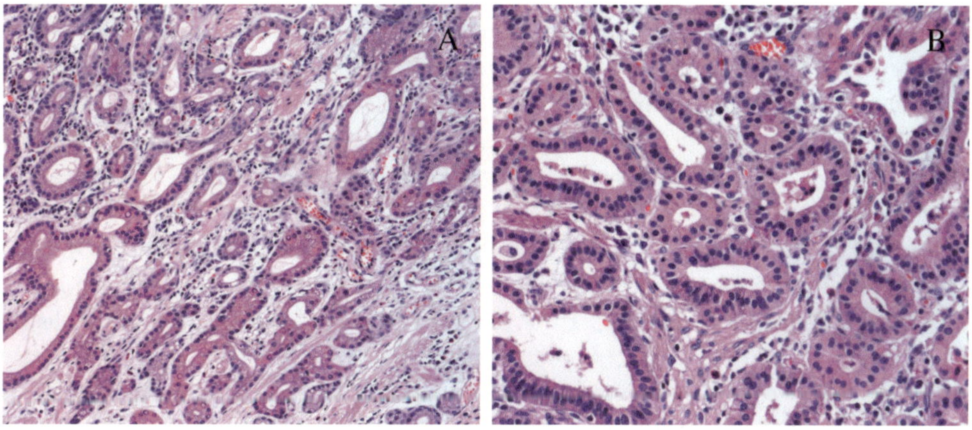

Figure 20. Microscopic photographs of gastric adenocarcinoma of fundic gland type. **A.** This variant is a well-differentiated adenocarcinoma mimicking the normal gastric fundic gland with irregular branching and angulated structures that invades in to the lamina propria. **B.** This adenocarcinoma predominantly consists of tumor cells mimicking chief cells with pale basophilic cytoplasm and basally located nuclei and scattered parietal cells with coarse granular eosinophilic cytoplasm.

11. Parietal cell carcinoma and oncocytic carcinoma

Since Capella et al originally described in 1984 as "gastric parietal cell carcinoma", less than 30 cases have been reported to date [194]. The reported mean age of the patients with this variant is 70.2 years (range 58-84 years) and it exclusively affects men (M:F ratio=9:1). Histologically, parietal cell carcinomas are usually composed of solid sheets of polygonal cells with round nuclei and abundant, finely granular eosinophilic cytoplasm that stain with phosphotungstic acid-hematoxylin and Luxol Fast Blue [194, 195]. Most of gastric parietal cell carcinomas are combined with well to moderately differentiated tubular or papillary adenocarcinoma. Parietal cell differentiation is confirmed by immunoreactivity for antibodies specific for parietal cell biomarkers H+/K+ ATPase and human milk fat globule-2. Ultrastructurally, the granular and eosinophilic cytoplasm, so call "oncocytic cytoplasm" corresponds to the abundance of mitochondria, intracytoplasmic secretory canaliculi, and cytoplasmic tubulovesicles [196, 197]. A few previous studies suggested that this variant of gastric adenocarcinoma is associated with a better prognosis than conventional gastric adenocarcinoma [194, 198-201]. Robey-Cafferty et al reported a case of parietal cell carcinoma with lymphoma-like morphologic features [197]. Takubo et al introduced ten cases of oncocytic adenocarcinoma, which are morphologically similar to parietal cell carcinoma but are negative for anti-parietal antibodies [195].

12. Miscellaneous carcinomas

Extremely rare variants of gastric carcinoma have been sporadically reported. Among them are (1) mucoepidermoid carcinoma of the stomach; one case was reported that this variant arose from preexisting ectopic mucous glands of stomach [202]. (2) Paneth cell carcinoma or gastric adenocarcinoma with Paneth cell differentiation; histologically, Paneth cell differentiation is characterized by cytoplasmic distinct coarse eosinophilic granules stained red with periodic acid-Schiff and Masson trichrome reagents and reddish brown with phosphotungstic acid hematoxylin, and electron microscopically by lysozyme in cytoplasmic electron dense granules [203]. Immunohistochemical staining for lysozyme, human defensin-5, and CDX2 is usually positive [204, 205]. and (3) gastric carcinoma with osteoclast-like giant cells; these variants contains a minor component of giant cells that contain 3 to 20 nuclei and are positive for CD68 and vimentin [206]. These findings suggest that giant cells are of monocytic/histiocytic origin and probably represent a host response to the tumor [207]. However, the clinicopathological significance of this variant has not been verified due to its rarity. Salient features of variants gastric adenocarcinoma are listed in Table 2.

HISTOLOGIC TYPE	SALIENT FEATURES OF GASTRIC CANCER VARIANTS
EBV-associated lymphoepithelioma-like carcinoma	EBV infection related tumor with a dense lymphoid stroma, positive EBER-ISH, aberrant methylation, and a better prognosis
Hepatoid adenocarcinoma	Subtype of AFP producing carcinoma resembling hepatocellular carcinoma and showing frequent liver metastasis, and a worse prognosis

http://dx.doi.org/10.5772/54342

HISTOLOGIC TYPE	SALIENT FEATURES OF GASTRIC CANCER VARIANTS
Neuroendocrine cell carcinoma	Aggressive tumor with distinct neuroendocrine cell features and a worse prognosis but good response to chemotherapy
Squamous and adenosquamous carcinoma	Pure or composite tumors with definite squamous features with a very strong male predominance and a worse prognosis
Choriocarcinoma	Tumors with variable choriocarcinomatous components, elevated β-HCG in the serum, frequent hematogenous spread and a worse prognosis
Sarcomatoid carcinoma	Biphasic neoplasm composed of a mixture of malignant epithelial and mesenchymal component with a poor prognosis
Acinar cell carcinoma	Adenocarcinoma resembling pancreatic acinar cells with production of pancreatic exocrine enzyme
Invasive micropapillary carcinoma	Adenocarcinoma with micropapillary features showing frequent lymphovascular invasion and lymph node metastasis
Gastric adenocarcinoma of fundic gland type (chief cell predominant)	Well differentiated adenocarcinoma mimicking a fundic gland polyp
Parietal cell carcinoma and oncocytic carcinoma	Well differentiated adenocarcinoma with Parietal cell differentiation and a better diagnosis

Table 2.

Author details

Sun-Mi Lee[1], Kyoung-Mee Kim[2] and Jae Y. Ro[3]

1 Departments of Pathology, University of Texas Health Science Center at San Antonio, San Antonio, TX, USA

2 SamSung Medical Center, SungKunKwan University School of Medicine, Seoul, Korea

3 The Methodist Hospital, Weill Medical College of Cornell University, Houston, TX, USA

References

[1] Giuffre, G., et al., HER2 status in unusual histological variants of gastric adenocarcinomas. J Clin Pathol, 2012. 65(3): p. 237-41.

[2] Horiuchi, K., et al., Carcinoma of stomach and breast with lymphoid stroma: localisation of Epstein-Barr virus. J Clin Pathol, 1994. 47(6): p. 538-40.

[3] Corvalan, A., et al., Epstein-Barr virus in gastric carcinoma is associated with location in the cardia and with a diffuse histology: a study in one area of Chile. Int J Cancer, 2001. 94(4): p. 527-30.

[4] Watanabe, H., M. Enjoji, and T. Imai, Gastric carcinoma with lymphoid stroma. Its morphologic characteristics and prognostic correlations. Cancer, 1976. 38(1): p. 232-43.

[5] Akiba, S., et al., Epstein-Barr virus associated gastric carcinoma: epidemiological and clinicopathological features. Cancer Sci, 2008. 99(2): p. 195-201.

[6] Lee, J.H., et al., Clinicopathological and molecular characteristics of Epstein-Barr virus-associated gastric carcinoma: a meta-analysis. J Gastroenterol Hepatol, 2009. 24(3): p. 354-65.

[7] Shibata, D. and L.M. Weiss, Epstein-Barr virus-associated gastric adenocarcinoma. Am J Pathol, 1992. 140(4): p. 769-74.

[8] Yanai, H., et al., Endoscopic and pathologic features of Epstein-Barr virus-associated gastric carcinoma. Gastrointest Endosc, 1997. 45(3): p. 236-42.

[9] Fukayama, M. and T. Ushiku, Epstein-Barr virus-associated gastric carcinoma. Pathol Res Pract, 2011. 207(9): p. 529-37.

[10] Ojima, H., et al., Discrepancy between clinical and pathological lymph node evaluation in Epstein-Barr virus-associated gastric cancers. Anticancer Res, 1996. 16(5B): p. 3081-4.

[11] Song, H.J., et al., Host inflammatory response predicts survival of patients with Epstein-Barr virus-associated gastric carcinoma. Gastroenterology, 2010. 139(1): p. 84-92 e2.

[12] Levine, P.H., et al., Elevated antibody titers to Epstein-Barr virus prior to the diagnosis of Epstein-Barr-virus-associated gastric adenocarcinoma. Int J Cancer, 1995. 60(5): p. 642-4.

[13] Tamura, T., et al., Lymphoepithelioma-Like Carcinoma of the Stomach with Epithelioid Granulomas. Case Rep Gastroenterol, 2010. 4(3): p. 361-368.

[14] Ushiku, T., et al., Gastric carcinoma with osteoclast-like giant cells. Lymphoepithelioma-like carcinoma with Epstein-Barr virus infection is the predominant type. Pathol Int, 2010. 60(8): p. 551-8.

[15] Arikawa, J., et al., Morphological characteristics of Epstein-Barr virus-related early gastric carcinoma: a case-control study. Pathol Int, 1997. 47(6): p. 360-7.

[16] Kaizaki, Y., et al., Atrophic gastritis, Epstein-Barr virus infection, and Epstein-Barr virus-associated gastric carcinoma. Gastric Cancer, 1999. 2(2): p. 101-108.

[17] Chapel, F., et al., Epstein-Barr virus and gastric carcinoma in Western patients: comparison of pathological parameters and p53 expression in EBV-positive and negative tumours. Histopathology, 2000. 36(3): p. 252-61.

[18] Kijima, Y., et al., The comparison of the prognosis between Epstein-Barr virus (EBV)-positive gastric carcinomas and EBV-negative ones. Cancer Lett, 2003. 200(1): p. 33-40.

[19] Saiki, Y., et al., Immunophenotypic characterization of Epstein-Barr virus-associated gastric carcinoma: massive infiltration by proliferating CD8+ T-lymphocytes. Lab Invest, 1996. 75(1): p. 67-76.

[20] Young, L.S. and A.B. Rickinson, Epstein-Barr virus: 40 years on. Nat Rev Cancer, 2004. 4(10): p. 757-68.

[21] Chen, J.N., et al., Epstein-Barr virus-associated gastric carcinoma: a newly defined entity. J Clin Gastroenterol, 2012. 46(4): p. 262-71.

[22] Ojima, H., et al., Infrequent overexpression of p53 protein in Epstein-Barr virus-associated gastric carcinomas. Jpn J Cancer Res, 1997. 88(3): p. 262-6.

[23] Gulley, M.L., et al., Epstein-Barr virus infection is an early event in gastric carcinogenesis and is independent of bcl-2 expression and p53 accumulation. Hum Pathol, 1996. 27(1): p. 20-7.

[24] Ohfuji, S., et al., Low frequency of apoptosis in Epstein-Barr virus-associated gastric carcinoma with lymphoid stroma. Int J Cancer, 1996. 68(6): p. 710-5.

[25] Delecluse, H.J., et al., Epstein Barr virus-associated tumours: an update for the attention of the working pathologist. J Clin Pathol, 2007. 60(12): p. 1358-64.

[26] Esteller, M., Epigenetics in cancer. N Engl J Med, 2008. 358(11): p. 1148-59.

[27] Kusano, M., et al., Genetic, epigenetic, and clinicopathologic features of gastric carcinomas with the CpG island methylator phenotype and an association with Epstein-Barr virus. Cancer, 2006. 106(7): p. 1467-79.

[28] Enomoto, S., et al., Lack of association between CpG island methylator phenotype in human gastric cancers and methylation in their background non-cancerous gastric mucosae. Cancer Sci, 2007. 98(12): p. 1853-61.

[29] Chong, J.M., et al., Global and non-random CpG-island methylation in gastric carcinoma associated with Epstein-Barr virus. Cancer Sci, 2003. 94(1): p. 76-80.

[30] Jung, E.J., et al., Lytic induction and apoptosis of Epstein-Barr virus-associated gastric cancer cell line with epigenetic modifiers and ganciclovir. Cancer Lett, 2007. 247(1): p. 77-83.

[31] Yamamoto, N., et al., Epstein-Barr virus and gastric remnant cancer. Cancer, 1994. 74(3): p. 805-9.

[32] Chang, M.S., et al., Microsatellite instability and Epstein-Barr virus infection in gastric remnant cancers. Pathol Int, 2000. 50(6): p. 486-92.

[33] Baas, I.O., et al., Helicobacter pylori and Epstein-Barr virus infection and the p53 tumour suppressor pathway in gastric stump cancer compared with carcinoma in the non-operated stomach. J Clin Pathol, 1998. 51(9): p. 662-6.

[34] Chen, J.N., et al., Epstein-Barr virus genome polymorphisms of Epstein-Barr virus-associated gastric carcinoma in gastric remnant carcinoma in Guangzhou, southern China, an endemic area of nasopharyngeal carcinoma. Virus Res, 2011. 160(1-2): p. 191-9.

[35] van Beek, J., et al., EBV-positive gastric adenocarcinomas: a distinct clinicopathologic entity with a low frequency of lymph node involvement. J Clin Oncol, 2004. 22(4): p. 664-70.

[36] Lee, H.L., et al., Treatment of Epstein-Barr virus-associated gastric carcinoma with endoscopic submucosal dissection. Gastrointest Endosc, 2011.

[37] Tang, S.J., et al., Endoscopic Mucosal Resection of an Epstein-Barr Virus-Associated Lymphoepithelioma-Like Gastric Carcinoma. Dig Dis Sci, 2012.

[38] Ishikura, H., et al., An AFP-producing gastric carcinoma with features of hepatic differentiation. A case report. Cancer, 1985. 56(4): p. 840-8.

[39] Nagai, E., et al., Hepatoid adenocarcinoma of the stomach. A clinicopathologic and immunohistochemical analysis. Cancer, 1993. 72(6): p. 1827-35.

[40] Gao, Y.B., et al., Preliminary study on the clinical and pathological relevance of gastric hepatoid adenocarcinoma. J Dig Dis, 2007. 8(1): p. 23-8.

[41] Ishikura, H., et al., Gastrointestinal hepatoid adenocarcinoma: venous permeation and mimicry of hepatocellular carcinoma, a report of four cases. Histopathology, 1997. 31(1): p. 47-54.

[42] Chang, Y.C., et al., alpha Fetoprotein producing early gastric cancer with liver metastasis: report of three cases. Gut, 1991. 32(5): p. 542-5.

[43] Gitlin, D., A. Perricelli, and G.M. Gitlin, Synthesis of -fetoprotein by liver, yolk sac, and gastrointestinal tract of the human conceptus. Cancer Res, 1972. 32(5): p. 979-82.

[44] Baek, S.K., et al., Clinicopathologic characteristics and treatment outcomes of hepatoid adenocarcinoma of the stomach, a rare but unique subtype of gastric cancer. BMC Gastroenterol, 2011. 11: p. 56.

[45] Kodama, T., et al., Production of alpha-fetoprotein, normal serum proteins, and human chorionic gonadotropin in stomach cancer: histologic and immunohistochemical analyses of 35 cases. Cancer, 1981. 48(7): p. 1647-55.

[46] Matsunou, H., et al., Alpha-fetoprotein-producing gastric carcinoma with enteroblastic differentiation. Cancer, 1994. 73(3): p. 534-40.

[47] Motoyama, T., et al., alpha-Fetoprotein producing gastric carcinomas: a comparative study of three different subtypes. Acta Pathol Jpn, 1993. 43(11): p. 654-61.

[48] Ooi, A., et al., Alpha-fetoprotein (AFP)-producing gastric carcinoma. Is it hepatoid differentiation? Cancer, 1990. 65(8): p. 1741-7.

[49] Kinjo, T., et al., Histologic and immunohistochemical analyses of alpha-fetoprotein--producing cancer of the stomach. Am J Surg Pathol, 2012. 36(1): p. 56-65.

[50] Liu, X., et al., Analysis of clinicopathologic features and prognostic factors in hepatoid adenocarcinoma of the stomach. Am J Surg Pathol, 2010. 34(10): p. 1465-71.

[51] Hishinuma, M., et al., Hepatocellular oncofetal protein, glypican 3 is a sensitive marker for alpha-fetoprotein-producing gastric carcinoma. Histopathology, 2006. 49(5): p. 479-86.

[52] Terracciano, L.M., et al., Hepatoid adenocarcinoma with liver metastasis mimicking hepatocellular carcinoma: an immunohistochemical and molecular study of eight cases. Am J Surg Pathol, 2003. 27(10): p. 1302-12.

[53] Iso, Y., et al., Solitary AFP- and PIVKA-II-producing hepatoid gastric cancer with giant lymph node metastasis. Hepatogastroenterology, 2005. 52(66): p. 1930-2.

[54] Lu, C.C., et al., Pure hepatoid adenocarcinoma of the stomach with spleen and lymph-node metastases. Am J Surg, 2010. 199(4): p. e42-4.

[55] Filmus, J. and S.B. Selleck, Glypicans: proteoglycans with a surprise. J Clin Invest, 2001. 108(4): p. 497-501.

[56] Kishimoto, T., et al., Hepatoid adenocarcinoma: a new clinicopathological entity and the hypotheses on carcinogenesis. Med Electron Microsc, 2000. 33(2): p. 57-63.

[57] Akiyama, S., et al., Histogenesis of hepatoid adenocarcinoma of the stomach: molecular evidence of identical origin with coexistent tubular adenocarcinoma. Int J Cancer, 2003. 106(4): p. 510-5.

[58] Kang, G.H. and Y.I. Kim, Alpha-fetoprotein-producing gastric carcinoma presenting focal hepatoid differentiation in metastatic lymph nodes. Virchows Arch, 1998. 432(1): p. 85-7.

[59] Trevisani, F., et al., Etiologic factors and clinical presentation of hepatocellular carcinoma. Differences between cirrhotic and noncirrhotic Italian patients. Cancer, 1995. 75(9): p. 2220-32.

[60] Okuda, K., R.L. Peters, and I.W. Simson, Gross anatomic features of hepatocellular carcinoma from three disparate geographic areas. Proposal of new classification. Cancer, 1984. 54(10): p. 2165-73.

[61] Kamata, S., et al., Expression and localization of ATP binding cassette (ABC) family of drug transporters in gastric hepatoid adenocarcinomas. Histopathology, 2008. 52(6): p. 747-54.

[62] Matsusaka, T., H. Watanabe, and M. Enjoji, Oat-cell carcinoma of the stomach. Fukuoka Igaku Zasshi, 1976. 67(2): p. 65-73.

[63] Kim, K.O., et al., Clinical overview of extrapulmonary small cell carcinoma. J Korean Med Sci, 2006. 21(5): p. 833-7.

[64] Matsubayashi, H., et al., Advanced gastric glandular-endocrine cell carcinoma with 1-year survival after gastrectomy. Gastric Cancer, 2000. 3(4): p. 226-233.

[65] Namikawa, T., et al., Primary gastric small cell carcinoma: report of a case and review of the literature. Med Mol Morphol, 2005. 38(4): p. 256-61.

[66] O'Byrne, K.J., et al., Extrapulmonary small cell gastric carcinoma. A case report and review of the literature. Acta Oncol, 1997. 36(1): p. 78-80.

[67] Chejfec, G. and V.E. Gould, Malignant gastric neuroendogrinomas. Ultrastructural and biochemical characterization of their secretory activity. Hum Pathol, 1977. 8(4): p. 433-40.

[68] Okita, N.T., et al., Neuroendocrine tumors of the stomach: chemotherapy with cisplatin plus irinotecan is effective for gastric poorly-differentiated neuroendocrine carcinoma. Gastric Cancer, 2011. 14(2): p. 161-5.

[69] Murakami, H., et al., Paraneoplastic neurological syndrome in a patient with gastric cancer. Gastric Cancer, 2010. 13(3): p. 204-8.

[70] Hirata, Y., et al., Gastric carcinoid with ectopic production of ACTH and beta-MSH. Cancer, 1976. 37(1): p. 377-85.

[71] Matsui, T., et al., A case of small cell carcinoma of the stomach. Hepatogastroenterology, 1997. 44(13): p. 156-60.

[72] Arakawa, A., et al., Small cell carcinoma of the stomach: a case report. Radiat Med, 1997. 15(5): p. 321-5.

[73] Arai, K. and M. Matsuda, Gastric small-cell carcinoma in Japan: a case report and review of the literature. Am J Clin Oncol, 1998. 21(5): p. 458-61.

[74] Matsui, K., et al., Small cell carcinoma of the stomach: a clinicopathologic study of 17 cases. Am J Gastroenterol, 1991. 86(9): p. 1167-75.

[75] Chiba, N., et al., Advanced gastric endocrine cell carcinoma with distant lymph node metastasis: a case report and clinicopathological characteristics of the disease. Gastric Cancer, 2004. 7(2): p. 122-7.

[76] Fukuda, T., et al., Early gastric cancer of the small cell type. Am J Gastroenterol, 1988. 83(10): p. 1176-9.

[77] Hanada, N., et al., [A case of partial response in liver metastatic lesion from gastric endocrine cell carcinoma treated with TS-1]. Gan To Kagaku Ryoho, 2006. 33(8): p. 1143-6.

[78] Tsushima, T., et al., [A case of metastatic gastric endocrine cell carcinoma which could be curably resected after chemotherapy with S-1/CDDP]. Gan To Kagaku Ryoho, 2008. 35(5): p. 817-20.

[79] Rindi, G., et al., ECL cell tumor and poorly differentiated endocrine carcinoma of the stomach: prognostic evaluation by pathological analysis. Gastroenterology, 1999. 116(3): p. 532-42.

[80] Huang, J., et al., Primary small cell carcinoma of the stomach: An experience of two decades (1990-2011) in a Chinese cancer institute. J Surg Oncol, 2012.

[81] Matsui, K., et al., Clinicopathologic features of neuroendocrine carcinomas of the stomach: appraisal of small cell and large cell variants. Arch Pathol Lab Med, 1998. 122(11): p. 1010-7.

[82] Tsuneyama, K., et al., A case report of gastric carcinosarcoma with rhabdomyosarcomatous and neuroendocrinal differentiation. Pathol Res Pract, 1999. 195(2): p. 93-7; discussion 98.

[83] Yamazaki, K., A gastric carcinosarcoma with neuroendocrine cell differentiation and undifferentiated spindle-shaped sarcoma component possibly progressing from the conventional tubular adenocarcinoma; an immunohistochemical and ultrastructural study. Virchows Arch, 2003. 442(1): p. 77-81.

[84] Kuroda, N., et al., Gastric carcinosarcoma with neuroendocrine differentiation as the carcinoma component and leiomyosarcomatous and myofibroblastic differentiation as the sarcomatous component. APMIS, 2006. 114(3): p. 234-8.

[85] Haratake, J., A. Horie, and S. Inoshita, Gastric small cell carcinoma with squamous and neuroendocrine differentiation. Pathology, 1992. 24(2): p. 116-20.

[86] Travis, W., T. Colby, and Y. Shimosato, Histological Classification of Lung and Pleural tumors. 1st ed. WHO/IASLC. 1999, Berlin, Germany: Springer.

[87] Brenner, B., et al., Small-cell carcinomas of the gastrointestinal tract: a review. J Clin Oncol, 2004. 22(13): p. 2730-9.

[88] Bartley, A.N., et al., Neuroendocrine and mucinous differentiation in signet ring cell carcinoma of the stomach: evidence for a common cell of origin in composite tumors. Hum Pathol, 2011. 42(10): p. 1420-9.

[89] Ho, K.J., et al., Small cell carcinoma of the esophagus: evidence for a unified histogenesis. Hum Pathol, 1984. 15(5): p. 460-8.

[90] Hussein, A.M., C.L. Otrakji, and B.T. Hussein, Small cell carcinoma of the stomach. Case report and review of the literature. Dig Dis Sci, 1990. 35(4): p. 513-8.

[91] Nishikura, K., et al., Carcinogenesis of gastric endocrine cell carcinoma: analysis of histopathology and p53 gene alteration. Gastric Cancer, 2003. 6(4): p. 203-9.

[92] Kusayanagi, S., et al., Primary small cell carcinoma of the stomach. J Gastroenterol Hepatol, 2003. 18(6): p. 743-7.

[93] Shpaner, A. and T.E. Yusuf, Primary gastric small-cell neuroendocrine carcinoma. Endoscopy, 2007. 39 Suppl 1: p. E310-1.

[94] Li, A.F., et al., Small cell carcinomas in gastrointestinal tract: immunohistochemical and clinicopathological features. J Clin Pathol, 2010. 63(7): p. 620-5.

[95] Hamilton, S. and L. Aaltonen, WHO Classification of Tumors of the Digestive System. IARC WHO Classification of Tumors. 2010, Lyon: IARC Press.

[96] Jiang, S.X., et al., Gastric large cell neuroendocrine carcinomas: a distinct clinicopathologic entity. Am J Surg Pathol, 2006. 30(8): p. 945-53.

[97] Shia, J., et al., Is nonsmall cell type high-grade neuroendocrine carcinoma of the tubular gastrointestinal tract a distinct disease entity? Am J Surg Pathol, 2008. 32(5): p. 719-31.

[98] Murayama, H., T. Imai, and M. Kikuchi, Solid carcinomas of the stomach. A combined histochemical, light and electron microscopic study. Cancer, 1983. 51(9): p. 1673-81.

[99] Ordonez, N.G., Value of thyroid transcription factor-1 immunostaining in distinguishing small cell lung carcinomas from other small cell carcinomas. Am J Surg Pathol, 2000. 24(9): p. 1217-23.

[100] Solcia, E., G. Kloppel, and L.H. Sobin, Histological Typing of Endocrine Tumors (WHO International Histological Classification of Tumours). 2nd ed. 2000, Berlin, Germany: Springer.

[101] Won, O.H., et al., Squamous cell carcinoma of the stomach. Am J Gastroenterol, 1978. 69(5): p. 594-8.

[102] Hoshi, K., et al., [Specific type stomach neoplasms: report based on the questionnaires of the 40th Stomach Cancer Research Group]. Nihon Gan Chiryo Gakkai Shi, 1983. 18(8): p. 2112-24.

[103] Lim, S.M., et al., A case of synchronous squamous cell carcinoma in the esophagus and stomach. Gut Liver, 2012. 6(1): p. 118-21.

[104] Dursun, M., et al., Primary squamous cell carcinoma of the stomach: a case report and review of the literature. Eur J Gastroenterol Hepatol, 2003. 15(3): p. 329-30.

[105] Hara, J., et al., Exophytic primary squamous cell carcinoma of the stomach. J Gastroenterol, 2004. 39(3): p. 299-300.

[106] Marubashi, S., et al., Primary squamous cell carcinoma of the stomach. Gastric Cancer, 1999. 2(2): p. 136-141.

[107] Oono, Y., et al., Primary gastric squamous cell carcinoma in situ originating from gastric squamous metaplasia. Endoscopy, 2010. 42 Suppl 2: p. E290-1.

[108] Parks, R.E., Squamous neoplasms of the stomach. Am J Roentgenol Radium Ther Nucl Med, 1967. 101(2): p. 447-9.

[109] Japanese classification of gastric carcinoma: 3rd English edition. Gastric Cancer, 2011. 14(2): p. 101-12.

[110] Schmidt, C., et al., Primary squamous cell carcinoma of the stomach. Report of a case and review of literature. Hepatogastroenterology, 2001. 48(40): p. 1033-6.

[111] Straus, R., S. Heschel, and D.J. Fortmann, Primary adenosquamous carcinoma of the stomach. A case report and review. Cancer, 1969. 24(5): p. 985-95.

[112] Mingazzini, P.L., P. Barsotti, and F. Malchiodi Albedi, Adenosquamous carcinoma of the stomach: histological, histochemical and ultrastructural observations. Histopathology, 1983. 7(3): p. 433-43.

[113] Tokuhara, K., et al., Primary squamous cell carcinoma in the gastric remnant. Surg Today, 2012. 42(7): p. 666-9.

[114] Davidsohn, C., Chorioepithelium und Magekrebs, eine seltene Verschmelzung zweier bosartiger Geschwulste. Charite Ann, 1905. 29: p. 12.

[115] Unakami, M., et al., [3 cases of malignant choriocarcinoma originating in the stomach]. Gan No Rinsho, 1982. 28(3): p. 204-10.

[116] Mori, H., et al., Choriocarcinomatous change with immunocytochemically HCG-positive cells in the gastric carcinoma of the males. Virchows Arch A Pathol Anat Histol, 1982. 396(2): p. 141-53.

[117] Saigo, P.E., et al., Primary gastric choriocarcinoma. An immunohistological study. Am J Surg Pathol, 1981. 5(4): p. 333-42.

[118] Jindrak, K., J.F. Bochetto, and L.I. Alpert, Primary gastric choriocarcinoma: case report with review of world literature. Hum Pathol, 1976. 7(5): p. 595-604.

[119] Satake, N., et al., Gastric cancer with choriocarcinoma and yolk sac tumor components: case report. Pathol Int, 2011. 61(3): p. 156-60.

[120] Hirano, Y., et al., Combined choriocarcinoma, neuroendocrine cell carcinoma and tubular adenocarcinoma in the stomach. World J Gastroenterol, 2008. 14(20): p. 3269-72.

[121] Motoyama, T., et al., Coexistence of choriocarcinoma and hepatoid adenocarcinoma in the stomach. Pathol Int, 1994. 44(9): p. 716-21.

[122] Garcia, R.L. and V.S. Ghali, Gastric choriocarcinoma and yolk sac tumor in a man: observations about its possible origin. Hum Pathol, 1985. 16(9): p. 955-8.

[123] Kobayashi, A., et al., Primary gastric choriocarcinoma: two case reports and a pooled analysis of 53 cases. Gastric Cancer, 2005. 8(3): p. 178-85.

[124] Senju, M., et al., [Case of advanced gastric cancer with remarkable gynecomastia and marked elevation of serum human chorionic gonadotropin (HCG)]. Nihon Shokakibyo Gakkai Zasshi, 1983. 80(6): p. 1331-5.

[125] Dye, D.W., R. Broadwater, and L.W. Lamps, Uncommon malignancies: case 2. Gastric choriocarcinoma. J Clin Oncol, 2005. 23(25): p. 6251-3.

[126] Krulewski, T. and L.B. Cohen, Choriocarcinoma of the stomach: pathogenesis and clinical characteristics. Am J Gastroenterol, 1988. 83(10): p. 1172-5.

[127] Noguchi, T., et al., A patient with primary gastric choriocarcinoma who received a correct preoperative diagnosis and achieved prolonged survival. Gastric Cancer, 2002. 5(2): p. 112-7.

[128] Tomita, K. and M. Kuwajima, Chorionic gonadotropin in gastric cancer tissue, especially its relation to the patient's prognosis. Gan No Rinsho, 1981. 27: p. 2.

[129] Yakeishi, Y., M. Mori, and M. Enjoji, Distribution of beta-human chorionic gonadotropin-positive cells in noncancerous gastric mucosa and in malignant gastric tumors. Cancer, 1990. 66(4): p. 695-701.

[130] Walker, L.R. and B. Erler, Gastric cancer in the setting of persistently elevated human chorionic gonadotropin: a case report. Case Rep Obstet Gynecol, 2011. 2011: p. 350318.

[131] Fujimoto, S., et al., The presence of an aberrant type of human chorionic gonadotropin in patients with gastric or colorectal cancer. Jpn J Surg, 1987. 17(5): p. 382-7.

[132] Arai, O., et al., [A case of advanced gastric cancer growing extramurally with gynecomastia and high hCG-beta serum level]. Gan To Kagaku Ryoho, 2010. 37(7): p. 1369-72.

[133] Matsunaga, N., et al., Primary choriocarcinoma of the stomach presenting as gastrointestinal hemorrhage: report of a case. Radiat Med, 1989. 7(5): p. 220-2.

[134] Masuda, R., et al., [A primary choriocarcinoma of the stomach with a review of 45 cases in Japan]. Gan No Rinsho, 1990. 36(9): p. 1025-30.

[135] Pick, L., Uber die chorioepthelahnlich metastsierende from desmagencarcinomas. Klin Wochenscher, 1926. 5: p. 1.

[136] Liu, A.Y., et al., Gastric choriocarcinoma shows characteristics of adenocarcinoma and gestational choriocarcinoma: a comparative genomic hybridization and fluorescence in situ hybridization study. Diagn Mol Pathol, 2001. 10(3): p. 161-5.

[137] Queckenstedt, H., Ueber Karzinsakome Leipzig. 1984.

[138] Tanimura, H. and M. Furuta, Carcinosarcoma of the stomach. Am J Surg, 1967. 113(5): p. 702-9.

[139] Nakayama, Y., et al., Gastric carcinosarcoma (sarcomatoid carcinoma) with rhabdomyoblastic and osteoblastic differentiation. Pathol Int, 1997. 47(8): p. 557-63.

[140] Sato, Y., et al., Gastric carcinosarcoma, coexistence of adenosquamous carcinoma and rhabdomyosarcoma: a case report. Histopathology, 2001. 39(5): p. 543-4.

[141] Ikeda, Y., et al., Gastric carcinosarcoma presenting as a huge epigastric mass. Gastric Cancer, 2007. 10(1): p. 63-8.

[142] Bansal, M., M. Kaneko, and R.E. Gordon, Carcinosarcoma and separate carcinoid tumor of the stomach. A case report with light and electron microscopic studies. Cancer, 1982. 50(9): p. 1876-81.

[143] Kumagai, K., et al., [A case of so-called carcinosarcoma of the stomach]. Gan No Rinsho, 1984. 30(15): p. 1931-6.

[144] Hanada, M., et al., Carcinosarcoma of the stomach. A case report with light microscopic, immunohistochemical, and electron microscopic study. Acta Pathol Jpn, 1985. 35(4): p. 951-9.

[145] Robey-Cafferty, S.S., et al., Sarcomatoid carcinoma of the stomach. A report of three cases with immunohistochemical and ultrastructural observations. Cancer, 1990. 65(7): p. 1601-6.

[146] Minamoto, T., et al., [So-called gastric carcinosarcoma--a case of chondrosarcomatous undifferentiated in the metastatic foci]. Gan No Rinsho, 1984. 30(10): p. 1321-6.

[147] Teramachi, K., et al., Carcinosarcoma (pure endocrine cell carcinoma with sarcoma components) of the stomach. Pathol Int, 2003. 53(8): p. 552-6.

[148] Melato, M., et al., Carcinosarcoma and separate neuroendocrine malignant tumor of a malignancy promoter, the gastric stump. Anticancer Res, 1993. 13(6B): p. 2485-8.

[149] Cho, K.J., et al., Carcinosarcoma of the stomach. A case report with light microscopic, immunohistochemical, and electron microscopic study. APMIS, 1990. 98(11): p. 991-5.

[150] Matsukuma, S., et al., Gastric stump carcinosarcoma with rhabdomyosarcomatous differentiation. Pathol Int, 1997. 47(1): p. 73-7.

[151] Olinici, C.D., et al., Heterotopic bone formation in gastric carcinoma. Case report and discussion of the literature. Rom J Gastroenterol, 2002. 11(4): p. 331-3.

[152] Yasuma, T., et al., Bone formation and calcification in gastric cancer--case report and review of literature. Acta Pathol Jpn, 1973. 23(1): p. 155-72.

[153] Sun, Y. and P.G. Wasserman, Acinar cell carcinoma arising in the stomach: a case report with literature review. Hum Pathol, 2004. 35(2): p. 263-5.

[154] Mizuno, Y., et al., Acinar cell carcinoma arising from an ectopic pancreas. Surg Today, 2007. 37(8): p. 704-7.

[155] Klimstra, D.S., et al., Acinar cell carcinoma of the pancreas. A clinicopathologic study of 28 cases. Am J Surg Pathol, 1992. 16(9): p. 815-37.

[156] Ordonez, N.G., Pancreatic acinar cell carcinoma. Adv Anat Pathol, 2001. 8(3): p. 144-59.

[157] Fukunaga, M., Gastric carcinoma resembling pancreatic mixed acinar-endocrine carcinoma. Hum Pathol, 2002. 33(5): p. 569-73.

[158] Chetty, R. and I. Weinreb, Gastric neuroendocrine carcinoma arising from heterotopic pancreatic tissue. J Clin Pathol, 2004. 57(3): p. 314-7.

[159] Emerson, L., et al., Adenocarcinoma arising in association with gastric heterotopic pancreas: A case report and review of the literature. J Surg Oncol, 2004. 87(1): p. 53-7.

[160] Jeong, H.Y., et al., Adenocarcinoma arising from an ectopic pancreas in the stomach. Endoscopy, 2002. 34(12): p. 1014-7.

[161] Song, D.E., et al., Adenocarcinoma arising in gastric heterotopic pancreas: a case report. J Korean Med Sci, 2004. 19(1): p. 145-8.

[162] Tsapralis, D., et al., Pancreatic intraductal papillary mucinous neoplasm with concomitant heterotopic pancreatic cystic neoplasia of the stomach: a case report and review of the literature. Diagn Pathol, 2010. 5: p. 4.

[163] Osanai, M., et al., Adenocarcinoma arising in gastric heterotopic pancreas: clinicopathological and immunohistochemical study with genetic analysis of a case. Pathol Int, 2001. 51(7): p. 549-54.

[164] Doglioni, C., et al., Pancreatic (acinar) metaplasia of the gastric mucosa. Histology, ultrastructure, immunocytochemistry, and clinicopathologic correlations of 101 cases. Am J Surg Pathol, 1993. 17(11): p. 1134-43.

[165] Faller, G. and T. Kirchner, Immunological and morphogenic basis of gastric mucosa atrophy and metaplasia. Virchows Arch, 2005. 446(1): p. 1-9.

[166] Wang, H.H., et al., Prevalence and significance of pancreatic acinar metaplasia at the gastroesophageal junction. Am J Surg Pathol, 1996. 20(12): p. 1507-10.

[167] Krishnamurthy, S., et al., Pancreatic acinar cell clusters in pediatric gastric mucosa. Am J Surg Pathol, 1998. 22(1): p. 100-5.

[168] Ambrosini-Spaltro, A., et al., Pancreatic-type acinar cell carcinoma of the stomach beneath a focus of pancreatic metaplasia of the gastric mucosa. Hum Pathol, 2009. 40(5): p. 746-9.

[169] Jain, D., et al., Composite glandular and endocrine tumors of the stomach with pancreatic acinar differentiation. Am J Surg Pathol, 2005. 29(11): p. 1524-9.

[170] Kusafuka, K., et al., Pancreatic-type mixed acinar-endocrine carcinoma with alpha-fetoprotein production arising from the stomach: a report of an extremely rare case. Med Mol Morphol, 2009. 42(3): p. 167-74.

[171] Shimoda, M., et al., Primary invasive micropapillary carcinoma of the stomach. Pathol Int, 2008. 58(8): p. 513-7.

[172] Roh, J.H., et al., Micropapillary carcinoma of stomach: a clinicopathologic and immunohistochemical study of 11 cases. Am J Surg Pathol, 2010. 34(8): p. 1139-46.

[173] De la Cruz, C., et al., Invasive micropapillary carcinoma of the breast: clinicopathological and immunohistochemical study. Pathol Int, 2004. 54(2): p. 90-6.

[174] Amin, M.B., et al., Micropapillary variant of transitional cell carcinoma of the urinary bladder. Histologic pattern resembling ovarian papillary serous carcinoma. Am J Surg Pathol, 1994. 18(12): p. 1224-32.

[175] Oh, Y.L. and K.R. Kim, Micropapillary variant of transitional cell carcinoma of the ureter. Pathol Int, 2000. 50(1): p. 52-6.

[176] Amin, M.B., et al., Micropapillary component in lung adenocarcinoma: a distinctive histologic feature with possible prognostic significance. Am J Surg Pathol, 2002. 26(3): p. 358-64.

[177] Michal, M., A. Skalova, and P. Mukensnabl, Micropapillary carcinoma of the parotid gland arising in mucinous cystadenoma. Virchows Arch, 2000. 437(4): p. 465-8.

[178] Verdu, M., et al., Clinicopathological and molecular characterization of colorectal micropapillary carcinoma. Mod Pathol, 2011. 24(5): p. 729-38.

[179] Kim, M.J., et al., Immunohistochemical and clinicopathologic characteristics of invasive ductal carcinoma of breast with micropapillary carcinoma component. Arch Pathol Lab Med, 2005. 129(10): p. 1277-82.

[180] Nassar, H., et al., Pathogenesis of invasive micropapillary carcinoma: role of MUC1 glycoprotein. Mod Pathol, 2004. 17(9): p. 1045-50.

[181] Lee, J.H., et al., The presence of a micropapillary component predicts aggressive behaviour in early and advanced gastric adenocarcinomas. Pathology, 2010. 42(6): p. 560-3.

[182] Sangoi, A.R., et al., Immunohistochemical comparison of MUC1, CA125, and Her2Neu in invasive micropapillary carcinoma of the urinary tract and typical invasive urothelial carcinoma with retraction artifact. Mod Pathol, 2009. 22(5): p. 660-7.

[183] Ohtsuki, Y., et al., KL-6 is another useful marker in assessing a micropapillary pattern in carcinomas of the breast and urinary bladder, but not the colon. Med Mol Morphol, 2009. 42(2): p. 123-7.

[184] Samaratunga, H. and K. Khoo, Micropapillary variant of urothelial carcinoma of the urinary bladder; a clinicopathological and immunohistochemical study. Histopathology, 2004. 45(1): p. 55-64.

[185] Eom, D.W., et al., Gastric micropapillary carcinoma: A distinct subtype with a significantly worse prognosis in TNM stages I and II. Am J Surg Pathol, 2011. 35(1): p. 84-91.

[186] Alvarado-Cabrero, I., et al., Micropapillary carcinoma of the urothelial tract. A clinicopathologic study of 38 cases. Ann Diagn Pathol, 2005. 9(1): p. 1-5.

[187] Kim, M.J., et al., Invasive colorectal micropapillary carcinoma: an aggressive variant of adenocarcinoma. Hum Pathol, 2006. 37(7): p. 809-15.

[188] Haupt, B., et al., Colorectal adenocarcinoma with micropapillary pattern and its association with lymph node metastasis. Mod Pathol, 2007. 20(7): p. 729-33.

[189] Comperat, E., et al., Micropapillary urothelial carcinoma of the urinary bladder: a clinicopathological analysis of 72 cases. Pathology, 2010. 42(7): p. 650-4.

[190] Lotan, T.L., et al., Immunohistochemical panel to identify the primary site of invasive micropapillary carcinoma. Am J Surg Pathol, 2009. 33(7): p. 1037-41.

[191] McQuitty, E., et al., Lymphovascular invasion in micropapillary urothelial carcinoma: a study of 22 cases. Arch Pathol Lab Med, 2012. 136(6): p. 635-9.

[192] Ueyama, H., et al., Gastric adenocarcinoma of fundic gland type (chief cell predominant type): proposal for a new entity of gastric adenocarcinoma. Am J Surg Pathol, 2010. 34(5): p. 609-19.

[193] Singhi, A.D., A.J. Lazenby, and E.A. Montgomery, Gastric adenocarcinoma with chief cell differentiation: a proposal for reclassification as oxyntic gland polyp/adenoma. Am J Surg Pathol, 2012. 36(7): p. 1030-5.

[194] Capella, C., et al., Gastric parietal cell carcinoma--a newly recognized entity: light microscopic and ultrastructural features. Histopathology, 1984. 8(5): p. 813-24.

[195] Takubo, K., et al., Oncocytic adenocarcinoma of the stomach: parietal cell carcinoma. Am J Surg Pathol, 2002. 26(4): p. 458-65.

[196] Yang, G.Y., et al., Parietal cell carcinoma of gastric cardia: immunophenotype and ultrastructure. Ultrastruct Pathol, 2003. 27(2): p. 87-94.

[197] Robey-Cafferty, S.S., J.Y. Ro, and E.G. McKee, Gastric parietal cell carcinoma with an unusual, lymphoma-like histologic appearance: report of a case. Mod Pathol, 1989. 2(5): p. 536-40.

[198] Barbosa, A.J., et al., Parietal cell carcinoma of the stomach and Menetrier's disease. Arq Gastroenterol, 1987. 24(1): p. 36-40.

[199] Byrne, D., M.P. Holley, and A. Cuschieri, Parietal cell carcinoma of the stomach: association with long-term survival after curative resection. Br J Cancer, 1988. 58(1): p. 85-7.

[200] Gaffney, E.F., Favourable prognosis in gastric carcinoma with parietal cell differentiation. Histopathology, 1987. 11(2): p. 217-8.

[201] Hedenbro, J.L., I. Hagerstand, and V. Rychterova, Parietal cell carcinoma. A new differential diagnosis for submucosal gastric tumors. Endoscopy, 1990. 22(1): p. 47-8.

[202] Hayashi, I., et al., Mucoepidermoid carcinoma of the stomach. J Surg Oncol, 1987. 34(2): p. 94-9.

[203] Ooi, A., et al., Predominant Paneth cell differentiation in an intestinal type gastric cancer. Pathol Res Pract, 1991. 187(2-3): p. 220-5.

[204] Lev, R. and T.D. DeNucci, Neoplastic Paneth cells in the stomach. Report of two cases and review of the literature. Arch Pathol Lab Med, 1989. 113(2): p. 129-33.

[205] Inada, K.I., et al., Paneth type gastric cancer cells exhibit expression of human defensin-5. Histopathology, 2005. 47(3): p. 330-1.

[206] Stracca-Pansa, V., et al., Gastric carcinoma with osteoclast-like giant cells. Report of four cases. Am J Clin Pathol, 1995. 103(4): p. 453-9.

[207] Baschinsky, D.Y., W.L. Frankel, and T.H. Niemann, Gastric carcinoma with osteoclast-like giant cells. Am J Gastroenterol, 1999. 94(6): p. 1678-81.

Chapter 9

DNA Methylation in Aggressive Gastric Carcinoma

Chung-Man Leung, Kuo-Wang Tsai and Hung-Wei Pan

Additional information is available at the end of the chapter

http://dx.doi.org/10.5772/52135

1. Introduction

Gastric cancer remains a common cancer type in humans to dates, especially in the Andean region of South America and in the Far East. Various factors contribute to cause of stomach cancer, including *Helicobacter pylori*, smoking and diet. Most patients are diagnosed with advanced gastric cancer, therefore, detailed elucidating mechanisms mediate gastric cancer progression and improving gastric cancer clinic strategies are helpful.

The complex interaction among different etiological factors leads to genetic and epigenetic alterations of proto-oncogenes and tumor-suppressor genes. Epigenetic regulation includes histone modification and DNA methylation, which involved in regulation of cell growth and development in mammals. Global DNA hypomethylation events were discovered in the human tumor in the early 1980s, and promoter hypermethylation of tumor suppressor genes were identified in cancer cells in mid 1990s.

Alteration of DNA methylation in the genome is found in almost types of cancer and can lead to change gene expression, such as over-expression of oncogenes and down-regulation of tumor suppressor genes during cancer progression. Promoter methylation is an alternative mechanism of gene silencing in human tumorigenesis. Although a number of methylated genes have been found in gastric cancer, useful methylation markers for early diagnosis and prognostic evaluation of cancer.

2. Clinical features, epidemiology, pathogenesis and progression of gastric cancer

2.1. Epidemiology

The incidence of stomach cancer is declining in most parts of the world, although it is ranked fourth after lung, breast, and colorectal cancer. A total of 989,600 new stomach cancer cases and 738,000 deaths are estimated to have occurred in 2008, accounting for 8% of total cancer cases and 10% of total cancer-related deaths [1]. The declining incidence is associated with factors related to the increased availability of refrigerated fresh foods and a decline in the consumption of those preserved using salt. The incidence rate varies substantially among countries. High incidence rates occur in East Asia, Eastern Europe, and South America. Regional variations reflect differences in dietary patterns (e.g., low intake of fruits and vegetables, and high intake of salt, nitrates, salt-cured fish, and smoked meat). Several other risk-implicated factors include *Helicobacter pylori* infection, hypochlorhydria, polyps, genetic alteration (e.g., type-A blood, pernicious anemia, *CDH1* mutation, familial gastric cancer, Li-Fraumeni syndrome, and *BRCA1* and *BRCA2*), previous radiation exposure, and prior gastrectomy.

2.2. Pathology

More than 95% of stomach cancers are adenocarcinomas. Other malignant tumors are rare and include carcinoid tumors, squamous cell carcinoma, adenoacanthoma, small cell carcinoma, mucinous carcinoma, and leiomyosarcoma. Although malignant lymphoma of the stomach is a relatively rare stomach neoplasm, it is the most common extranodal site for lymphomas of the gastrointestinal tract. It is potentially associated with *H. pylori* infection because the lymphoid tissue is often stimulated in response to colonization of the lining by *H. pylori* [2]. Furthermore, almost all patients with gastric MALT lymphoma exhibit signs of *H. pylori* infection.

2.3. Staging

There are currently 2 classification systems in use for staging stomach cancer. The Japanese classification is based on anatomic locations and the extent of the regional lymph [3]. The other staging system was developed by the International Union against Cancer and the American Joint Commission on Cancer. Tumor stage is determined based on tumor invasion depth, whereas nodal stage is determined by the number of positive lymph nodes [4]. Advances in diagnostic modalities such as endoscopic ultrasound, computed tomography (CT), positron emission tomography, magnetic resonance imaging (MRI) and laparoscopy have improved preoperative clinical staging. Classification provides useful information for tailoring initial treatment strategies.

2.4. Treatment

Surgery–Complete surgical resection is the primary treatment of early-stage stomach cancer. Gastrectomy and lymphadenopathy are the most widely used approaches, although superficial cancers can occasionally be treated by local endoscopical excision. Resection type (total or subtotal gastrectomy) and the extent of lymphadenectomy depend on the extent, location, and stage of the disease.

Adjuvant treatment–Even patients who present the most favorable condition and undergo curative surgical resection frequently expire from disease recurrence. Adjuvant therapy is commonly conducted using chemotherapy, radiation therapy, or a combination of the two. A significant survival benefit of postoperative adjuvant combined modality therapy using radiotherapy and fluorouracil-based chemotherapy has been shown in several randomized trials [5-7].

Neoadjuvant treatment–Data from several uncontrolled series indicate that some patients with initially unresectable locally advanced disease may respond sufficiently to chemotherapy or chemoradiotherapy and are able to undergo potentially curative surgery. The benefits of preoperative therapy include an increased resectability rate, reduced rate of local and distant recurrences, and improved survival. However, this approach has not been widely adopted, primarily because of a lack of randomized trials that examine its advantages.

2.5. Prognosis

Gastric cancer (GC) is frequently diagnosed at an advanced stage. The prognosis of advanced cancer remains poor. Prognosis has improved only modestly during the previous two decades, attributable to advances in surgical treatment, postoperative care, and multimodal therapy. In the United States, the 5-year survival rate for all stages was 27% between 2001 and 2007, compared to 15% between 1975 and 1977 [8]. Local recurrence and distant metastases are the 2 primary areas of treatment failure in patients. After attempting curative resection, recurrence was local or regional in 40% of cases and distant in 60% [9].

Recent advances in genomic science have enabled the identification of detailed molecular mechanisms of stomach carcinogenesis and its progression. These techniques have been used to identify markers for early detection of stomach cancer. A better knowledge of the molecular bases will lead to new paradigms and potential therapeutic improvements. It can provide better information on potential tumor aggressiveness and assist in the personalization of treatment strategies for better outcomes.

3. Principle of DNA epigenetic modification, DNA methylation and detection

3.1. Genomic DNA methylation/demethylation

3.1.1. DNA methylation

Epigenetic regulation, including histone modification and DNA methylation, has a critical role in regulating cell growth and development in mammals [10, 11]. DNA methylation involves the regulation of gene expression by establishing and maintaining DNA methylation status at the promoter of critical genes. DNA methyltransferases (DNMTs) catalyze the covalent addition of methyl groups to 5-position of cytosine (5-methylcytosine; 5mC) bases in newly synthesized DNA (Fig. 1. Cytosine of CpG dinucleotides can be methylated by

DNMTs to form 5mC, which use S-adenosyl methionine as a donor for the methyl group. In mammalian cells, DNMTs genes are classified into de novo (DNMT3A and DNMT3B) and maintenance (DNMT1), and function in printing methylation genome maps [11]. DNMT1 is highly expressed in differentiated cells and efficiently hemi-methylated DNA during DNA replication. DNMT3A and DNMT3B are most abundant in embryonic stem cells and have low expressions in differentiated cells [12].

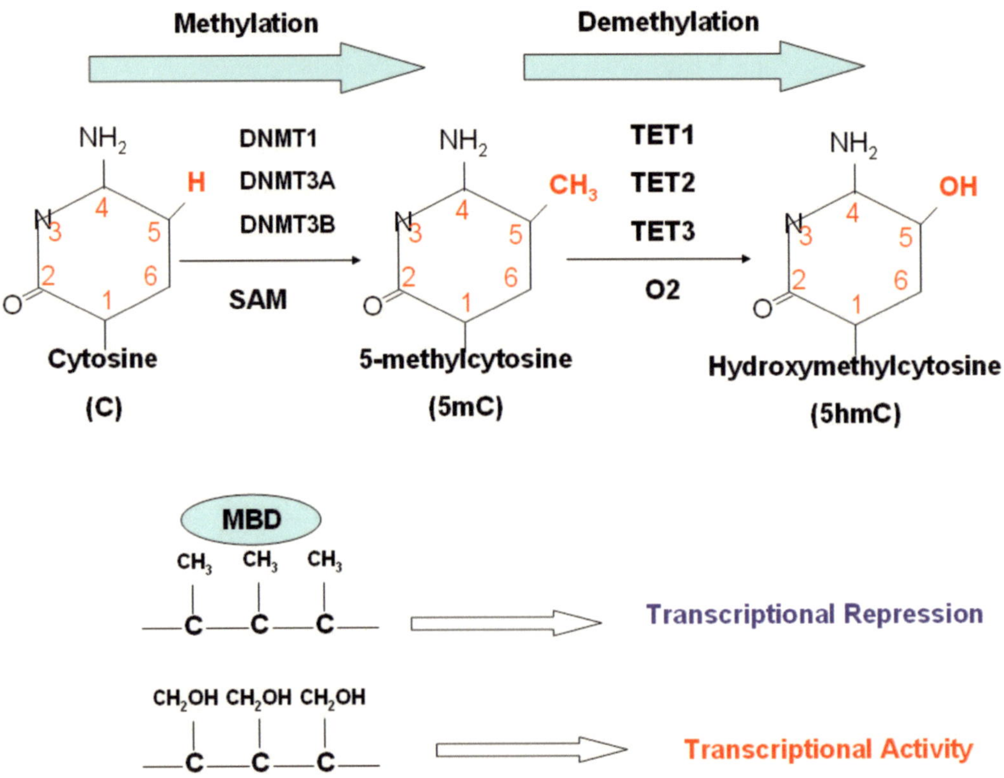

Figure 1. Schematic diagram depicting genomic DNA methylation and demethylation in cytosine

3.1.2. DNA demethylation

Tahiliani et al. [13] identified the leading enzyme (ten-eleven-translocation, TET) that can convert 5mC to 5-hydroxymethylcytosine (5hmC). Three TET proteins (TET1, TET2, and TET3) can convert 5mC to (5hmC), leading to DNA demethylation [14]. 5hmC is a potentially key intermediate in a possible active DNA demethylation process through DNA repair mechanisms. 5hmC is generated from oxidized 5mC, and has a critical role in stem/progenitor cell differentiation [11, 15-23]. The role of 5hmC in gene regulation is a crucial issue that is potentially associated with gastric cancer progression; however, its biological function in gastric cancer is unknown.

3.2. DNA methylation-regulated genes in gastric cancer

3.2.1. Protein coding genes

Global DNA hypomethylation events that occur primarily at DNA-repetitive regions and hypermethylation at specific promoter CpG islands of tumor suppressor genes are frequently observed in human tumors [10]. In gastric cancer, DNA methylation contributes to cancer progression and leads to aberrantly silencing expression of tumor suppressor genes, or oncogene reactivation [24]. Park et al.[25] profiled a global DNA methylation of gastric cancer using a methylated DNA enrichment technique and performed an analysis using a next-generation sequence approach. Gastric cancer was associated with hypermethylation of 5' CpG islands and the 5'-end of protein-coding genes, as well as hypomethylation of DNA-repetitive elements. During recent decades, a gain or loss of DNA methylation at the promoter of protein-coding gene events has been continuously studied. Numerous studies have implicated an aberrant expression of methylation-associated genes involved in the pathogenesis of gastric cancer (Table 1). E (epithelial)-cadherin gene promoter hypermethylation has frequently been observed in human gastric cancers, and methylation status has been associated with deceased expression in gastric carcinogenesis [26]. Sudo et al. also reported that promoter methylation-mediated silencing of the E-cadherin gene was closely associated with the development of Epstein-Barr virus-associated gastric carcinoma [27]. Similarly, several studies have shown that the accumulation of DNA methylation in promoter regions of tumor suppressor genes may alter cell cycle, growth, and motility, as well as adhesion molecules by silencing critical gene expression (including p16, p15, DAPK, RUNX3, MLH1, Table 1). In contrast to tumor suppressor genes, loss of DNA methylation has frequently occurred in oncogene promoter regions and leads to aberrant overexpression in gastric cancer, such as S100A6, S100A4, VEGF-C, PAR2, SNCG, and MAGE-A1-3 (Table 1).

	Gene name	Ref.
Protein-coding genes	CXCL12, CDH1, ZNF331, EDNRB, SOX9, PTPN6, MOS, DCC, CRK, VAV1, MLF1, MGMT, p16, RASSF2, hMLH1, HAND1, HRASLS, TM, FLNc, ALX4, TMEFF2, CHCHD10, IGFBP3, NPR1, GKN1, RASAL1, PAX5, SFRP1, GPX3, ADAMTS9, S100A6, EphA1, p14, DAPK, WWOX, TCF4, RUNX3, CHFR, RECK, BMP3, HACE1, PGP9.5, APC, VIM, MGMT, PTCH1a, RASSF2A, S100A4, PKD1, TMS1, RUNX3, ER, p15, EphA7, NID1, NID2, HHIP, VEGF-C, FHIT, MTAP, PLAGL1, PAR2, DFNA5, RASSF1A, CTNNB1, MTSS1, LIMS2, SNCG, MAGE-A1, MAGE-A2, MAGE-A3, CASP1, COX-2, Syk, ITGA1, SOCS-1, SERPINB5, PTEN	[40, 45-47, 51, 54, 57, 60, 61, 65, 75-112]
Small nonprotein-coding genes	miR-1,miR-9, miR-10b, miR-18b, miR-34b/c, miR-124a, miR-129, miR-137, miR-148a, miR-152, miR-155, miR-181c, miR-196b, miR-203, miR212, miR512, miR-516a	[29, 34, 35, 38, 39, 113-123]

The underline indicates that genes overexpressed with promoter hypomethylation in gastric cancer.

Table 1. Genes aberrantly expressed with hypo/hypermethylated promoter in gastric cancer.

3.2.2. microRNA

MicroRNAs (miRNAs) are endogenous non-protein-coding RNAs of short 21-23 nucleotides [28]. Abnormal miRNA expression has a critical role in gastric cancer progression. However, miRNA transcription mechanisms are similar to classic protein-coding genes; the hypermethylated promoter region of tumor-suppressive miRNAs may result in gastric cancer formation and progression. Our previous studies identified several methylation-associated miRNAs through AGS treated with a demethylation agent [29, 30]. Among these miRNAs, we first observed a primate-specific miRNA cluster (C19MC) comprising 46 pre-miRNAs, which could be co-regulated depending on the methylation status of its distal CpG-rich domain in placenta tissue [30, 31]. C19MC expression has been shown to display a maternal-specific methylation imprint acquired in oocytes [31]. We also recently identified several tumor-suppressive miRNA that were regulated with aberrant DNA methylation in gastric cancer (Figure 2). Expression of miR-1, miR-9, miR-129, and miR-34b/c was suppressed by DNA hypermethylation, and miR-196b was overexpressed with hypomethylation in gastric cancer [29, 32-35]. Numerous other studies have shown that several tumor-suppressive miRNAs contain the aberrant hypermethylation of their promoter regions in gastric cancer, including miR-9, miR-34b/c, miR-129, miR-137, miR-181c, miR-199a, miR-212, miR-512, and miR-516 [29, 30, 34-40].

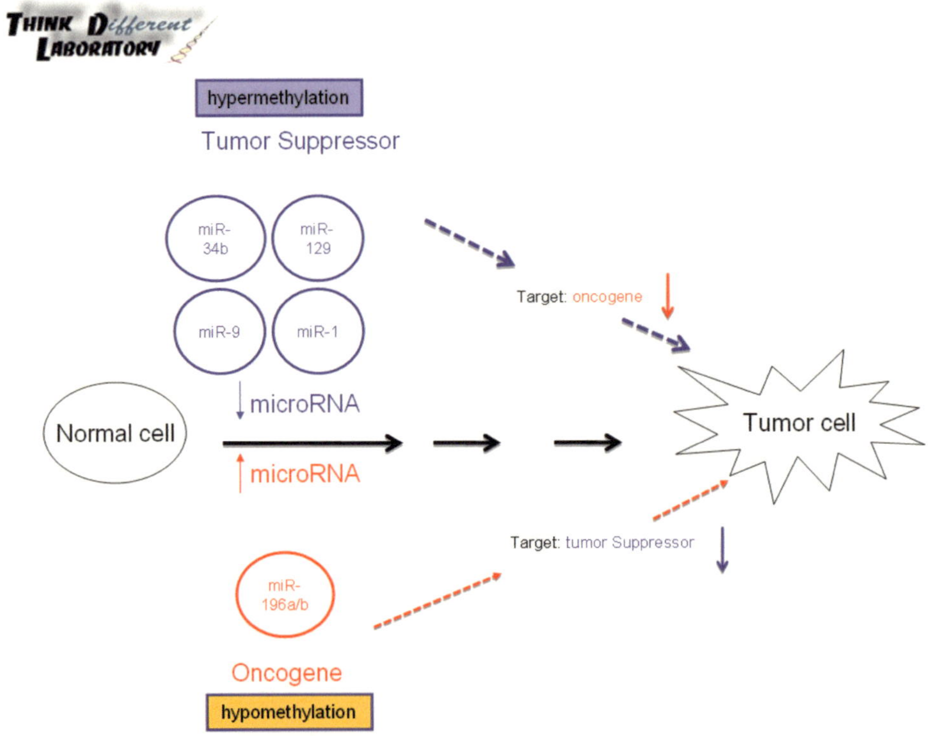

Figure 2. Schematic diagram depicting DNA hypo-/hypermethylation resulted miRNAs dysregulation in gastric cancer according our recent studies.

4. Promoter methylation of given genes versus clinical significance and prognostic values and therapeutic applications

Promoter methylation is an alternative mechanism of gene silencing in human tumorigenesis. Although a number of methylated genes have been observed in gastric cancer, useful methylation markers for early diagnosis and prognostic evaluation of gastric cancer remain unknown [41, 42]. Although the clinical outcome of gastric cancer has gradually improved, the prognosis of patients at the advanced stage remains poor. The prognosis varies widely in gastric cancer patients for undetermined biologic reasons. Thus, a greater understanding of the pathogenesis and molecular mechanisms of gastric cancer may lead to novel diagnostic, therapeutic, and preventive strategies [41, 43]. Gastric carcinogenesis is a multistep process that includes numerous genetic and epigenetic alterations, such as activation of oncogenes, overexpression of growth factors and receptors, and inactivation of tumor suppressor genes. In addition to genetic alterations, epigenetic alterations such as DNA methylation of CpG islands are involved in cancer development and progression. Promoter methylation is regarded as one of the primary mechanisms to inactivate tumor-related genes, along with gene mutation and deletions, ultimately leading to carcinogenesis. Promoter methylation is a critical hallmark of cancer cells, and has a significant role in tumor transformation and progression, impacting the clinical course of the disease. Although promoter methylation of a number of cancer-related genes, including tumor suppressor genes, has been observed in gastric cancer and precancerous lesions, epigenetic inactivation of genes related to tumor initiation and progression has not been well studied in gastric cancer outcome [41].

4.1. Gene methylation and its impact on clinical outcome in gastric cancer

Using methylation-specific polymerase chain reactions (MSP) and quantitative methylation-specific polymerase chain reactions (Q-MSP), the promoter methylation of specific genes is examined, as well as their association with clinical outcomes of gastric cancer. Inactivation of tumor suppressor genes and activation of oncogenes caused by genetic and epigenetic alterations are known to play a significant role in carcinogenesis. An increasing amount of evidence shows that epigenetic silencing of the tumor suppressor genes, particularly caused by hypermethylation of CpG islands in promoters, is critical to carcinogenesis and metastasis. Here, we detail recent progress in the study of methylations of tumor suppressor genes involved in the pathogenesis of gastric cancer.

CDH1 E-cadherin is a cell adhesion molecule considered a potential invasion/metastasis suppressor and is mutationally inactivated in almost half of all undifferentiated-scattered (diffuse-type) gastric carcinomas. In addition, silencing of E-cadherin by CpG methylation within its promoter region has been reported in several gastric carcinoma cell lines. Hypermethylation of the E-cadherin promoter was evident in 30%-55% of primary gastric carcinomas [26, 44-47] and occurred more frequently in carcinomas of the undifferentiated-scattered type (in 15 of 18, 83%) than in other histologic subtypes (34%), and it was present at similar rates in early (60%) versus advanced (49%) carcinomas [26]. E-cadherin methylation was present in 31% of gastric mucosae from dyspeptic patients, and was associated with *H. pylori* infection, although this is independent of the age of the patient or presence or absence of gastritis. E-cadherin methylation was present in 0% of normal mucosa, 57% of intestinal metaplasias, and 58% of primary and 65% of metastatic cancers. E-cadherin methylation status was concordant in 92% of intestinal metaplasias and primary cancers, and in 85% of primary and metastatic cancers from the same resected specimen. E-cadherin methylation in gastric cancer was associated with depth of tumor invasion and regional nodal metastasis [48]. By examining the relationship between molecular changes in E-cadherin and metastasis in early gastric carcinoma (EGC), Yi Kim et al. showed that 45.0% of 60 primary EGCs exhibited methylation in the CpG island of E-cadherin. Abnormal expression of E-cadherin was significantly correlated with patient age, tumor size, Lauren classification, differentiation, and lymph node metastasis [49]. Therefore, the E-cadherin promoter frequently undergoes hypermethylation in human gastric cancers, particularly those of the undifferentiated-scattered histologic subtype. E-cadherin promoter hypermethylation is associated with decreased expression and may occur during early stages of gastric cancer. Inactivation of E-cadherin might be involved in metastasis in EGC and play an important role in microscopic differentiation.

DAPK Death-associated protein kinase (DAP-kinase) is a serine/threonine kinase and a positive mediator of apoptosis. Downregulation of DAP-kinase is associated with an increased metastatic potential of tumors. Gene promoter hypermethylation could lead to downregulation of DAP-kinase. Methylation status was assessed by MSP. In total, 69.2% of GC demonstrated promoter methylation of DAP-kinase. Methylation of DAP-kinase was observed in intestinal, diffuse, and mixed types of GC. It also occurred in similar frequencies among antral, body, and cardiac gastric cancer. No association between methylation status and age or sex was demonstrated. However, the methylated cases were correlated with the presence of nodal metastasis, advance stage of disease, and a poorer event-free survival. DAP-kinase promoter methylation as a potential prognostic marker for gastric cancer patients deserved further evaluation [50]. Aberrant methylation of DAPK genes was detected in 22% of tumors. Kato et al. examined 43 patients treated by 5-fluorouracil-based chemotherapy, who had distant metastasis or recurrence after radical resection, to determine the relation between chemosensitivity and methylation. The response rate was lower in patients with either DAPK methylation than without (21% vs. 45%). Overall survival tended to be shorter in patients with both methylations compared with either or no methylation. The time to progression of patients with methylation of DAPK was significantly shorter than of patients without methylation. In conclusion, DAPK methylation might predict the prognosis and response to chemotherapy in gastric cancer [51].

CHFR Checkpoint with fork head-associated and ring finger (CHFR) governs the transition from prophase to prometaphase in response to mitotic stress. MSP and combined bisulfite restriction analysis (COBRA) are both used in detecting aberrant methylation of the CHFR gene in gastric cancer. The methylation rates of the CHFR gene promoter were significantly higher in gastric cancer samples than in the corresponding para cancer normal gastric mucosa by MSP (52% vs. 19%). However, there was no significant correlation between methylation status of the CHFR gene and the clinicopathologic parameters of gastric cancer, including age, sex, tumor size, clinical stage, Borrmann type, tumor invasion depth, differentiation, and lymph node metastasis. Aberrant methylation of the CHFR gene was detected in 42% of gastric cancer specimens using COBRA and MSP. Therefore, aberrant methylation of the CHFR gene is a frequent event in the carcinogenesis of gastric cancer. Detecting the methylation of the CHFR gene in gastric mucosa may be conducive to the diagnosis of gastric cancer [52, 53]. However, the frequency of DAPK and CHFR methylation in cancer tissues was significantly associated with the extent of differentiation and lymph node metastasis. DAPK and CHFR promoter hypermethylation may be critical in evaluating the differentiation grade and lymph node status of gastric cancer. Weak gene expression and loss of gene expression caused by promoter hypermethylation may be a cancer-specific event [54, 55].

RUNX3 Runt-related transcription factor 3 (RUNX3) is a novel tumor suppressor gene that is frequently silenced by promoter hypermethylation in gastric cancer. Sakakura et al. observed significant downregulation of RUNX3 through methylation on the promoter region in primary tumors (75%), as well as in all clinical peritoneal metastases of gastric cancers (100%), compared with normal gastric mucosa. Stable transfection of RUNX3 inhibited cell proliferation slightly, and modest transforming growth factor-beta (TGF-beta)-induced antiproliferative and apoptotic effects were observed. RUNX3 significantly inhibited peritoneal metastases of gastric cancers in animals. Microarray analysis identified approximately 28 candidate genes under the possible downstream control of RUNX3, some of which were considered to be potentially involved in peritoneal metastases, which were related to signal transduction, apoptosis, immune responses, and cell adhesion. Some of the genes are involved in the TGF-beta signaling pathway. These results indicate that silencing of RUNX3 affects the expression of important genes involved in aspects of metastasis, including cell adhesion, proliferation, apoptosis, and promoting the peritoneal metastasis of gastric cancer. Identification of such genes could indicate novel therapeutic modalities and therapeutic targets [56]. In other studies, overall, 55% of GC demonstrated methylation of the RUNX3 promoter; 82% of GC was classified as stable microsatellite instability, 5% as low-level microsatellite instability and 13% as high-level microsatellite instability (MSI-H); and mitochondrial microsatellite instability (mtMSI) was detected in 11% of GC. A significant association was found between mtMSI and tumor-node-metastasis staging. Furthermore, an interesting association among the MSI-H status, mtMSI, and RUNX3 methylation. These data suggest that RUNX3 is an important target of methylation in the evolution of mtMSI and nuclear microsatellite instability (nMSI-H) [57].

p16 The INK4a/ARF locus encodes 2 cell cycle-regulatory proteins: p16INK4a and p14ARF. Silencing of p16INK4a and p14ARF expressions by aberrant methylation of the CpG islands in the promoter regions has recently been observed to be an alternative mechanism that inactivates possible tumor suppressor functions in various tumors. Of 10 cell lines studied, silencing of the expression of p16INK4a and p14ARF caused by the detection of promoter methylation by MSP and RT-PCR in 6 (60%) and 2 (20%) cell lines, respectively. p14ARF silencing was detected only in cell lines derived from gastric cancer of the diffuse type, whereas p16INK4a silencing was found in cell lines derived from both diffuse and intestinal types. In primary gastric cancers, promoter methylation of p16INK4a and p14ARF was found in 17% and 24% of the tumors independently. Whereas p14ARF methylation was observed more frequently in intestinal type cancers in an early stage and in diffuse type cancers in an advanced stage, MSI tended to be related especially to p14ARF methylation in cancers of the intestinal type. Thus, the significance of p14ARF methylation differed between intestinal and diffuse types, and such a difference was not observed in p16INK4a methylation [58]. Aberrant p16 methylation was observed in 38% of primary gastric cancers, but in none of the corresponding gastric mucosae [59]. When carcinoma specimens were compared with adjacent normal gastric mucosa samples, a significant increase in promoter methylation of p16, Runx3, DAPK, and CHFR was observed, whereas all 30 histologically normal gastric specimens were methylation-free for all 4 genes. The methylation rate of the 4 genes increased from normal stomach tissue to tumor-adjacent gastric mucosa to gastric cancer tissue [54].

4.2. Hypermethylation profiling

DNA methylation has been studied extensively in gastric cancer. However, most studies have focused on aberrant methylation in a single gene. Because methylated genes rarely occur more frequently in groups than in isolation, the concept of a CpG island methylator phenotype (CIMP) in gastric. CIMP has been defined as a subset of malignancies that show widespread hypermethylation of multiple promoter CpG island loci [60].

More recently, microarray technology has made it possible to comprehensively analyze gene expression profiles [56, 61-64]. Representational difference analysis (RDA) is also used to screen differentially methylated DNA sequences between gastric primary tumor and metastatic lymph nodes [65, 66]. By using these techniques, the expression levels of thousands of genes can be analyzed in a single experiment. These technologies are a powerful tool for analyzing gene expression profiles related to the development and progression of specific diseases. Although there have been significant improvements in the analysis of genetic alterations for gastric cancer, there is insufficient information on understanding a common pathway for the development and progression of gastric cancer. Gastric cancer has diverse clinical properties such as histological type, metastatic status, race, and sex. Thus, further exploration to search for genetic alterations in gastric cancer is required.

5. Cirulating DNA methylation as biomarkers

Previous studies have demonstrated that tumor cells can release DNA to peripheral blood and enriched circulating DNA level can be observed in the serum of cancer patients, several times higher than the reference range. Previous studies have detected methylated DNA of multiple gene promoters in blood plasma, urine, sputum and peritoneal washes in several different cancers, and high-frequency hypermethylation of tumor suppression is mostly cancer-specific; therefore, it may be used as a molecular diagnostic marker of cancer [67-74].

Numerous studies have attempted to detect circulating methylated DNA from body fluid as a good biomarker for prognosis and diagnosis of gastric carcinoma (Table 2). Detection of promoter regions hypermethylation of candidate genes FAM5C, MYLK, RUNX3, TFP12, RASSF1A, p16 and CDH1 in the serum have been applied to predict the clinical features of gastric cancer patients. Furthermore, DNA methylation of BNIP3, CHFR, CYP1B1, MINT25, SFRP2, RASSF2, p16, RUNX3, CDH1, hMLH1, ABCG2, BNIP3, and RECK in peritoneal fluid form gastric cancer patients has been analyzed using quantitative methylation-specific polymerase chain reaction and as a good biomarker for the diagnosis and detection of gastric cancer. Thus, circulating methylated DNA can reflect the real methylation status of candidate gene promoters in gastric cancer tissue by examining body fluid. Therefore, releasing methylated DNA fragments has a high potential as a novel biomarker for the detection and recurrence monitoring of gastric cancer.

Body fluid	Gene name	Ref.
serum	FAM5C, MYLK, RUNX3, TFP12, RASSF1A, p16, CDH1, DAPK, GSTP1, p15	[120, 124-127]
Peritoneal fluid	BNIP3, CHFR, CYP1B1, MINT25, SFRP2, RASSF2, p16, RUNX3, CDH1, hMLH1, ABCG2, BNIP3, RECK	[55, 120, 128, 129]

Table 2. The aberrant DNA methylation of gene promoter in body fluid is a promising biomarker for gastric cancer

6. Conclusion

Gastric cancer is one of the leading causes of cancer-related death in China. Although the molecular mechanisms of gastric carcinogenesis are unclear, epigenetic silencing of tumor-related genes by promoter hypermethylation has recently emerged as a crucial mechanism of tumorigenesis. The promoter hypermethylation profile differs among cancer types and within each gene, providing tumor type- and gene-specific hypermethylation profiles that may be involved in the corresponding molecular mechanism of tumorigenesis. The identification of a novel gene targeted by promoter hypermethylation may provide insights into mechanisms for the inactivation of tumor-suppressive pathways and is critical for the identification of tumor markers in gastric cancer [42, 43]. Currently, DNA methylation markers have been used in early detection, prognosis, and prediction of response to cancer therapy.

Acknowledgements

This work was supported by the grants from the Kaohsiung Veterans General Hospital Research Program, Kaohsiung, Republic of China, Taiwan (VGHKS100-124 to Hung-Wei Pan, VGHKS100-058 to Chung-Man Leung, and VGHKS101-010 to Kuo-Wang Tsai).

Author details

Chung-Man Leung[1], Kuo-Wang Tsai[2] and Hung-Wei Pan[2*]

*Address all correspondence to: E-mail: hwpan@vghks.gov.tw

1 Department of Radiation Oncology, Kaohsiung Veterans General Hospital, Kaohsiung, Taiwan, Republic of China

2 Department of Medical Education and Research, Kaohsiung Veterans General Hospital, Kaohsiung, Taiwan, Republic of China

References

[1] Jemal, A., et al., Global cancer statistics. CA Cancer J Clin, 2011. 61(2): p. 69-90.

[2] Kusters, J.G., A.H. van Vliet, and E.J. Kuipers, Pathogenesis of Helicobacter pylori infection. Clin Microbiol Rev, (2006). , 449-490.

[3] Japanese classification of gastric carcinoma: 3rd English edition. Gastric Cancer, (2011). , 101-112.

[4] Edge, S.B. and C.C. Compton, The American Joint Committee on Cancer: the 7th edition of the AJCC cancer staging manual and the future of TNM. Ann Surg Oncol, (2010). , 1471-1474.

[5] Dent, D.M., et al., Prospective randomized trial of combined oncological therapy for gastric carcinoma. Cancer(1979). , 385-391.

[6] Macdonald, J.S., et al., Chemoradiotherapy after surgery compared with surgery alone for adenocarcinoma of the stomach or gastroesophageal junction. N Engl J Med, (2001). , 725-730.

[7] Moertel, C.G., et al., Combined 5-fluorouracil and radiation therapy as a surgical adjuvant for poor prognosis gastric carcinoma. J Clin Oncol, (1984). , 1249-1254.

[8] Siegel, R., D. Naishadham, and A. Jemal, Cancer statistics, 2012. CA Cancer J Clin, 2012. 62(1): p. 10-29.

[9] Wanebo, H.J., et al., Cancer of the stomach. A patient care study by the American College of Surgeons. Ann Surg, 1993. 218(5): p. 583-92.

[10] Esteller, M., Cancer Epigenetics for the 21st Century: What's Next? Genes Cancer, (2011). , 604-606.

[11] Dahl, C., K. Gronbaek, and P. Guldberg, Advances in DNA methylation: 5-hydroxymethylcytosine revisited. Clin Chim Acta, 2011. 412(11-12): p. 831-6.

[12] Goll, M.G. and T.H. Bestor, Eukaryotic cytosine methyltransferases. Annu Rev Biochem, (2005). , 481-514.

[13] Tahiliani, M., et al., Conversion of 5-methylcytosine to 5-hydroxymethylcytosine in mammalian DNA by MLL partner TET1. Science(2009). , 930-935.

[14] Cliffe, L.J., et al., JBP1 and JBP2 are two distinct thymidine hydroxylases involved in J biosynthesis in genomic DNA of African trypanosomes. Nucleic Acids Res, 2009. 37(5): p. 1452-62.

[15] Cimmino, L., et al., TET family proteins and their role in stem cell differentiation and transformation. Cell Stem Cell(2011). , 193-204.

[16] Ficz, G., et al., Dynamic regulation of 5-hydroxymethylcytosine in mouse ES cells and during differentiation. Nature(2011). , 398-402.

[17] Gu, T.P., et al., The role of Tet3 DNA dioxygenase in epigenetic reprogramming by oocytes. Nature(2011). , 606-610.

[18] Guo, J.U., et al., Emerging roles of TET proteins and 5-hydroxymethylcytosines in active DNA demethylation and beyond. Cell Cycle(2011). , 2662-2668.

[19] Zhao, J.J., et al., Identification of LZAP as a new candidate tumor suppressor in hepatocellular carcinoma. PLoS One, (2011). , e26608.

[20] Ito, S., et al., Role of Tet proteins in 5mC to 5hmC conversion, ES-cell self-renewal and inner cell mass specification. Nature(2011). , 1129-1133.

[21] Ito, S., et al., Tet proteins can convert 5-methylcytosine to 5-formylcytosine and 5-carboxylcytosine. Science(2011). , 1300-1303.

[22] Jin, S.G., et al., Genomic mapping of 5-hydroxymethylcytosine in the human brain. Nucleic Acids Res, (2011). , 5015-5024.

[23] Pastor, W.A., et al., Genome-wide mapping of 5-hydroxymethylcytosine in embryonic stem cells. Nature(2011). , 394-397.

[24] Gigek, C.O., et al., Epigenetic mechanisms in gastric cancer. Epigenomics, 2012. 4(3): p. 279-94.

[25] Park, J.H., et al., Identification of DNA methylation changes associated with human gastric cancer. BMC Med Genomics, (2011). , 82.

[26] Tamura, G., et al., E-Cadherin gene promoter hypermethylation in primary human gastric carcinomas. J Natl Cancer Inst, (2000). , 569-573.

[27] Sudo, M., et al., Promoter hypermethylation of E-cadherin and its abnormal expression in Epstein-Barr virus-associated gastric carcinoma. Int J Cancer, (2004). , 194-199.

[28] Kim, V.N., Small RNAs: classification, biogenesis, and function. Mol Cells, 2005. 19(1): p. 1-15.

[29] Tsai, K.W., et al., Epigenetic regulation of miR-196b expression in gastric cancer. Genes Chromosomes Cancer, (2010)., 49(11):969-980.

[30] Tsai, K.W., et al., Epigenetic control of the expression of a primate-specific micro-RNA cluster in human cancer cells. Epigenetics (2009)., 4(8):587-592.

[31] Noguer-Dance, M., et al., The primate-specific microRNA gene cluster (C19MC) is imprinted in the placenta. Hum Mol Genet, (2010)., 3566-3582.

[32] Chen, W.S., et al., Silencing of miR-1-1 and miR-133a-2 cluster expression by DNA hypermethylation in colorectal cancer. Oncol Rep, (2012)., 1069-1076.

[33] Liao, Y.L., et al., Transcriptional regulation of miR-196b by ETS2 in gastric cancer cells. Carcinogenesis(2012)., 760-769.

[34] Tsai, K.W., et al., Aberrant hypermethylation of miR-9 genes in gastric cancer. Epigenetics, (2011). 6(10):1189-97

[35] Tsai, K.W., et al., Epigenetic regulation of miR-34b and miR-129 expression in gastric cancer. Int J Cancer, (2011)., 2600-2610.

[36] Cheung, H.H., et al., Methylation of an intronic region regulates miR-199a in testicular tumor malignancy. Oncogene(2011).

[37] Saito, Y., et al., Chromatin remodeling at Alu repeats by epigenetic treatment activates silenced microRNA-512-5p with downregulation of Mcl-1 in human gastric cancer cells. Oncogene(2009)., 2738-2744.

[38] Shen, R., et al., Epigenetic repression of microRNA-129-2 leads to overexpression of SOX4 in gastric cancer. Biochem Biophys Res Commun, (2010)., 1047-1052.

[39] Suzuki, H., et al., (2010). Methylation-associated silencing of microRNA-34b/c in gastric cancer and its involvement in an epigenetic field defect. Carcinogenesis, 2066-2073.

[40] Chen, X.R., et al., Role of BMP3 in progression of gastric carcinoma in Chinese people. World J Gastroenterol, (2010)., 1409-1413.

[41] Yao, D., et al., Quantitative assessment of gene methylation and their impact on clinical outcome in gastric cancer. Clin Chim Acta, (2012)., 787-794.

[42] Lee, J.H., et al., Frequent CpG island methylation in precursor lesions and early gastric adenocarcinomas. Oncogene(2004)., 4646-4654.

[43] Kang, G.H., et al., Profile of aberrant CpG island methylation along multistep gastric carcinogenesis. Lab Invest, (2003)., 519-526.

[44] Corn, P.G., et al., Frequent hypermethylation of the 5' CpG island of E-cadherin in esophageal adenocarcinoma. Clin Cancer Res, 2001. 7(9): p. 2765-9.

[45] Du, P., et al., Methylation of PTCH1a gene in a subset of gastric cancers. World J Gastroenterol, (2009)., 3799-3806.

[46] Tahara, T., et al., CpG island promoter methylation (CIHM) status of tumor suppressor genes correlates with morphological appearances of gastric cancer. Anticancer Res, (2010). , 239-244.

[47] Tahara, T., et al., Chronic aspirin use suppresses CDH1 methylation in human gastric mucosa. Dig Dis Sci, (2010). , 54-59.

[48] Chan, A.O., et al., Promoter methylation of E-cadherin gene in gastric mucosa associated with Helicobacter pylori infection and in gastric cancer. Gut, (2003). , 502-506.

[49] Yi Kim, D., et al., E-cadherin expression in early gastric carcinoma and correlation with lymph node metastasis. J Surg Oncol, (2007). , 429-435.

[50] Chan, A.W., et al., Promoter hypermethylation of Death-associated protein-kinase gene associated with advance stage gastric cancer. Oncol Rep, (2005). , 937-941.

[51] Kato, K., et al., Methylated TMS1 and DAPK genes predict prognosis and response to chemotherapy in gastric cancer. Int J Cancer, (2008). , 603-608.

[52] Cheng, Z.D., et al., Promoter methylation of CHFR gene in gastric carcinoma tissues detected using two methods. Chin J Cancer, (2010). , 163-166.

[53] Hiraki, M., et al., Aberrant gene methylation in the lymph nodes provides a possible marker for diagnosing micrometastasis in gastric cancer. Ann Surg Oncol, (2010). , 1177-1186.

[54] Hu, S.L., et al., Promoter methylation of p16, Runx3, DAPK and CHFR genes is frequent in gastric carcinoma. Tumori, (2010). , 726-733.

[55] Hiraki, M., et al., Aberrant gene methylation in the peritoneal fluid is a risk factor predicting peritoneal recurrence in gastric cancer. World J Gastroenterol, (2010). , 330-338.

[56] Sakakura, C., et al., Possible involvement of RUNX3 silencing in the peritoneal metastases of gastric cancers. Clin Cancer Res, (2005). , 6479-6488.

[57] Gargano, G., et al., Aberrant methylation within RUNX3 CpG island associated with the nuclear and mitochondrial microsatellite instability in sporadic gastric cancers. Results of a GOIM (Gruppo Oncologico dell'Italia Meridionale) prospective study. Ann Oncol, (2007). Suppl 6: , vi103-vi109.

[58] Tsujimoto, H., et al., Promoter methylations of p16INK4a and p14ARF genes in early and advanced gastric cancer. Correlations of the modes of their occurrence with histologic type. Pathol Res Pract, (2002). , 785-794.

[59] Kanyama, Y., et al., Detection of p16 promoter hypermethylation in serum of gastric cancer patients. Cancer Sci, (2003). , 418-420.

[60] Chen, H.Y., et al., High CpG island methylator phenotype is associated with lymph node metastasis and prognosis in gastric cancer. Cancer Sci, (2012). , 73-79.

[61] Zhang, X., et al., An 8-gene signature, including methylated and down-regulated glutathione peroxidase 3, of gastric cancer. Int J Oncol, 2010. 36(2): p. 405-14.

[62] Chen, J., et al., Microarray analysis of gene expression in metastatic gastric cancer cells after incubation with the methylation inhibitor 5-aza-2'-deoxycytidine. Clin Exp Metastasis, (2004). , 389-397.

[63] Yamashita, S., et al., Chemical genomic screening for methylation-silenced genes in gastric cancer cell lines using 5-aza-2'-deoxycytidine treatment and oligonucleotide microarray. Cancer Sci, (2006). , 64-71.

[64] Terashima, M., et al., Gene expression profiles in human gastric cancer: expression of maspin correlates with lymph node metastasis. Br J Cancer, (2005). , 1130-1136.

[65] Wang, J.F. and D.Q. Dai, Metastatic suppressor genes inactivated by aberrant methylation in gastric cancer. World J Gastroenterol, (2007). , 5692-5698.

[66] Wang, J.F. and D.Q. Dai, [Difference in methylation of genomic DNA between gastric primary cancer and lymph nodes with metastatic gastric cancer]. Zhonghua Yi Xue Za Zhi(2006). , 536-539.

[67] Balch, C., et al., Minireview: epigenetic changes in ovarian cancer. Endocrinology, 2009. 150(9): p. 4003-11.

[68] Bremnes, R.M., R. Sirera, and C. Camps, Circulating tumour-derived DNA and RNA markers in blood: a tool for early detection, diagnostics, and follow-up? Lung Cancer, 2005. 49(1): p. 1-12.

[69] Fleischhacker, M. and B. Schmidt, Circulating nucleic acids (CNAs) and cancer--a survey. Biochim Biophys Acta, 2007. 1775(1): p. 181-232.

[70] Giasuddin, A.S., K.A. Jhuma, and A.M. Haq, Applications of free circulating nucleic acids in clinical medicine: recent advances. Bangladesh Med Res Counc Bull, (2008). , 26-32.

[71] Patel, A., J.D. Groopman, and A. Umar, DNA methylation as a cancer-specific biomarker: from molecules to populations. Ann N Y Acad Sci, 2003. 983: p. 286-97.

[72] Vlassov, V.V., P.P. Laktionov, and E.Y. Rykova, Circulating nucleic acids as a potential source for cancer biomarkers. Curr Mol Med, (2010). , 142-165.

[73] Xue, X., Y.M. Zhu, and P.J. Woll, Circulating DNA and lung cancer. Ann N Y Acad Sci, 2006. 1075: p. 154-64.

[74] Ziegler, A., U. Zangemeister-Wittke, and R.A. Stahel, Circulating DNA: a new diagnostic gold mine? Cancer Treat Rev, 2002. 28(5): p. 255-71.

[75] Tao, K., et al., Quantitative analysis of promoter methylation of the EDNRB gene in gastric cancer. Med Oncol, (2012). , 107-112.

[76] Shi, J., et al., Prognostic significance of aberrant gene methylation in gastric cancer. Am J Cancer Res, (2012). , 116-129.

[77] Yoon, J.H., et al., Inactivation of the Gastrokine 1 gene in gastric adenomas and carcinomas. J Pathol, (2011). , 618-625.

[78] Seto, M., et al., Reduced expression of RAS protein activator like-1 in gastric cancer. Int J Cancer, (2011). , 1293-1302.

[79] Li, X., et al., Epigenetic inactivation of paired box gene 5, a novel tumor suppressor gene, through direct upregulation of p53 is associated with prognosis in gastric cancer patients. Oncogene, 2012. 31(29): p. 3419-30.

[80] Kinoshita, T., et al., Decreased expression and aberrant hypermethylation of the SFRP genes in human gastric cancer. Hepatogastroenterology, (2011). , 1051-1056.

[81] Zhang, C., et al., High-resolution melting analysis of ADAMTS9 methylation levels in gastric, colorectal, and pancreatic cancers. Cancer Genet Cytogenet, (2010). , 38-44.

[82] Wang, X.H., et al., S100A6 overexpression is associated with poor prognosis and is epigenetically up-regulated in gastric cancer. Am J Pathol, (2010). , 586-597.

[83] Wang, J., et al., Expression of EphA1 in gastric carcinomas is associated with metastasis and survival. Oncol Rep, (2010). , 1577-1584.

[84] Maeda, N., et al., Loss of WW domain-containing oxidoreductase expression in the progression and development of gastric carcinoma: clinical and histopathologic correlations. Virchows Arch, (2010). , 423-432.

[85] Joo, J.K., et al., CpG methylation of transcription factor 4 in gastric carcinoma. Ann Surg Oncol, (2010). , 3344-3353.

[86] Goto, T., et al., Methylation of the p16 gene is frequently detected in lymphatic-invasive gastric cancer. Anticancer Res, (2010). , 2701-2703.

[87] Du, Y.Y., D.Q. Dai, and Z. Yang, Role of RECK methylation in gastric cancer and its clinical significance. World J Gastroenterol, 2010. 16(7): p. 904-8.

[88] Sakata, M., et al., (2009). Methylation of HACE1 in gastric carcinoma. Anticancer Res, . 29(6): p. ., 2231-3.

[89] Mizukami, H., et al., PGP9.5 was less frequently methylated in advanced gastric carcinoma. Hepatogastroenterology, (2009). , 1576-1579.

[90] Kitamura, Y.H., et al., (2009). Frequent methylation of Vimentin in well-differentiated gastric carcinoma. Anticancer Res, . 29(6): , 2227-2229.

[91] Hibi, K., et al., Methylation of the MGMT gene is frequently detected in advanced gastric carcinoma. Anticancer Res, (2009). , 5053-5055.

[92] Wang, Y.C., et al., Detection of RASSF1A promoter hypermethylation in serum from gastric and colorectal adenocarcinoma patients. World J Gastroenterol, (2008). , 3074-3080.

[93] Li, Y., et al., Frequent S100A4 Expression with Unique Splicing Pattern in Gastric Cancers: A Hypomethylation Event Paralleled with E-cadherin Reduction and Wnt Activation. Transl Oncol, 2008. 1(4): p. 165-76.

[94] Kim, M., et al., Epigenetic inactivation of protein kinase D1 in gastric cancer and its role in gastric cancer cell migration and invasion. Carcinogenesis(2008). , 629-637.

[95] Zhao, C.H., X.M. Bu, and N. Zhang, Hypermethylation and aberrant expression of Wnt antagonist secreted frizzled-related protein 1 in gastric cancer. World J Gastroenterol, 2007. 13(15): p. 2214-7.

[96] Wang, J., et al., Differential expression of EphA7 receptor tyrosine kinase in gastric carcinoma. Hum Pathol, (2007). , 1649-1656.

[97] Ulazzi, L., et al., Nidogen 1 and 2 gene promoters are aberrantly methylated in human gastrointestinal cancer. Mol Cancer, (2007). , 17.

[98] Taniguchi, H., et al., Transcriptional silencing of hedgehog-interacting protein by CpG hypermethylation and chromatic structure in human gastrointestinal cancer. J Pathol, (2007). , 131-139.

[99] Matsumura, S., et al., DNA demethylation of vascular endothelial growth factor-C is associated with gene expression and its possible involvement of lymphangiogenesis in gastric cancer. Int J Cancer, (2007). , 1689-1695.

[100] Leal, M.F., et al., Promoter hypermethylation of CDH1, FHIT, MTAP and PLAGL1 in gastric adenocarcinoma in individuals from Northern Brazil. World J Gastroenterol, (2007). , 2568-2574.

[101] Arisawa, T., et al., Promoter hypomethylation of protease-activated receptor 2 associated with carcinogenesis in the stomach.J Gastroenterol Hepatol, (2007). , 943-948.

[102] Akino, K., et al., Identification of DFNA5 as a target of epigenetic inactivation in gastric cancer.Cancer Sci, (2007). , 88-95.

[103] Kim, S.K., et al., The epigenetic silencing of LIMS2 in gastric cancer and its inhibitory effect on cell migration.Biochem Biophys Res Commun, (2006). , 1032-1040.

[104] Chang, M.S., et al., CpG island methylation status in gastric carcinoma with and without infection of Epstein-Barr virus.Clin Cancer Res, (2006). , 2995-3002.

[105] Liu, H., et al., Loss of epigenetic control of synuclein-gamma gene as a molecular indicator of metastasis in a wide range of human cancers.Cancer Res, (2005). , 7635-7643.

[106] Jung, E.J., et al., Expression of family A melanoma antigen in human gastric carcinoma. Anticancer Res, 2005. 25(3B): p. 2105-11.

[107] Jee, C.D., et al., Loss of caspase-1 gene expression in human gastric carcinomas and cell lines.Int J Oncol, (2005). , 1265-1271.

[108] Wang, S., et al., (2004). Hypermethylation of Syk gene in promoter region associated with oncogenesis and metastasis of gastric carcinoma.World J Gastroenterol, 10(12): , 1815-1818.

[109] Park, J., et al., Aberrant methylation of integrin alpha4 gene in human gastric cancer cells.Oncogene(2004). , 3474-3480.

[110] Oshimo, Y., et al., Epigenetic inactivation of SOCS-1 by CpG island hypermethylation in human gastric carcinoma.Int J Cancer, (2004). , 1003-1009.

[111] Ito, R., et al., Loss of maspin expression is associated with development and progression of gastric carcinoma with p53 abnormality.Oncol Rep, (2004). , 985-990.

[112] Honda, T., et al., Demethylation of MAGE promoters during gastric cancer progression.Br J Cancer, (2004). , 838-843.

[113] Pavicic, W., et al., Altered Methylation at MicroRNA-Associated CpG Islands in Hereditary and Sporadic Carcinomas: MS-MLPA-Based Approach. Mol Med, (2011).

[114] Luo, H., et al., Down-regulated miR-9 and miR-433 in human gastric carcinoma. J Exp Clin Cancer Res, (2009). , 82.

[115] Rotkrua, P., et al., MiR-9 down-regulates CDX2 expression in gastric cancer cells. Int J Cancer, (2011).

[116] Kim, K., et al., Epigenetic regulation of microRNA-10b and targeting of oncogenic MAPRE1 in gastric cancer.Epigenetics(2011). , 740-751.

[117] Ando, T., et al., (2009). DNA methylation of microRNA genes in gastric mucosae of gastric cancer patients: its possible involvement in the formation of epigenetic field defect.Int J Cancer, 124(10): , 2367-2374.

[118] Zhu, A., et al., MicroRNA-148a is silenced by hypermethylation and interacts with DNA methyltransferase 1 in gastric cancer.Med Oncol, (2011).

[119] Hashimoto, Y., et al., Involvement of epigenetically silenced microRNA-181c in gastric carcinogenesis.Carcinogenesis(2010). , 777-784.

[120] Craig, V.J., et al., Epigenetic silencing of microRNA-203 dysregulates ABL1 expression and drives Helicobacter-associated gastric lymphomagenesis.Cancer Res, (2011). , 3616-3624.

[121] Wada, R., et al., miR-212 is downregulated and suppresses methyl-CpG-binding protein MeCP2 in human gastric cancer.Int J Cancer, (2010). , 1106-1114.

[122] Takei, Y., et al., The Metastasis-Associated microRNA miR-516a-3p Is a Novel Therapeutic Target for Inhibiting Peritoneal Dissemination of Human Scirrhous Gastric-Cancer. Cancer Res, (2011). , 1442-1453.

[123] Chen, Q., et al., (2011). miR-137 is frequently down-regulated in gastric cancer and is a negative regulator of Cdc42.Dig Dis Sci, 56(7): , 2009-2016.

[124] Lee, T.L., et al., Detection of gene promoter hypermethylation in the tumor and serum of patients with gastric carcinoma.Clin Cancer Res, (2002). , 1761-1766.

[125] Chen, L., et al., Hypermethylated FAM5C and MYLK in serum as diagnosis and prewarning markers for gastric cancer.Dis Markers, (2012). , 195-202.

[126] Zheng, Y., et al., (2011). Analysis of the RUNX3 gene methylation in serum DNA from esophagus squamous cell carcinoma, gastric and colorectal adenocarcinoma patients.Hepatogastroenterology, 58(112): , 2007-2011.

[127] Tan, S.H., et al., Detection of promoter hypermethylation in serum samples of cancer patients by methylation-specific polymerase chain reaction for tumour suppressor genes including RUNX3.Oncol Rep, (2007). , 1225-1230.

[128] Yu, Q.M., et al., CDH1 methylation in preoperative peritoneal washes is an independent prognostic factor for gastric cancer.J Surg Oncol, (2012).

[129] Hiraki, M., et al., Aberrant gene methylation is a biomarker for the detection of cancer cells in peritoneal wash samples from advanced gastric cancer patients. Ann Surg Oncol, (2011). , 3013-3019.

Section 4

Diagnostic Tools, Prognosis and Management

Chapter 10

Imaging Findings of Gastric Carcinoma

Eriko Maeda, Masaaki Akahane, Kuni Ohtomo,
Keisuke Matsuzaka and Masashi Fukayama

Additional information is available at the end of the chapter

http://dx.doi.org/10.5772/52076

1. Introduction

Surgery is the only certain treatment for gastric carcinoma, so early detection and accurate staging is a key to successive treatment and mortality reduction. In this chapter, we would like to explain radiologic imaging of gastric carcinoma by

1. Reviewing the evidences for gastric carcinoma screening
2. Demonstrating the TNM classification of gastric carcinoma and the relevant imaging findings for each stages and
3. Introducing unusual imaging findings of gastric carcinoma and differential diagnoses.

1.1. Gastric carcinoma screening

Gastric carcinoma is the fourth most common cancer worldwide, behind lung, breast and colorectal carcinomas, and is the second leading cause of death in both sexes worldwide and in Asia [1, 2]. There is about twice male predominance.Gastric carcinoma is particularly common in countries such as Korea (incidence 62.2 per 100,000 males; mortality 22.8 per 100,000 males), Japan (46.8; 20.5), China (41.3; 30.5), Chile (27.3; 23.1), Russia (26.9; 24.0) but not as common in a large part of western societies such as the United States (5.7; 2.7) and United Kingdom (8.0; 4.8) [1].

The high mortality is mainly due to late presentation, therefore early detection and treatment is an important way to reduce death from gastric cancer [2].There are four major methods for screening gastric carcinoma; fluoroscopy, endoscopy, serum pepsinogen testing, and *Helicobacter pylori* antibody testing [3]. Because of a large difference in burden of gastric carcinoma among nations, benefit of gastric cancer screening cannot be debated on the same ground for societies throughout the world. However, there have been no randomized trials evaluating the impact of screening on mortality from gastric carcinoma [2,3].For societies where gastric carcinoma is uncommon, National Cancer Institute of the United States state that for screening would not result in a decrease in mortality fromgastric carcinoma [4].

In Japan, there is a government-sponsored mass screening program with barium meal fluorography. Participants are recommended to undergo endoscopy of the upper gastrointestinal tract when positive findings are detected at fluorography. Asymptomatic individuals older than 40 years are eligible for this program, but only around 20% of the eligible subjects actually participates the program [3]. Most case-control studies from Japan show a 40-60% decrease in mortality from gastric carcinoma in the subjects who participated the program [2,5-8]. In contrast, Japanese prospective series setting death from gastric cancer as an endpoint have inconsistent results [2,9-13].Even in combination with serum pepsinogen, a large Japanese study screening 17,647 men aged 40-60 years the positive predictive value over the 7-year period was 0.85% [14].Thus even in societies with high incidence, identification of high-risk groups that benefit from screening may be necessary to perform cost-effective screening.The subgroups might include elderly patients with atrophic gastritis or pernicious anemia, patients with partial gastrectomy, patients with Epstein-Barr virus associated gastric carcinoma or history of multiple carcinomas, patients with the diagnosis of sporadic adenomas, familial adenomatous polyposis or hereditary nonpolyposis colon cancer [15-19].

Endoscopy has advantage over fluoroscopy, especially in detection of flat and non-ulcerative lesions. A Japanese study comparing finding ratio of gastric carcinoma with fluoroscopy and endoscopy reports 2.7 to 4.6-times higher ratio for endoscopy [20]. However, effective screening with endoscopy relies on the skill of the endoscopists and availability of endoscopes, and it is likely to be unfeasible to perform mass screening using endoscopy.

2. TNM classification of gastric carcinomas and the relevant imaging findings

Owing to recent advances in CT technology, we have been able to visualize early carcinomas and to stage tumors with considerable accuracy, with the use of appropriate contrast technique and effervescent agent or water [21]. Recent CT with conventional transverse images, multiplanar reconstruction (MPR) images and virtual endoscopy can detect gastric carcinomas efficiently with the detection rates of 91%, 96% and 98%, respectively [22].

Gastric carcinomas appear as a focal area of mural thickening with or without ulceration, as a polypoid lesion, or as generalized mural thickening. Lesions occurring in the antrum, in the body, and in the fundus comprise 30% of all gastric carcinomas respectively, and the remaining 10% involve the whole stomach [23].

CT criteria for T staging of gastric carcinoma is as follows [22].

T1 lesion = focal thickening of the inner layer, almost well enhanced, and has visible low-attenuation-strip outer layer of gastric wall and clear fat plane around tumor

http://dx.doi.org/10.5772/52076

T2 lesion = focal or diffuse thickening of the wall with transmural enhancement, almost well enhanced, and has smooth outer wall border and clear fat plane around tumor

T3 lesion = transmural tumor with irregular or nodular outer border and/or perigastric fat infiltration

T4 lesion = Obliteration of fat plane betweengastric tumor and adjacent organ or invasion of adjacent organ

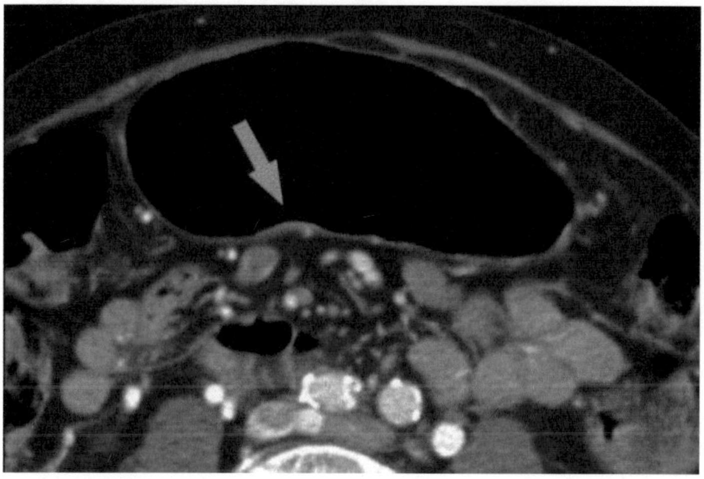

Figure 1. T1a gastric carcinoma in a 76-year old man. Contrast CT shows a subtle thickening and enhancement of the inner layer (arrow) with low-attenuation-strip outer layer of gastric wall and clear fat plane around tumor.

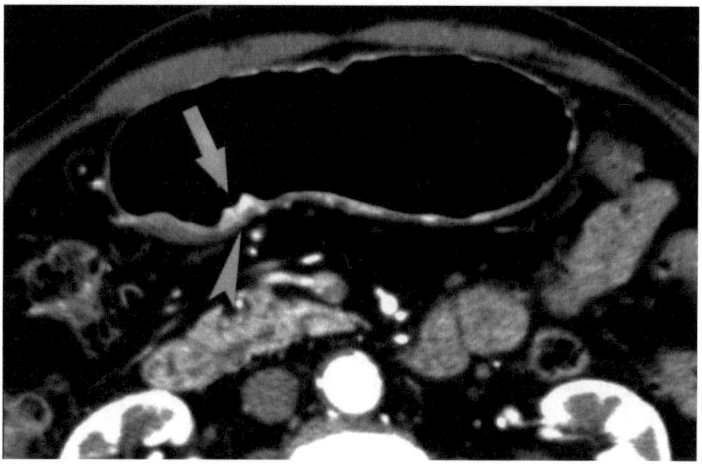

Figure 2. T2 gastric carcinoma in a 82-year old man. Contrast CT shows a well-enhanced focal mural thickening (arrow)andfocal enhancement of the outer layer (arrowhead).The tumor has smooth outer wall border and clear fat plane around tumor.

Accuracy of CT in T-staging with transverse images only is 73%, but it rises to 89% with the use of MPR [22]. Therefore it is important to perform appropriate reconstruction techniques in CT diagnosis of gastric carcinoma.

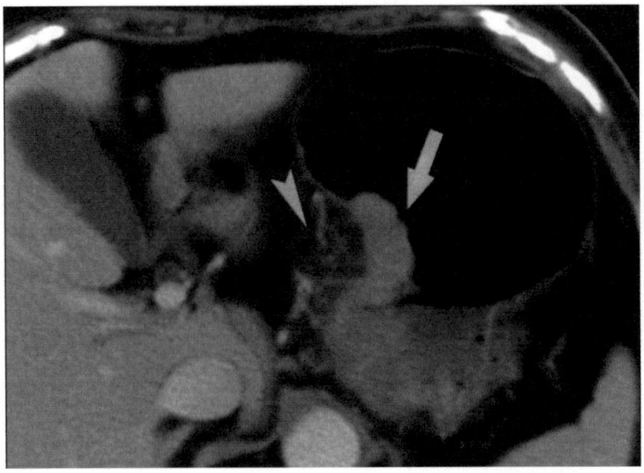

Figure 3. T3 gastric carcinoma in a 64-year old woman. Contrast CT shows a mass in the lesser curvature (arrow), obliterating the outer layer of the stomach. The outer border of the tumor is irregular, and perigastric fat stranding is visualized (arrowhead).

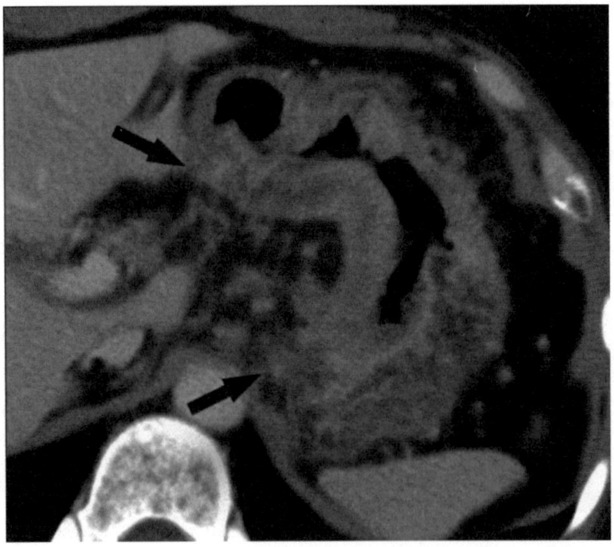

Figure 4. Type IV gastric carcinoma in a 47-yer old man. Contrast CT shows diffuse mural thickening obliterating thefolds and the inner structure of the gastric wall (arrows). The enhancement "running" through the gastric wall is characteristic of scirrhous tumors.

T1 tumors are classified into T1a and T1b tumors; a T1a lesion stay within the mucosal layer, while a T1b lesion stay within the submucosal layer (Figure 1).

A T2 tumor infiltrates into the muscularis propria layer and stays within the layer (Figure 2).

A T3 tumor extends over the muscularis propria layer, but its border stays within the subserosal layer (Figure 3).

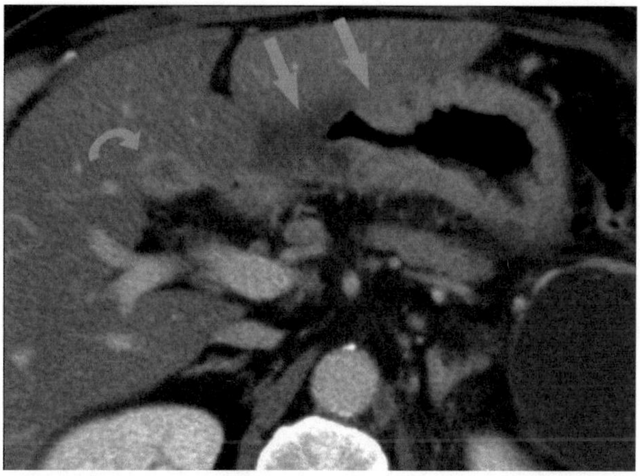

Figure 5. Advanced gastric carcinoma in a 60-year old man. Contrast CT shows diffuse mural thickening of the antrum (arrows). The fat plane between the tumor and the liver is obliterated. Liver metastasis can be found as well (curved arrow).

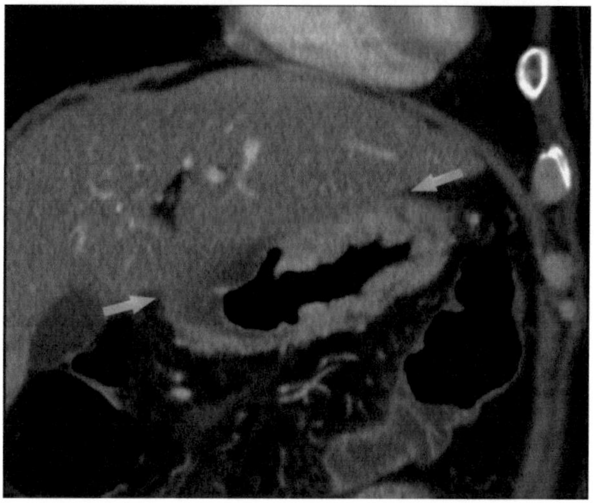

Figure 6. Advanced gastric carcinoma in a 60-year old man (the same patient as Figure 5). The clear and smooth border between the tumor and the liver (between two arrows) can be shown with coronal MPR. This tumor can be staged as T4a.

T4 tumors are classified into T4a and T4b tumors; A T4a lesion invades the serosa, exposing its surface to the peritoneal cavity in many cases. The tumor is classified as T4b when it invades the adjacent organs, such as the transverse colon, pancreas, spleen, liver and the diaphragm.Signet-ring cell carcinoma, often found at T4a stage, usually manifests as a scirrhous tumor, and appears as diffuse thickening of the gastric wall with obliteration of gastric folds, usually extending from the antrum into the body and fundus (Figure 4) [23].

T4b tumor requires resection of adjacent organs with the primary tumor, and discrimination of T4a tumors from "T4b-looking tumor" is an important function of preoperative imaging. An advanced tumor can be recognized as T4a when the fat plane between the tumor and the adjacent organ is visualized, or when the fat plane is invisible or compressed by the tumor, the tumor is considered to be T4a if it has a clear and smooth border (Figures 5-7).MPR in appropriate plane is especially effective in differentiating between T4a and T4b; MPR is reported to improve the specificity without compensation in sensitivity in diagnosis of invasion into the transverse colon or mesocolon and the pancreas [24].

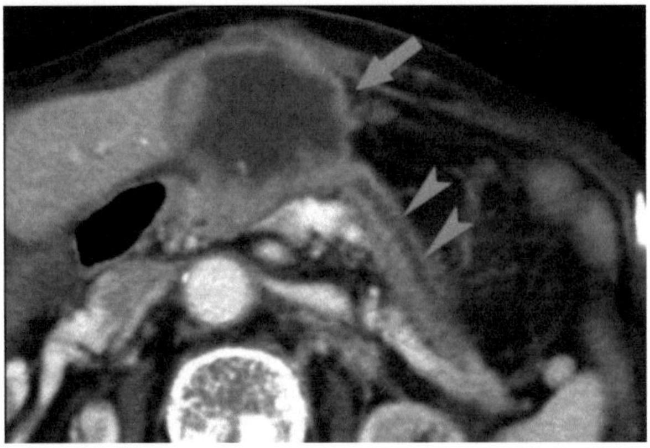

Figure 7. Advanced gastric carcinoma in a 88-year old woman. The tumor extends downwards toward the pancreas (arrow), and causes dilatation of the main pancreatic duct as a result of pancreatic infiltration (arrowheads). This tumor is staged as T4b.

Criteria for N staging for gastric carcinoma is as follows:

N0 = no lymph nodes involved

N1 = metastases in 1-2 regional lymph nodes

N2 = metastases in 3-6 regional lymph nodes

N3a = metastases in 7-15 regional lymph nodes

N3b = metastases in more than 15 regional lymph nodes

Gastric carcinoma is often accompanied with nodal metastases even at relatively earlier stages. Micrometastases and normal-sized metastatic nodes are common in gastric carcinoma, and this makes accurate N staging difficult. Ring enhancement,inhomogeneous enhancementand strong enhancement at arterial phase are known as possible signs of metastases in a normal sized lymph node. Therefore it is important to point out nodes with these atypical findings, even when the node is smaller than 10mm.Since accurate counting of lymph node metastases is the key to accurate N staging,active reconstruction with MPR is warranted for accurate measurement and interpretation of conglomerated lymph nodes (Figures 8,9).

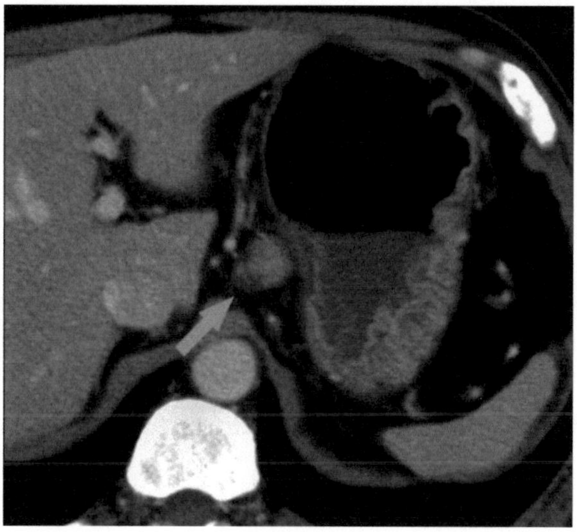

Figure 8. A 50-year old man with gastric carcinoma. Contrast CT shows a mass at the lesser curvature (arrow).

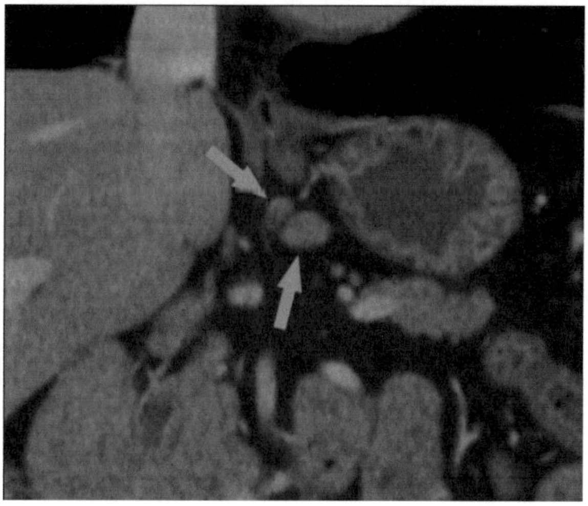

Figure 9. A 50-year old man with gastric carcinoma (the same patient as Figure 8). MPR in the coronal plane shows this mass consists of two lymph nodes.

The liver is the most common metastatic sites for gastric carcinoma because the gastric veins drain into the hepatic portal system.Metastatic hepatic tumors are often accompanied with ring enhancement at earlier phase, and portal phase in addition to the equilibrium phase. Some tumors lose contrast to the liver parenchyma after the delivery of the contrast material, and we obtain the plane CT images as well in the metastasis survey protocolof our institution.Other common sites for distant metastases include the lungs, adrenal glands, and the ovaries (Krukenberg tumors).Positron emission tomography (PET) with 2-[fluorine-18]fluoro-2-deoxy-d-glucose (FDG) is not appropriated for local tumor staging, but is effective for detection of distant metastases [25].

CT does not have enough sensitivity for detection of peritoneal dissemination. Even with recent 16- or 64-row detector scanners, the sensitivity and specificity of CT diagnosis of peritoneal dissemination are 28.3% and 98.9% respectively when definite criteria are adopted, and 50.9% and 96.2% when the criteria included the suspicious findings [26]. This report mentions greater tumor size and advanced T stage as predictive factors for dissemination, and recommends staging laparoscopy for tumors with these factors, even when CT results are negative for peritoneal dissemination. The value of FDG-PET in detection of peritoneal dissemination is still controversial [25].

3. Unusual imaging findings of gastric carcinoma and differential diagnoses

Rarely, gastric carcinomas present with gross or psammomatous calcifications. Calcified gastric carcinomas are usually found in mucinous adenocarcinoma; a carcinoma characterized by prominent glandular formations and abundant mucin deposition. Calcifications in mucinous carcinoma are military and punctate [27,28]. Rarely, calcification within gastric carcinoma lesion occurs as a result of secretion of parathyroid hormone-like substance [29]. Other reported atypical features of gastric carcinomas include transpyloric spread, giant gastric folds and hypervascular masses [27,30,31].

Epstein-Barr virus associated gastric carcinoma (EBVaGC) is a clinicopathologically and molecularly distinct type of gastric carcinoma.EBV-associated gastric carcinoma (EBVaGC) occurs worldwide, with the reported incidence varying from 1.3% to 20.1%, affects 70,000-80,000 people per year (estimate), constituting the largest group of EBV-associated malignancies [16,32,33].EBVaGC is associated with male predominance, location in the proximal stomach, multiplicity and carcinomas affecting remnant stomachs [33,34].Although there are some conflicting evidences, lower rate of lymph node involvement and relatively favorable prognosis is suggested [32,33,35].EBVaGC is associated with two types of histology: lymphoepithelioma (LE) -like type which is almost identical to the subgroup reported as "gastric carcinoma with lymphoid stroma (GCLS)", and ordinary type [36,37].Imaging findings of LE-like type or GCLS is characterized by a large thickness-to-length ratio, and is sometimes accompanied with a bulky portion projecting from the gastric wall [38] (Figure 10).

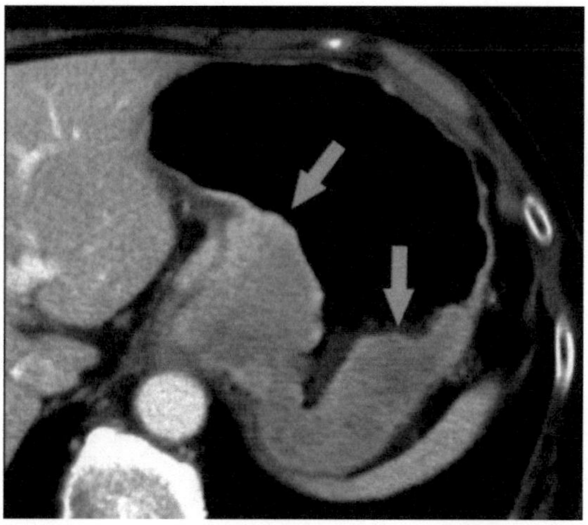

Figure 10. LE-type EBVaGC in a 69-year old woman. Contrast CT shows massive mural thickening involving the gastric fundus and the esophagogastric junction (arrows).

Gastric carcinoma need to be differentiated from other malignant tumors involvingthe stomach, whichincludes carcinoid, carcinosarcoma, lymphoma, mucosa-associated lymphoid tissue lymphoma (MALToma) and gastrointestinal stromal tumor (GIST) (Figures 11-13) [27]. Benign tumors of the stomach include hyperplastic or adenomatous polyps, leiomyoma, schwannoma, lipoma, hemangioma and glomus tumor. Heterotopic pancreas can also be mistaken as a gastric carcinoma (Figure 14).

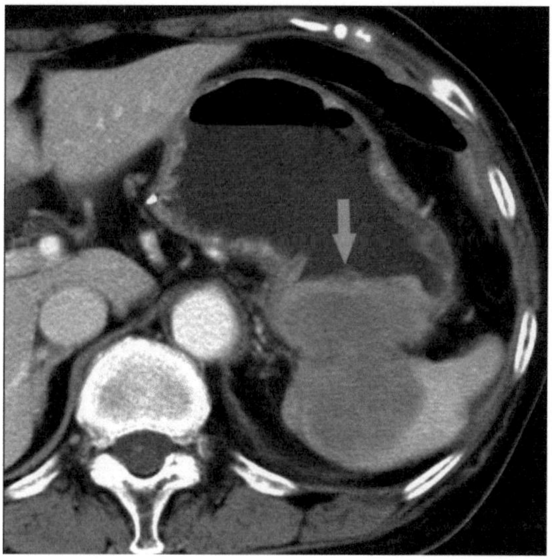

Figure 11. Diffuse large B-cell lymphoma in a 73-year old woman. Contrast CT shows a dumbbell-shaped mass extending from the fundus into the spleen (arrow).

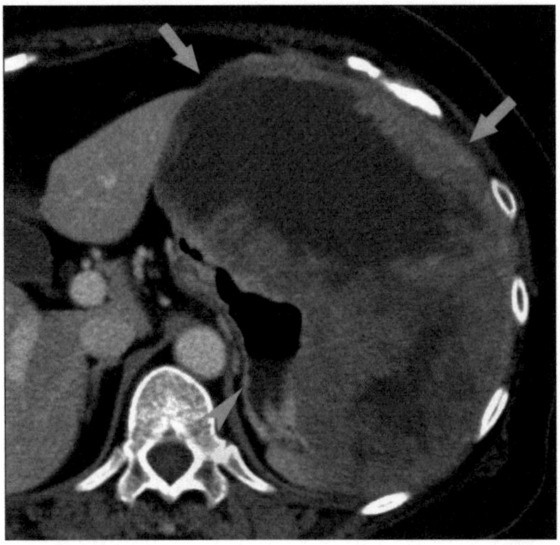

Figure 12. High-grade GIST in a 53-year old man. Contrast CT shows an enormous tumor extending along the outer gastric wall (arrows).The tumor has a smooth border but the enhancement is very heterogeneous, with a large area of necrosis showing homogeneous low attenuation. Note the compressed cavity of the stomach (arrowhead).

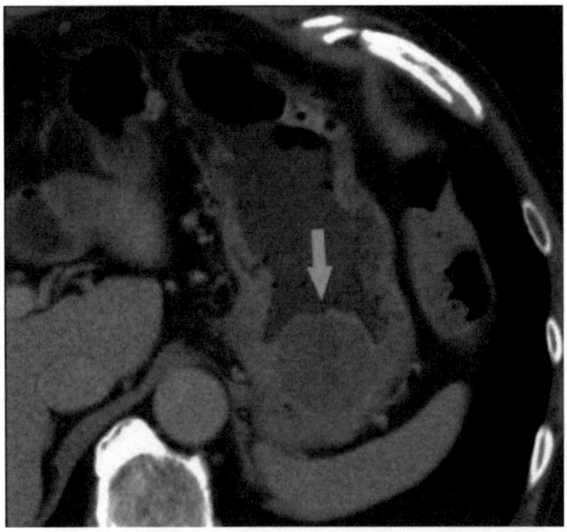

Figure 13. Low-grade GIST in a 74-year old man. Contrast CT shows a smooth round tumor with homogeneous enhancement within the fundus (arrow).

http://dx.doi.org/10.5772/52076

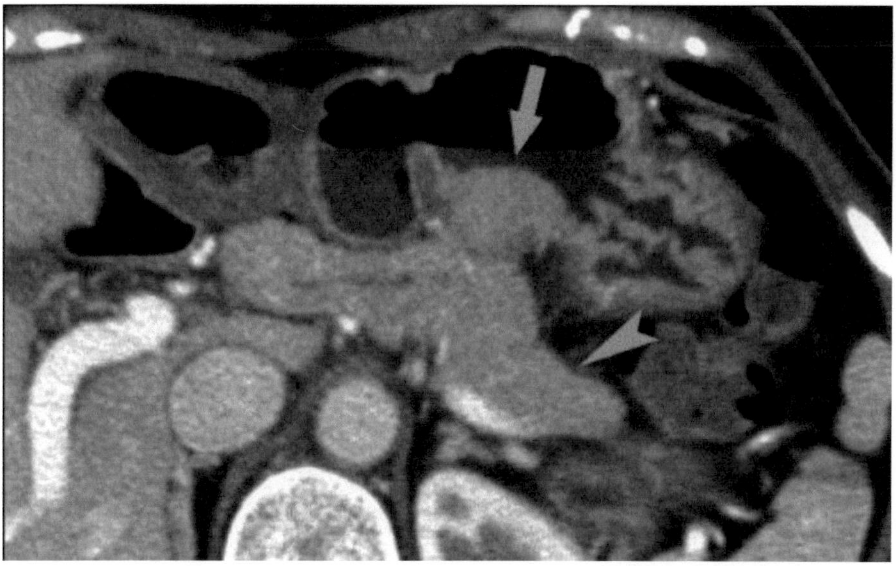

Figure 14. A 46-year old woman with a submucosal mass. Contrast CT shows a mass (arrow) presenting similar enhancement as the pancreas (arrowhead). Heterotopic pancreas was suspected on CT and at endoscopic ultrasonography, and was confirmed by fine-needle biopsy.

4. Conclusion

Although early detection is the key to the mortality reduction of gastric carcinoma, the benefit of screening is still under debate even in the societies with high incidence. Recent CT with appropriate reconstruction technique can detect and locally stage gastric carcinomas sufficiently. It remains a challenge to accurately diagnose lymph node metastasis and peritoneal dissemination with imaging. Imaging can also depict unusual manifestationsof gastric carcinomas such as calcification and a large thickness-to-width ratio or projecting mass in EBVaGC.

Author details

Eriko Maeda[1*], Masaaki Akahane[1], Kuni Ohtomo[1], Keisuke Matsuzaka[2] and Masashi Fukayama[2]

*Address all correspondence to: emaeda-tky@umin.ac.jp

1 Department of Radiology, Graduate School of Medicine, University of Tokyo, Japan

2 Department of Pathology, Graduate School of Medicine, University of Tokyo, Japan

References

[1] Ferlay, J., Shin, H.R., Bray, F., Forman, D., Mathers, C., & Parkin, D.M. (2008). GLOBOCAN v1.2, Cancer Incidence and Mortality Worldwide: IARC Cancer Base No. 10Lyon, France: *International Agency for Research on Cancer*.

[2] Leung, W. K., Wu, M. S., Kakugawa, Y., et al. (2008). Asia Pacific Working Group on Gastric Cancer. Screening for gastric cancer in Asia: current evidenceand practice. *Lancet Oncol.*, 9(3), 279-87.

[3] Hamashima, C., Shibuya, D., Yamazaki, H., et al. (2008). The Japanese guidelines for gastric cancer screening. *Jpn J Clin Oncol.*, 38(4), 259-67.

[4] National Cancer Institute. (2012). Stomach (Gastric) cancer screening (PDQ) cancer. *Health Professional*, http://cancer.gov/cancertopics/pdq/screening/gastric/ .

[5] Kunisaki, C., Ishino, J., Nakajima, S., et al. (2006). Outcomes of mass screening for gastric carcinoma. Ann Surg Oncol, 13(2), 221-28.

[6] Oshima, A., Hirata, N., Ubukata, T., et al. (1986). Evaluation of a mass screening program for stomach cancer with a case-control study design. *Int J Cancer*, 38(6), 829-33.

[7] Fukao, A., Tsubono, Y., Tsuji, I., et al. (1995). The evaluation of screening for gastric cancer in Miyagi Prefecture, Japan: a population-based case-control study. *Int L Cancer*, 60(1), 45-48.

[8] Abe, Y., Mitsushima, T., Nagatani, K., et al. (1995). Epidemiological evaluation of the protective effect for dying of stomach cancer by screening programme for stomach cancer with applying a method of case-control study-a study of an efficient screening programme for stomach cancer. *Nippon Shokakibyo Gakkai Zasshi*, 92(5), 836-45.

[9] Oshima, A., Hanai, A., & Fujimoto, I. (1979). Evaluation of a mass screening program for stomach cancer. *Natl Cancer Inst Monogr.*, 53, 181-86.

[10] Hisamichi, S., & Sugawara, N. (1984). Mass screening for gastric cancer by X-ray examination. *Jpn J Clin Oncol.*, 14(2), 211-13.

[11] Inaba, S., Hirayama, H., Nagata, C., et al. (1999). Evaluation of a screening program on reduction of gastric cancer mortality in Japan: preliminary results from a cohort study. *Prev Med.*, 20(2), 9-102.

[12] Mizoue, T., Yoshimura, T., Tokui, N., et al. (2003). Prospective study of screening for stomach cancer in Japan. *Int J Cancer:*, 106(1), 103-07.

[13] Lee, K. J., Inoue, M., Otani, T., et al. (2006). Gastric cancer screening and subsequent risk of gastric cancer: a large-scale population-based cohort study, with a 13-year follow up in Japan. *Int J Cancer*, 118(9), 2315-21.

[14] Ohata, H., Oka, M., Yanaoka, K., et al. (2005). Gastric cancer screening of a high-risk population in Japan using serum pepsinogen an barium digital radiography. *Cancer Sci.*, 96(10), 713-20.

[15] Staël, von., Holstein, C., Eriksson, S., Huldt, B., et al. (1991). Endoscopic screening during 17 years for gastric stump carcinoma. *A prospective clinical trial. Scand J Gastroenterol*, 26(10), 1020-6.

[16] Fukayama, M. (2010). Epstein-Barr virus and gastric carcinoma, *Pathol Int.*, 60(5), 337-50.

[17] Ming, S., & Goldman, H. (1965). Gastric polyps: a histogenetic classification and its relation to carcinoma. *Cancer*, 18(6), 721-726.

[18] Utsunomiya, J., Maki, T., Iwama, T., et al. (1974). Gastric lesion of familial polyposis coli. *Cancer*, 34(3), 745-54.

[19] Aarnio, M., Salovaara, R., Aaltonen, L. A., et al. (1997). Features of gastric cancer in hereditary non-polyposis colorectal cancer syndrome. *Int J Cancer*, 74(5), 551-5.

[20] Tashiro, A., Sano, M., Kinameri, K., et al. (2006). Comparing mass screening techniques for gastric cancer in Japan. *World J Gastroenterol*, 12(30), 4874-75.

[21] Shimizu, K., Ito, K., Matsunaga, N., et al. (2005). Diagnosis of gastric cancer with MDCT using the water-filling method and multiplanar reconstruction: CT-histologic correlation. *AJR Am J Roentgenol*, 185(5), 1152-58.

[22] Chen, C. Y., Hsu, J. S., Wu, D. C., et al. (2007). Gastric cancer: preoperative local staging with 3D multi-detector row CT: correlation with surgical and histopathologic results. *Radiology*, 242(2), 472-82.

[23] Ba-Ssalamah, A., Prokop, M., Uffmann, M., et al. (2003). Dedicated multidetector CT of the stomach: spectrum of diseases. *Radio Graphics*, 23(3), 625-644.

[24] Kim, Y. H., Lee, K. H., Park, S. H., et al. (2009). Staging of T3 and T4 gastric carcinoma with multidetector CT: added value of multiplanar reformation for prediction of adjacent organ invasion. *Radiology*, 250(3), 767-775.

[25] Lim, J. S., Yun, M. J., Kim, M. J., et al. (2006). CT and PET in stomach cancer: preoperative staging and monitoring of response to therapy. *Radio Graphics* 26(1), 143-156.

[26] Kim, S. J., Kim, H. H., Kim, Y. H., et al. (2009). Peritoneal metastasis: detection with 16- or 64-detector row CT in patients undergoing surgery for gastric cancer. *Radiology*, 253(2), 407-415.

[27] Park, S. H., Han, J. K., Kim, T. K., et al. (1999). Unusual gastric tumors: radiologic-pathologic correlation. *Radio Graphics*, 19(6), 1435-1446.

[28] Dickson, A. M., Schuss, A., Goyal, A., et al. (2004). Radiology-Pathology Conference:Calcified untreated gastric cancer. *Clin Imaging*, 28(6), 418-21.

[29] Murayama, H., Kamio, A., Imai, T., et al. (1982). Gastric carcinoma with psammomatous calcification: report of a case, with reference to calcinogenesis. *Cancer*, 49(4), 788-96.

[30] Mei, M., Jingmei, N., Zongming, C., et al. (2012). Diffuse type gastric carcinoma presenting as giant gastric folds: Lessons learned from six miss diagnosed cases. *Clin Res Hepatol Gastroenterol*, http://dx.doi.org/10.1016/j.clinre,2012.04.009.

[31] Johnson, P. T., Horton, K. M., & Fishman, E. K. (2010). Hypervascular gastric masses: CT findings and clinical correlates. *AJR Am J Roentgenol* 2010 Dec. 195(6):W, 415-20.

[32] van Beek, J., zur Hausen, A., Klein Kranenbarg, E., et al. (2004). EBV-positive gastric adenocarcinomas: a distinct clinicopathologic entity with a low frequency of lymph node involvement, *J Clin Oncol.*, 22(4), 664-70.

[33] Lee, J. H., Kim, S. H., Han, S. H., et al. (2009). Clinicopathological and molecular characteristics of Epstein-Barr virus-associated gastric carcinoma: a meta-analysis, *J Gastroenterol Hepatol*, 24(3), 354-65.

[34] Murphy, G., Pfeiffer, R., Camargo, M. C., et al. (2009). Meta-analysis shows that prevalence of Epstein-Barr virus-positive gastric cancer differs based on sex and anatomic location, *Gastroenterology*, 137(3), 824-33.

[35] Tokunaga, M., & Land, C. E. (1998). Epstein-Barr virus involvement in gastric cancer: biomarker for lymph node metastasis, *Cancer Epidemiol Biomarkers Prev.*, 7(5), 449-50.

[36] Fukayama, M., & Ushiku, T. (2011). Epstein-Barr virus-associated gastric carcinoma, *Pathol Res Pract.*, 207(9), 529-37.

[37] Watanabe, H., Enjoji, M., & Imai, T. (1976). Gastric carcinoma with lymphoid stroma. Its morphologic characteristics and prognostic correlations, *Cancer*, 38(1), 232-43.

[38] Maeda, E., Akahane, M., Uozaki, H., et al. (2009). CT appearance of Epstein-Barr virus-associated gastric carcinoma, *Abdom Imaging*, 34(5), 618-25.

[39] Randjelovic, T., Filipovic, B., Babic, D., et al. (2007). Carcinosarcoma of the stomach: a case report and review of the literature. *World J Gastroenterol*, 13(41), 5533-6.

Chapter 11

Prognosis in the Cancer of the Stomach

Okan Akturk and Cemal Ulusoy

Additional information is available at the end of the chapter

http://dx.doi.org/10.5772/52655

1. Introduction

Although the incidence of gastric cancer has been declining in most industrialized countries over the past two decades, it still remains the second leading cause of cancer related deaths worldwide [1]. The incidence is highest in Japan, Korea, China, Latin America and Eastern Europe. In western countries like the United States, the incidence is lower, with 21,000 new cases diagnosed each year [2]. Gastric carcinoma is one of the most frequent malignancies in the world and its clinical behavior especially depends on the metastatic potential of the tumor. In particular, lymphatic metastasis is one of the main predictors of tumor recurrence and survival, and current pathological staging systems reflect the concept that lymphatic spread is the most relevant prognostic factor in patients undergoing curative resection [3]. This is compounded by the observation that two-thirds of gastric cancer in the Western world presents at an advanced stage, with lymph node metastasis at diagnosis [4].

2. Patterns of relapse and metastasis

Gastric cancer can spread via direct extension, lymphatic and hematogenous routes and also peritoneal invasion. There are 5 ways of recurrence following surgical removal of gastric carcinoma: lymph node, remnant stomach, local, peritoneal and hematogenous recurrence. Sixty percent to 72% of gastric cancer patients succumb to recurrences within the first 2 years. Hematogenous or lymphatic spreads without intra abdominal metastases occur rarely. It may be postulated that gastric cancer prefers to spread intra abdominally, and that locoregional control is therefore an important issue in treatment strategy [5]. Locoregional recurrence rates vary from 25% to 96% depending on different detection methods and study populations. Several prognostic factors have been identified.

3. Stage

The pathologic stage has consistently been shown to be of prognostic significance for both 5year survival and local recurrence rates [6]. The best prognosis is seen in patients with early stage of the cancer. The survival rates that come from the National Cancer Institute's SEER database and which are based on people diagnosed with stomach cancer and treated with surgery between 1991 and 2000 are as follows. (Table 1)

Stage IA	71%
Stage IB	57%
Stage IIA	45%
Stage IIB	33%
Stage IIIA	20%
Stage IIIB	14%
Stage IIIC	9%
Stage IV	4%

Table 1. Add caption

4. Histology and recurrence

Gastric cancer can recur in different pathways. The possibility of predicting the risk and type of recurrence in patients with resectable gastric cancer could have important implications for therapy, both in the surgical approach (extent of lymphadenectomy, partial or total resection) and in complementary therapies. Marelli et al. found out that the main difference was found on the onset of peritoneal recurrence in a study of 412 patients in which they compared the recurrence patterns of intestinal type and diffuse type [7]. Shiriashi et al. confirmed that most recurrences were within the first two years after surgery and rare after 5 years [8].

For intestinal type of the tumor lymph node positivity, depth of invasion, advanced age and male gender significantly increases the risk of recurrence. The patterns of relapse were mainly locoregional or hematogenous and peritoneal recurrence was limited. For diffuse type of tumors very high rates of peritoneal recurrence were observed in neoplasms with infiltration of the serosa, involvement of second level lymph nodes, and large tumor size. Locoregional recurrences were frequent in advanced forms, lymph node–positive cases, and tumors larger than 4 cm. The rate of hematogenous recurrence was generally smaller than that of peritoneal or locoregional disease. Early forms and tumors smaller than 4 cm recurred primarily via hematogenous route.

The main difference was found in the onset of peritoneal recurrence; this was observed in 34% of diffuse-type cases compared to 9% of intestinal-type cases, and was the main pathway of spread in the former. Compared to intestinal-type cells, the diffuse type showed a greater predisposition to proliferate in the peritoneum, considering that 50% of the cases with infiltration of the serosa led to peritoneal carcinomatosis, which was observed in only 16% of T3 and T4 intestinal-type cases. On the contrary, recurrences of intestinal-type tumors were mainly locoregional or hematogenous. The incidence of hematogenous recurrence did not show significant differences between the intestinal and the diffuse types; in both groups of patients, they observed a higher frequency of this recurrence in lymph node– positive cases, a finding in accord with other reports. However, the degree of involvement in the various organs was different, because the intestinal type metastasized primarily to the liver, whereas in the diffuse type the liver was involved in only half of the cases; in the other cases, hematogenous metastases involved distant organs. The data may suggest that in the diffuse type, but not in the intestinal type, superextended lymphadenectomy may play a more important role in reducing the risk of recurrence. The diffuse type may show a greater propensity than the intestinal type to metastasize to third- and fourth-level lymph nodes [7].

In a large series Nakamura et al. demonstrated that there is some correlation between the tumor histological type and the gross type. Seventy nine percent of diffusely infiltrating tumors and 69% of ulcerative infiltrating tumors were poorly differentiated and 60% of polipoid tumors were well differentiated in advanced carcinomas. In early carcinomas 89% of Type 1 and 77% of Type IIa lesions were well differentiated. Type llc tumors were either well (31%), moderate (19%) or poorly differentiated (50%). In their large series of 10 thousand patients the most frequently encountered macroscopic type of advanced carcinoma was the ulcerative infiltrating tumor (41%), followed by ulcerating circumscribed type (31%). In early carcinomas type IIc (70%) was the most frequently encountered type, followed by Type II a. In advanced forms well differentiated types showed fairer prognosis [9].

Adachi et al. demonstrated that patients with poorly differentiated type show a poorer prognosis especially when the tumor is bigger than 10 cm or serosal involvement is positive. If the tumor did not invade serosa but had lymph node metastasis, survival rate was significantly lower in the well differentiated group [10]. Moriguchi et al. also demonstrated that when the tumor invasion was restricted within mucosa or submucosa the well differentiated type of tumor were associated with poorer prognosis [11]. This difference can be explained by the characteristics of well differentiated type which readily develops blood-bourne metastases irrespective of the degree of penetration by tumor cells [10].

5. Grade

The difficulty of assessing the prognosis of gastric cancer using histological methods is well known and this is also reflected in the essentially descriptive character of presently used classifications [12]. In a study by Chiaravalli et al. which they reviewed the effect of the grade on prognosis among patients with T2-T4 cancer, the more favorable behavior of grade 1 compared to grade 2 tumors and of the latter compared to grade 3 cases was confirmed. Among diffuse type cancers a low low-grade desmoplastic type with a significantly better prognosis and worse prognosis of a high-grade anaplastic subtype were identified histologically from the bulk of diffuse gastric cancers owing to their distinctive histologic, clinicopathologic, and prognostic aspects. [13]. However, the stage itself, with special reference to lymph-node metastases and invasion level beyond subserosa, remains the most important prognostic clue for gastric cancer [14].

Tumor size: In a study by Yokota et al., which they reviewed 697 patients with gastric cancer, the patients were divided into three groups: 102 patients with tumors of less than 2 cm in diameter, 392 patients with tumors of 2-7 cm in diameter, and 203 patients with tumors of more than 7 cm in diameter. Patients with larger tumors had more invasion into the gastric wall in terms of depth of invasion and more frequent lymph node metastasis than did patients with smaller tumors. Histologically, diffuse, scirrhous-type was more common in the larger tumor group. The frequency of lymphatic and vascular permeation in the larger tumor group was higher than that in the other groups. The 5-year survival rates according to tumor size were 94.3% in cases of tumors of less than 2 cm, 75.1% in cases of tumors of 2-7 cm, and 26.3% in cases of tumors of more than 7 cm. Multivariate analysis revealed that the prognosis of gastric cancer patients was affected most by depth of invasion, followed by lymph node metastasis and tumor location. Tumor size is not an independent prognostic factor. In conclusion, according to the results of univariate analysis, tumor size is clinically a predictor of survival of patients with gastric cancer. In multivariate analysis, however, it is not an independent factor, and the presence of lymph node metastasis, depth of invasion and tumor location are more important than tumor size (15). However in another study of clinicopathologic data of 479 patients who underwent curative operation for gastric carcinoma, the patients were divided into three groups: 182 with tumors measuring <4 cm (group I), 252 with tumors of 4–10 cm (group II), and 45 with tumors of 10 cm (group III). The 10year survival rates for group I, II, and III patients were 92%, 66%, and 33%, respectively (p<0.01), and the three groups were significantly different with regard to depth of invasion (p<0.01), number and level of lymph node metastasis (p<0.01), and stage of disease (p<0.01). Multivariate analysis indicated that tumor size independently influenced the survival of patients. [16] Among patients with gastric cancer larger than 10 cm, independent prognostic factors were serosal invasion, extragastric lymph node metastasis, and liver metastasis. Prognosis after gastrectomy was determined by these tumor factors and was not associated with the patient or operation factors [17].

6. Tumor location

Middle third and distal cancers tend to decline worldwide. However, in the western populations proximal gastric cancers tend to increase even though the incidence of those cancers stays the same in Japan [18]. In a study by Saito et al, tumors of the cardia had a mean size of 6.8 cm, which was significantly larger than the mean size of 5.9 cm for tumors found in the middle- and lower third of the stomach. The incidence of serosal invasion, lymph node metastasis, and lymphatic and blood vessel invasion was higher in association with adenocarcinoma of the cardia than with adenocarcinoma in remaining parts of the stomach. In the analysis of patients who had undergone curative resection, the 5-year survival rates were 61.6%, 79.1%, and 82.6% in patients with carcinoma of the cardia, upper one-third, and remaining middle- and lower one-third of the stomach, respectively, and the differences were statistically significant. Multivariate analysis indicated that adenocarcinoma of the gastric cardia is an independent prognostic factor. With regard to the site of recurrence, both lymph node and hematogenous recurrence were observed more frequently in the cardia than in the remaining parts of the stomach [19]. A multivariate analysis demonstrates that R0 resection is independent of other strong predictors of survival, like T, N and M [20].

7. Lymphatic and vascular invasion

Hyung et al. reviewed a total of 280 patients who underwent curative gastrectomy for advanced gastric cancer without lymph node metastasis. Lymphatic vessel invasion (LVI) was noted in 20.0%, blood vessel invasion (BVI) in 5.4%, and either LVI or BVI in 22.5%. None of the clinicopathologic features was related to LBVI. Patients with LBVI had a recurrence rate of 26.8%, whereas patients without LBVI had a recurrence rate of 13.5%. The 5-year survival rates were 82.4% for patients without LBVI and 67.1% for patients with LBVI. LBVI was shown to be an independent risk factor for recurrence [21]. Del Casar et al. reviewed 144 patients with primary gastric adenocarcinoma, who consecutively underwent surgery with a mean follow up of 33 months. LBVI was present in 46 patients (31.9%). The presence of LBVI correlated significantly with tumor stage, lymph node involvement, surgical resectability, histological type and histological grade, being present in a higher percentage among II-IV tumor stage, poorly differentiated, diffuse type, R1-R2 and lymph node-positive tumors. In addition, statistical analysis demonstrated that LBVI was significantly associated with a poorer overall patients' survival in the univariate analysis as well as in the multivariate analysis. However, their results failed to show any significant relationship between LBVI and any of the intratumoral biological parameters studies [22].

LBVI is an adverse prognostic indicator and the presence of LBVI seems to provide useful information for the prognosis and clinical management of patients with node-negative advanced and also early gastric carcinoma [23].

8. Peritoneal cytology

Mezhir et al. demonstrated that a positive peritoneal cytology, even in the absence of gross peritoneal disease, indicates a poor outcome [24, 25]. In the Dutch Gastric Cancer Group, positive cytological findings were found in 4.4% of the patients and were indicative of a poor prognosis, with a median survival of 13 months [26]. Thus, the Japanese Society for Gastric Cancer has included peritoneal cytology as part of the staging procedure, while the TNM classification system has classified cytology-positive gastric cancer patients as stage IV patients since 1997 [27,28].

9. Lymph node ratio

Xiao et al. reviewed the significance of metastatic lymph node ratio in gastric cancer and compared it to N staging of 7th edition of UICC [29]. Lymph node metastasis is one of the most important gastric cancer prognostic factors [30]. The identified number of involved lymph nodes depends on the number of lymph nodes removed and examined, which in turn depends on the surgical and pathologic procedures. Although TNM classification is a convenient and reproducible method for precise staging, it demands the examination of at least 15 lymph nodes. If the number of dissected and examined lymph nodes is small, down-migration of N stage may occur, and conversely, if the number is large, upmigration of N stage may occur, which is also referred to as stage migration in some references [31,32]. To improve prognosis prediction, the number of positive lymph nodes should be considered in the context of the number of nodes examined. The metastatic lymph node ratio (MLNR), defined as the number of positive lymph nodes divided by the number of lymph nodes retrieved, has been proposed as an alternative to classification systems that assess the absolute number of positive lymph nodes [29]. In a study by Nitti et al. the 5-year survivals according to the metastatic/examined lymph nodes ratio (N ratio) were 14%, 50%, 61%, and 82% in the group of patients with N ratio >25%, 11%-25%, 1%-10%, and 0%, respectively (P <.0001). At multivariate analysis, the N ratio was the best single independent prognostic factor [33]. In a study by Kulig et al., it was said that even though the LNR cannot be used as a substitute for staging with adequate lymphadenectomy, it may help to stratify patients in terms of prognosis when the number of resected lymph nodes is limited and therefore the stage is inadequately defined [34]. The metastatic lymph node ratio system reduces stage migration in patients undergoing D1 lymphadenectomy for gastric adenocarcinoma [35]. Xu et al. stated that positive N ratio classification is a better prognostic tool compared with N staging system after D2 resection in patients with gastric cancer. It can prevent stage migration and can be used regardless of the examined number of lymph nodes [36].

10. Age

In a review by Wang et al., it is stated that the prognostic value of age in gastric cancer patients remains controversial [37]. Some researchers thought that it was not an independent prognostic factor [38-40], whereas others thought that younger patients has worse prognoses than elderly due to the worse biological behaviors of tumors and histological type [41]. However, Saito et al. held that elderly patients had worse prognosis because they had limited lymph node dissection and lower tolerance of chemotherapy [42].

11. Genomics and prognosis

Gastric cancer is said to be a chronic proliferative disease with multiple genetic and epigenetic alterations [43-44]. The specific combination of alterations differs in the 2 histological types of gastric cancer, suggesting that intestinal-type and diffuse-type carcinomas have distinct carcinogenetic pathways. Chromosomal instability (CIN); in particular, loss of heterozygosity (LOH), genomic amplifications, and DNA aneuploidy, are frequently observed in intestinal-type gastric carcinoma [45, 46]. Intestinal type of gastric cancer is thought to be generated after a multistep process of intestinal metaplasia-dysplasia-carcinoma [47]. This process of intestinal type gastric cancer development mimics the progression from adenoma to colon carcinoma, which results from the accumulation of molecular genetic alterations involving activation of oncogenes and inactivation of tumor suppressor genes [48]. Microsatellite instability and p53 mutation, reduced p27 expression, cyclin E overexpression and 6.0kb transcripts of the c-met gene are involved in malignant transformation from precancerous lesions to intestinal-type gastric cancer. In addition, DCC loss, APC mutations, 1q loss of heterozygosity (LOH), p27 loss, reduced expression of tumor growth factor (TGF)β type I receptor and HER2 gene amplification are frequently associated with an advanced stage of intestinal-type gastric carcinoma [49]. Diffuse type gastric cancer is considered to be de novo cancer, and precursor cells have not yet been identified [47]. In contrast, LOH at chromosome 17p (p53) and mutation or loss of E-cadherin are more often implicated in the development of diffuse-type gastric cancer, while loss of p27 and gene amplification of Ksam and c-met lead to disease progression and metastatic spread [49].

Author details

Okan Akturk[1] and Cemal Ulusoy[2]

1 Ankara Numune Education and Research Hospital, Ankara, Turkey

2 Istanbul Kanuni Sultan Suleyman Education and Research Hospital, Istanbul, Turkey

References

[1] Bickenbach, K, & Strong, V. E. Comparisons of Gastric Cancer Treatments: East vs. West. J Gastric Cancer. (2012). Jun; , 12(2), 55-62.

[2] Kunisaki, C, Makino, H, Kimura, J, Takagawa, R, Kosaka, T, Ono, H. A, et al. Impact of lymphovascular invasion in patients with stage I gastric cancer. Surgery (2010). , 147, 204-211.

[3] Biondi, A, Persiani, R, Cananzi, F, Zoccali, M, Vigorita, V, Tufo, A, & D'Ugo, D. D. R0 Resection in the treatment of gastric cancer: room for improvement. World JGastroenterol. (2010). Jul 21; , 16(27), 3358-70.

[4] Hundahl, S. A, Phillips, J. L, & Menck, H. R. The National Cancer ata Base Report on poor survival of U.S. gastric carcinoma patients treated with gastrectomy: Fifth Edition

American Joint Committee on Cancer staging, proximal disease, and the "different disease" hypothesis. Cancer. (2000). , 88, 921-932.

[5] Wu, C. W, Lo, S. S, Shen, K. H, Hsieh, M. C, Chen, J. H, Chiang, J. H, Lin, H. J, Li, A. F, & Lui, W. Y. Incidence and factors associated with recurrence patterns after intended curative surgery for gastric cancer. World J Surg. (2003). Feb; , 27(2), 153-8.

[6] Dicken, B. J, Bigam, D. L, Cass, C, Mackey, J. R, Joy, A. A, & Hamilton, S. M. Gastric adenocarcinoma: review and considerations for future directions. Ann Surg. (2005). Jan; , 241(1), 27-39.

[7] Marelli, D, Roviello, F, & De Manzoni, G. (2002). Different Patterns of Recurrence in Gastric Cancer Depending on Lauren's Histological Type: Longitudinal Study. World Journal of Surgery, 26 9 (September2002), 116011650

[8] Shiraishi, N, Inomata, M, Osawa, N, Yasuda, K, Adachi, Y, & Kitano, S. Early and late recurrence after gastrectomy for gastric carcinoma. Univariate and multivariate analyses. Cancer. (2000). Jul 15; , 89(2), 255-61.

[9] Nakamura, K, Ueyama, T, Yao, T, Xuan, Z. X, Ambe, K, Adachi, Y, & Yakeishi, Y. Matsukuma A, Enjoji M. Pathology and prognosis of gastric carcinoma. Findings in 10,000patients who underwent primary gastrectomy. Cancer. (1992). Sep 1; , 70(5), 1030-7.

[10] Adachi, Y, Oshiro, T, Mori, M, Maehara, Y, & Sugimachi, K. Tumor size as a simple prognostic indicator for gastric carcinoma. Ann SurgOncol. (1997). Mar; , 4(2), 137-40.

[11] Moriguchi, S, Kamakura, T, Odaka, T, Nose, Y, Maehara, Y, Korenaga, D, & Sugimachi, K. Clinical features of the differentiated and undifferentiated types of advanced gastric carcinoma: univariate and multivariate analyses. J SurgOncol. (1991). Nov; , 48(3), 202-6.

[12] Chiaravalli, AM, Klersy, C, Vanoli, A, Ferretti, A, & Capella, C. .Solcia E Histotype-based prognostic classification of gastric cancer. World J Gastroenterol. 2012 Mar 7; 18(9): 896-904.

[13] Chiaravalli, AM, Klersy, C, Tava, F, Manca, R, Fiocca, R, Capella, C, & Solcia, . .Lower- and higher-grade subtypes of diffuse gastric cancer. Hum Pathol. 2009Nov; 40(11): 1591-9.

[14] Chiaravalli, A. M, Cornaggia, M, Furlan, D, Capella, C, Fiocca, R, Tagliabue, G, Klersy, C, & Solcia, E. The role of histological investigation in prognostic evaluation of advanced gastric cancer. Analysis of histological structure and molecular changes

[15] Yokota, T, Ishiyama, S, Saito, T, Teshima, S, Yamada, Y, Iwamoto, K, & Takahashi, M. Murata K, Yamauchi H. Is tumor size a prognostic indicator for gastric carcinoma? Anticancer Res. (2002). Nov-Dec; 22(6B):, 3673-7.

[16] Adachi, Y, Oshiro, T, Mori, M, Maehara, Y, & Sugimachi, K. Tumor size as a simple prognostic indicator for gastric carcinoma. Ann SurgOncol. (1997). Mar; , 4(2), 137-40.

[17] Shiraishi, N, Sato, K, Yasuda, K, Inomata, M, & Kitano, S. Multivariate prognostic study on large gastric cancer. J SurgOncol. (2007). Jul 1; , 96(1), 14-8.

[18] Yuksel, B. C, Akturk, O. M, & Ozel, I. H. Lymph node dissection in gastric carcinoma. Intech (2012).

[19] Saito, H, Fukumoto, Y, Osaki, T, Fukuda, K, Tatebe, S, Tsujitani, S, & Ikeguchi, . .Distinct recurrence pattern and outcome of adenocarcinoma of the gastric cardiain comparison with carcinoma of other regions of the stomach. World J Surg. 2006 Oct; 30(10): 1864-9.

[20] Siewert, J. R, Feith, M, Werner, M, & Stein, H. J. Adenocarcinoma of the esophagogastric junction. Results of surgical therapy based on anatomical/topographic classification in 1,002 consecutive patients. Ann Surg (2000). , 232, 353-361.

[21] Hyung, W. J, Lee, J. H, Choi, S. H, Min, J. S, & Noh, S. H. Prognostic impact of lymphatic and/or blood vessel invasion in patients with node-negative advanced gastric cancer. Ann SurgOncol. (2002). Jul; , 9(6), 562-7.

[22] del Casar JM, Corte MD, Alvarez A, García I, Bongera M, González LO,García-Muñiz JL, Allende MT, Astudillo A, Vizoso FJ. Lymphatic and/or blood vessel invasion in gastric cancer: relationship with clinicopathological parameters, biological factors and prognostic significance. J Cancer Res ClinOncol. (2008). Feb; , 134(2), 153-61.

[23] Du, C. Y, Chen, J. G, Zhou, Y, Zhao, G. F, Fu, H, Zhou, X. K, & Shi, Y. Q. Impact of lymphatic and/or blood vessel invasion in stage II gastric cancer. World J Gastroenterol. Jul 21; , 18(27), 3610-6.

[24] Griniatsos, J, Michail, O, Dimitriou, N, & Karavokyros, I. Lymph node, peritoneal and bone marrow micrometastases in gastric cancer: Their clinical significance. World J GastrointestOncol. (2012). Feb 15; , 4(2), 16-21.

[25] Mezhir, J. J, Shah, M. A, Jacks, L. M, Brennan, M. F, Coit, D. G, & Strong, V. E. Positive peritoneal cytology in patients with gastric cancer: natural history and outcome of 291 patients. Ann SurgOncol. (2010). Dec; , 17(12), 3173-80.

[26] Bonenkamp, J. J, Songun, I, & Hermans, J. van de Velde CJ. Prognostic value of positive cytology findings from abdominal washings in patients with gastric cancer. Br J Surg. (1996). May; , 83(5), 672-4.

[27] Japanese Gastric Cancer AssociationJapanese classification of gastric carcinoma: 3rd English edition. Gastric Cancer. (2011). Jun; , 14(2), 101-12.

[28] Sobin, L. H, & Fleming, I. D. TNM Classification of Malignant Tumors, fifth edition ((1997). Union InternationaleContre le Cancer and the American Joint Committee on Cancer. Cancer. 1997 Nov 1;, 80(9), 1803-4.

[29] Xiao, L. B, Yu, J. X, Wu, W. H, Xu, F. F, & Yang, S. B. Superiority of metastatic lymph noderatio to the 7th edition UICC N staging in gastric cancer. World J Gastroenterol. (2011). Dec 14;, 17(46), 5123-30.

[30] Yokota, T, Ishiyama, S, Saito, T, Teshima, S, Narushima, Y, Murata, K, & Iwamoto, K. Yashima R, Yamauchi H, Kikuchi S. Lymph node metastasis as a significant prognostic factor in gastric cancer: a multiple logistic-regression analysis. Scand J Gastroenterol. (2004). Apr;, 39(4), 380-4.

[31] Yoo, C. H, Noh, S. H, Kim, Y. I, & Min, J. S. Comparison of prognostic significance of nodal-staging between old (4th edition) and new (5th edition) UICC TNM classification for gastric carcinoma. International Union against Cancer. World J Surg. (1999). May;discussion 497-8., 23(5), 492-7.

[32] Aurello, P, Angelo, D, Rossi, F, Bellagamba, S, Cicchini, R, Nigri, C, & Ercolani, G. . Classification of lymph node metastases from gastric cancer: comparison between N-site and N-number systems. Our experience and review of the literature. Am Surg. 2007 Apr;73(4):359-66.

[33] Nitti, D, Marchet, A, Olivieri, M, Ambrosi, A, Mencarelli, R, Belluco, C, & Lise, M. Ratio between metastatic and examined lymph nodes is an independent prognostic factor after D2 resection for gastric cancer: analysis of a large European mono institutional experience. Ann SurgOncol. 2003 Nov;10(9):1077-85.

[34] Kulig, J, Sierzega, M, & Kolodziejczyk, P. Popiela T; Polish Gastric Cancer StudyGroup. Ratio of metastatic to resected lymph nodes for prediction of survival in patients with inadequately staged gastric cancer. Br J Surg. (2009). Aug;, 96(8), 910-8.

[35] Maduekwe, U. N, Lauwers, G. Y, Fernandez-del-castillo, C, Berger, D. L, Ferguson, C. M, Rattner, D. W, & Yoon, S. S. New metastatic lymph node ratio system reduces stage migration in patients undergoing D1 lymphadenectomy for gastric adenocarcinoma. AnnSurgOncol. (2010). May;, 17(5), 1267-77.

[36] Xu, D. Z, Geng, Q. R, Long, Z. J, Zhan, Y. Q, Li, W, Zhou, Z. W, Chen, Y. B, Sun, X. W, Chen, G, & Liu, Q. Positive lymph node ratio is an independent prognostic factor in gastric cancer after d2 resection regardless of the examined number of lymph nodes. AnnSurgOncol. (2009). Feb;, 16(2), 319-26.

[37] Wang, W, Li, Y. F, Sun, X. W, Chen, Y. B, Li, W, Xu, D. Z, Guan, X. X, Huang, C. Y, Zhan, Y. Q, & Zhou, Z. W. Prognosis of 980 patients with gastric cancer after surgical resection. Chin J Cancer. (2010). Nov;PubMed PMID: 20979691., 29(11), 923-30.

[38] Deng, J, Liang, H, Sun, D, et al. Suitability of 7th UICC N Stage for predicting the overall survival of gastric cancer patients after curative resection in China [J]. Ann Surg Oncol, (2010).

[39] An, J. Y, Baik, Y. H, Choi, M. G, et al. The prognosis of gastric cardia cancer after R0 resection [J]. Am J Surg, (2010).

[40] Zhang, X. F, Huang, C. M, Lu, H. S, et al. Surgical treatment and prognosis of gastric cancer in 2,613 patients [J]. World J Gastroenterol, (2004).

[41] Park, J. C, Lee, Y. C, Kim, J. H, et al. Clinicopathological aspects and prognostic value with respect to age: an analysis of 3,362 consecutive gastric cancer patients [J]. J Surg On-col, (2009).

[42] Saito, H, Osaki, T, & Murakami, D. Effect of age on prognosis in patients with gastric cancer [J]. ANZ J Surg, (2006).

[43] Yasui, W, Oue, N, Aung, P. P, Matsumura, S, Shutoh, M, & Nakayama, H. Molecular-pathological prognostic factors of gastric cancer: a review. Gastric Cancer. (2005). , 8(2), 86-94.

[44] Yasui, W, Oue, N, Ito, R, Kuraoka, K, & Nakayama, H. Search for new biomarkers of gastric cancer through serial analysis of gene expression and its clinical implications. Cancer Sci. (2004). , 95(5), 385-92.

[45] Kim, Y. H, Kim, N. G, Lim, J. G, Park, C, & Kim, H. Chromosomal alterations in paired gastric adenomas and carcinomas. Am JPathol. (2001). , 158(2), 655-62.

[46] [46] Sugai, T, Nakamura, S, Uesugi, N, Habano, W, Yoshida, T, Tazawa, H, et al. Role of DNA aneuploidy, overexpression of geneproduct, and cellular proliferation in the progression of gastric cancer. Cytometry. (1999). , 53.

[47] Lauwers, G. Y. Defining the pathologic diagnosis of metaplasia, atrophy, dysplasia, and gastric adenocarcinoma. J Clin Gastroenterol (2003). S, 37-43.

[48] Kinzler, K. W, & Vogelstein, B. Lessons from hereditary colorectal cancer. Cell (1996). , 87, 159-70.

[49] Nobili, S, Bruno, L, Landini, I, Napoli, C, Bechi, P, Tonelli, F, Rubio, C. A, Mini, E, & Nesi, G. Genomic and genetic alterations influence the progression of gastric cancer. World J Gastroenterol. (2011). Jan 21;, 17(3), 290-9.

Chapter 12

Gastric Carcinoma: A Review on Epidemiology, Current Surgical and Chemotherapeutic Options

Rokkappanavar K. Kumar, Sajjan S. Raj,
Esaki M. Shankar, E. Ganapathy,
Abdul S. Ebrahim and Shukkur M. Farooq

Additional information is available at the end of the chapter

http://dx.doi.org/10.5772/45896

1. Introduction

Malignancies associated with the upper gastrointestinal (GI) tract are reported to be extremely lethal. Most patients with gastric cancer (GC) in the United States are symptomatic and already have complex untreatable disease at the time of presentation. GC in general, is a senile malignancy (cancer of the aged) and is reportedly twice as common in blacks as in whites. Routine screening is not extensively performed, except in countries, which have a very high incidence of GC, such as Japan, Venezuela, and Chile. The three most common primary malignant gastric neoplasms are adenocarcinoma (95%), lymphoma (4%), and malignant GIST (Gastrointestinal stromal tumor)(1%). Fortunately, dedicated research into its pathogenesis and detection of new risk factors, treatment, and advanced endoscopic techniques have led to early diagnosis of GC in the modern era.

2. Adenocarcinoma

Adenocarcinoma of the gastric epithelium is the most common form of malignancies of the gut (90% of cases). Carcinoma of the connective tissue (sarcoma) and lymphatics (lymphoma) is reportedly less common. Adenocarcinomas (Figures 1, 2) most commonly occur in the gastric cardia (31%), followed by the antrum (26%), and body of the stomach (14%). The 5-year overall survival rate is 25.7%, which has not changed drastically over the past 30 to 40 years. Surgery remains the mainstay of treatment for GC, the survival can be improved with multimodal approach.

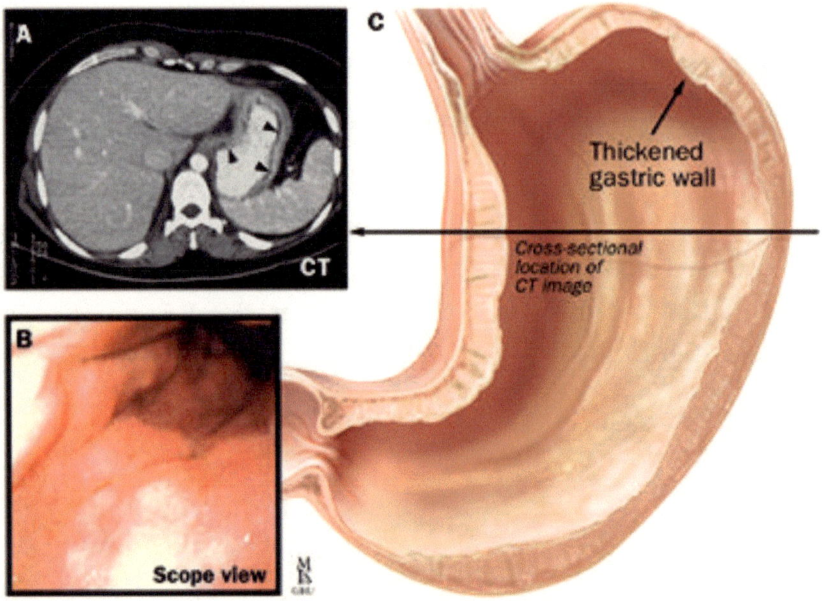

Figure 1. Showing A. CT image of Linitis plastic (arrows denotes a thickened gastric wall). B. endoscopic image. C. illustration of linits plastic. Picture courtesy: John Hopkins Medicine- Gastroenterology and Hepatology department. 'An introduction to Gastric cancer', 2012.

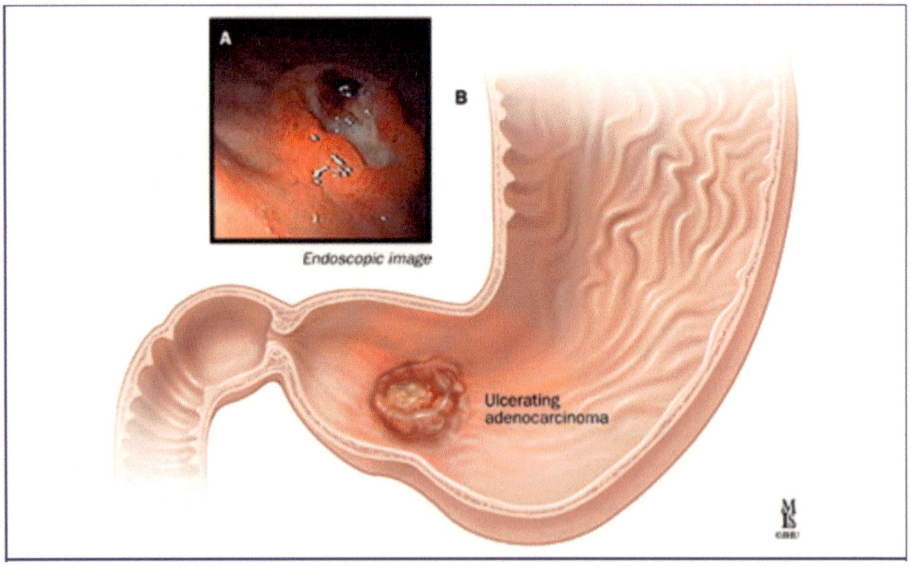

Figure 2. Showing A. the Endoscopic image of an ulcerating adenocarcinoma. B. Ulcerating adenocarcinoma, pictorial representation. Picture courtesy: John Hopkins Medicine- Gastroenterology and Hepatology department. 'An introduction to Gastric cancer', 2012.

2.1. Incidence and prevalence

GC is one of the most common cancers worldwide, causing almost 738,000 deaths annually. The incidence of GC varies widely, both globaly and within individual country. High-incidence has been reported from parts of Latin America, Eastern Asia, Europe and the Middle East [1]. The overall incidence rates are different, but they are increased among certain ethnic and racial groups, such as Hispanics and African-Americans [2] in the US. More recently, for reasons unknown, a growing rate in the incidence of GC has been reported among young adults in the US [3]. The incidence of early GC (EGC), as well as the percentage of gastric adenocarcinomas that are EGCs, vary depending on the population: In Japan and Eastern Asia, up to one-half of resections for gastric adenocarcinoma represent EGC. In Japan, the proportion rose from 15 to as high as 57 percent with the introduction of routine screening programs; In Korea, 25 to 30 percent of gastric adenocarcinomas are EGCs [4]; In Western countries, EGCs account for 15 to 21 percent of gastric adenocarcinomas [4]

GC tends to occur 1.5 to 2.5 times more frequently in African Americans, Hispanic Americans, and Native Americans than whites. GC occurs at a median age of 69 years for men and 73 for women [5], and has an elevated incidence in groups of lower socioeconomic status. In the US, an estimated 21,130 new cases of GC were diagnosed in 2009, with 10,620 deaths [2]. According to the Surveillance Epidemiology and End Results (SEER) [5] (2000–2006) database, only 24% of GCs are confined to the stomach (localized); 31 to 32% of newly diagnosed cases have spread beyond the stomach into the peripheral lymph nodes (regional) or other organs (distant), respectively [5]. GC predominantly affects men compared to women, at a ratio of 2:1. On the basis of SEER 2002-2006 data, the age-adjusted incidence of GC is 7.9 per 100,000 men and women per year [5]. In younger patients, tumors are more often of the diffuse variety and tend to be large, aggressive, and more poorly differentiated, sometimes infiltrating the entire stomach (linitis plastica). The 5-year OS (overall survival) rate is 25.7%, which has not changed significantly over the past 30 to 40 years [5]. Surgical intervention is still the only available option to effectively cure GC, and endurance could be improved with multimodal therapy.

2.2. Etiology

Gastric adenocarcinoma is a multifactorial disease. It is observed that when people migrate from a place with high incidence to a place with low incidence the occurrence of cancer in new generations is lesser. This suggests an unknown environmental factor contributing to the development of GC. It is widely believed that consumption of salt-preserved and smoked food is associated with onset of GC. Achlorhydric stomach predisposes to growth of bacteria wherein nitrate is converted into nitrite, a proven carcinogen. Bacteria may be introduced exogenously through the ingestion of partially decayed foods, which are consumed generously worldwide by the lower socioeconomic classes. Serial endoscopic examinations of the stomach in patients with atrophic gastritis have documented replacement of the usual gastric mucosa by intestinal-type cells. This process of intestinal metaplasia may lead to cellular atypia and eventual neoplasia. The theoretical sequence of development of gastric adenocarcinoma is illustrated in figure 3 [7].

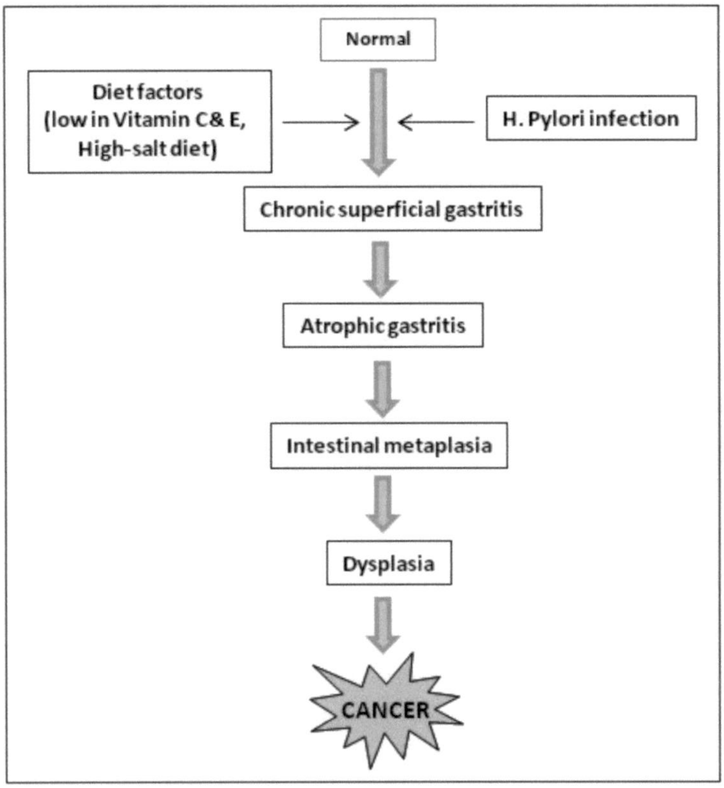

Figure 3. Showing the sequence of development of GC (*Adopted from: Swartz's principles of surgery, 9th edition, September 2009*).

2.3. *Helicobacter pylori* [7, 8]

Helicobacter pylori has been classified as a group 1 (i.e. definite) carcinogen by the World Health organization (WHO) report. Recent lines of evidence showed that persistent *H.pylori* infection increases the risk of GC in patients to about three-fold. Patients with history of gastric ulcers are more likely to develop GC as compared to uninfected individuals, (incidence ratio 1.8, 95% confidence interval 1.6 to 2.0), and patients with a history of duodenal ulcer are at decreased risk for GC (incidence ratio 0.6, 95% CI 0.4 to 0.7). *H. pylori* causes chronic gastritis, loss of gastric acidity, and bacterial growth in the gastric antrum. The effect of *H. pylori* eradication on the subsequent risk for GC in high-incidence areas is under investigation.

2.4. Epstein-Barr virus

EBV, a virus belonging to the herpesviridae family of DNA viruses is reported to be associated with the development of late stages of cancer. EBV accounts for ~10% of all GCs.

2.5. Genetic factors

Numerous genetic abnormalities have been implicated in the development of GC, and most of them are aneuploid. Genetic abnormalities in the tumor suppressor gene *p53*, and COX-2 are the two most common causes observed among the sporadic cases of GC. More than two thirds of GCs have deletion or suppression mutations in the *p53* message.

2.6. Fruits, vegetables and fiber

Consumption of fruits and vegetables, especially fruits is believed to protect against GC. Case-control studies from Europe, Asia, and North America have shown that intake of fruits and vegetables could confer protection against GC, reducing the risk by ~40 percent for fruits, and ~30 percent for vegetables for the highest versus lowest categories of intake, respectively. Diets low in vitamin C show the strongest association with GC. The protection attributed to consumption of vegetables and fruits is most likely related to vitamin C content, which is believed to lower the formation of carcinogenic N-nitroso compounds in the gut. However, cooked vegetables do not show the equal degree of protection as uncooked vegetables.

2.7. Other factors

Prospective investigations have highlighted the importance of intake of cereal fibers in alleviating the risk of development of diffuse type GC, but not the intestinal type. Individuals with blood group A are reported to develop ~20 percent increased risk of GC than those with group O, B, or AB [6]. Interestingly, excessive body weight and obesity are associated with an increased risk of development of GC [9]. According to a study, the strength of association between body weight and cancer increased with increasing BMI. Several studies have investigated the relationship between tobacco smoking and GC. A meta-analysis of 40 different investigations has estimated that the risk was increased by ~1.5 to 1.6-fold and was higher in men. A prospective study found that, compared with non-smokers, active smokers were at increased risk for cancer at the gastric cardia (HR 2.9, 95% CI 1.7, 4.7), and gastric noncardia (HR 2.0, 95% CI 1.3, 3.2] [10]. Finally, regular use of NSAIDs has been inversely associated with the risk of distal gastric adenocarcinoma [11, 12].

2.8. Premalignant conditions of the stomach

Certain premalignant conditions of the stomach are reported to predispose to the development of GC. A study conducted in Tokyo and Japan involving 1900 cases has shown that the prevalence of certain premalignant conditions (figure 4) is associated with the development of EGC.Atrophic gastritis is by far the most commonly reported precancerous condition of the stomach predisposing to development of GC.

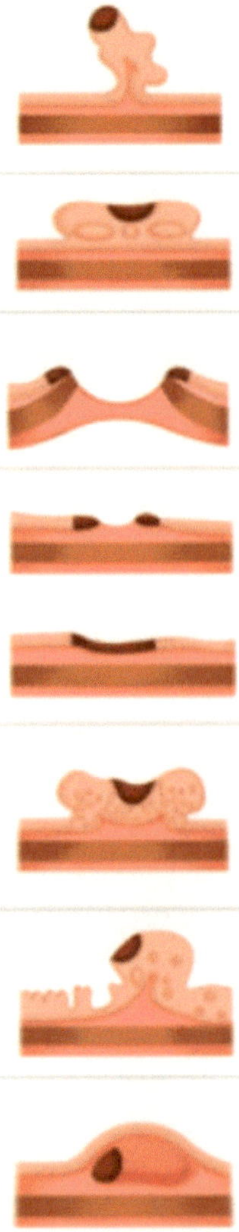

1900 Cases		
Precancerous lesion	Number of cases	%
Hyperplastic polyp	10	0.53
Adenoma	47	2.47
Chronic ulcer	13	0.68
Atrophic gastritis	1802	94.84
Verrucous gastritis	26	1.37
Stomach remnant	2	0.11
Aberrant pancreas	0	0
	Total 1900	100

Figure 4. Showing the premalignant lesions of the stomach (Source: Swartz's principles of surgery, 9th edition. September 2009)

2.9. Molecular pathogenesis of GC

Almost half of the intestinal types of GCs is associated with mutations in tumor suppressor genes. *TP53* is one key regulatory molecule that protects cells in the chronic inflammatory stress microenvironment, and any event leading to the loss of *TP53* expression by LOH (i.e. Loss Of Heterozygosity or mutational inactivation) culminates in frequent gastric alterations and development of GC, occurring in >60% of invasive tumors [13]. Another molecular factor associated with GC is the *c-met* oncogene expression that is reportedly amplified in 19% of intestinal type and 39% of diffuse type of GCs. Especially, expression of 6.0 kb *c-met* transcript is associated with more advanced disease stage at the time of presentation. Likewise, there are other molecular mechanisms suggested for GC. *k-ras* mutations are detected in intestinal metaplasia, dysplasia and invasive cancers. *TP73* is found to be either overexpressed or not expressed at all. Over expression of *p73* and the oncogenic isoform *Delta Np73* suppresses *p73* transcriptional and apoptotic activity in gastroepithelial cancer cells and increases intracellular β-catenin levels, an effect that is inhibited in the presence of wild-type but not mutant *p53*. Loss of expression has been reported via epigenetic mechanisms in EBV-associated GCs [14]. Mutations in APC (adenomatous polyposis coli) gene are identified in significantly more intestinal-type than diffuse-type GCs (33 versus 13 percent). These mutations are also found in *H. pylori*-associated dysplasia and intestinal metaplasia [14]. Loss of *TFF1* (trefoil factor family1) expression has been observed in intestinal metaplasia of the incomplete type and in GCs. The trefoil factor family (TFF) of proteins comprises a group of gastrointestinal peptides that are involved in the protection of the mucous epithelium. Cell cycle regulatory molecules — Cyclin E and cyclin-dependent kinase inhibitor 1B (CDKN1B, p27) are the two important cell-cycle regulators that take part in G1/S transition. Cyclin E overexpression is a frequent event in GCs, and might be an indicator for malignant transformation of dysplasia, and/or tumor aggressiveness following development of an invasive cancer. E-cadherin, a key protein on cell surfaces responsible for intercellular connections, is absent in diffuse type of carcinoma enabling tumor cells to invade and metastasize.

2.10. Pathology

Dysplasia, the earliest stage in the development of cancer, is regarded as the precursor of GC. Mildly dysplastic cases are followed up with endoscopic surveillance plus *H.pylori* eradication. Nonetheless, severely dysplastic cases need gastric resection if tumor is widespread or multifocal; or may need Endoscopic Mucosal Resection (EMR) if the tumor is localized.

2.11. Early and late GC

Early GC is defined as adenocarcinoma limited to the mucosa and submucosa of the stomach, irrespective of lymph node status. Late GC defined as a gastric carcinoma that has invaded the muscle wall. It is the stage at which the tumor is commonly diagnosed in the US. Different types of Early GCs (EGC) have been illustrated in figure 5.

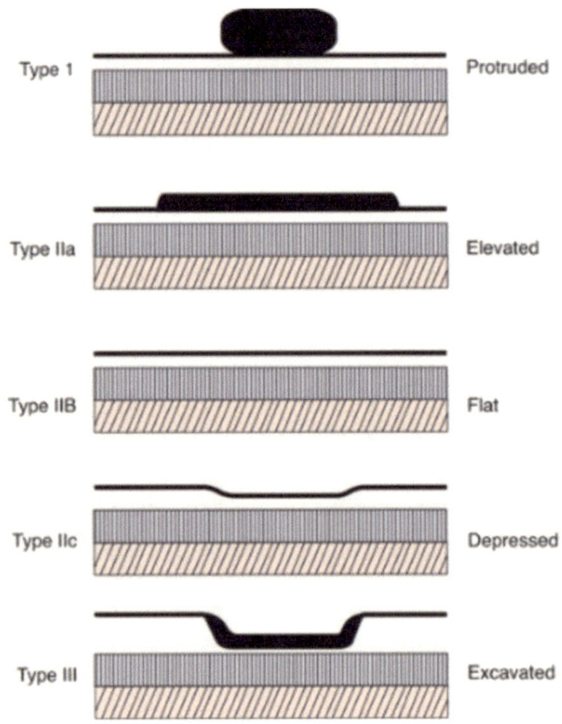

Figure 5. Different types of EGC (Source: Swartz's principles of surgery, 9th edition, September 2009)

2.12. Gross morphology and histologic subtypes

Morphologically, there are four varieties of GCs: polypoid, fungating, ulcerative, and scirrhous. In polypoidal and fungating, the bulk of the tumor mass is found intraluminally. In case of ulcerative and scirrhous type the bulk of the tumor is found in the wall of the stomach. Whilst polypoid type of tumors are not ulcerated, fungating tumors are elevated intraluminally, and ulcerated. As the name implies, ulcerative variety morphologically resembles ulcers. On contrary, the scirrhous tumors tend to infiltrate the entire thickness of the stomach and cover a very large surface area. Scirrhous tumors involve the entire stomach and have a very poor prognosis. This is classically described as 'Linitis plastica' or leather bottle appearance which is characterized by loss of distensibility of the gastric wall. Regarding the anatomic location of GC, in the US, 30% of GCs originate in the distal, 20% arise in the mid portion, and 37% originate in the proximal third of the stomach. The remaining 13% involve the entire stomach.

2.13. Histology

Histologic characterization of the GC is important as histologic type and the depth of invasion are the most important prognostic indicators. There are many histologic classifications of GC. The histologic classification described by WHO involves: Adenocarcinoma (papillary, tubular, mucinous, signet-ring), adenosquamous, squamous, small cell, undifferentiat-

http://dx.doi.org/10.5772/45896

ed, and others. Further, there is a Japanese classification which is similar to the one described by WHO, but more descriptive. There is also a Lauren classification which classifies GCs into intestinal (53%), diffuse (33%), and unclassified (14%) GC types.

2.14. Pathologic staging

Prognosis depends on the pathologic stage of the disease, and TNM (i.e. tumor-node-metastasis) (Table 1) staging is the most widely used system based on the depth of tumor invasion, extent of lymph node metastases [38], and presence of distant metastases. This system was initially developed by the American Joint Committee on Cancer and the International Union Against Cancer, and has undergone several modifications since then.

Primary tumor (T)		**Regional lymph nodes (N)**	
TX	Primary tumor cannot be assessed	**NX**	Regional lymph node(s) cannot be assessed
T0	No evidence of primary tumor	**N0**	No regional lymph node metastasis
Tis	Carcinoma in situ: intraepithelial tumor without invasion of the lamina propria	**N1**	Metastasis in 1-2 regional lymph nodes
T1	Tumor invades lamina propria, muscularis mucosae, or submucosa	**N2**	Metastasis in 3-6 regional lymph nodes
T1a	Tumor invades lamina propria or muscularis mucosae	**N3**	Metastasis in seven or more regional lymph nodes
T1b	Tumor invades submucosa	**N3a**	Metastasis in 7-15 regional lymph nodes
T2	Tumor invades muscularispropria	**N3b**	Metastasis in 16 or more regional lymph nodes
T3	Tumor penetrates subserosal connective tissue without invasion of visceral peritoneum or adjacent structures		
T4	Tumor invades serosa (visceral peritoneum) or adjacent structures	**Distant metastasis (M)**	
T4a	Tumor invades serosa (visceral peritoneum)	**M0**	No distant metastasis
T4b	Tumor invades adjacent structures	**M1**	Distant metastasis

Primary tumor (T)		**Regional lymph nodes (N)**	
TX	Primary tumor cannot be assessed	**NX**	Regional lymph node(s) cannot be assessed
T0	No evidence of primary tumor	**N0**	No regional lymph node metastasis
Tis	Carcinoma in situ: intraepithelial tumor without invasion of the lamina propria	**N1**	Metastasis in 1-2 regional lymph nodes
T1	Tumor invades lamina propria, muscularis mucosae, or submucosa	**N2**	Metastasis in 3-6 regional lymph nodes
T1a	Tumor invades lamina propria or muscularis mucosae	**N3**	Metastasis in seven or more regional lymph nodes
T1b	Tumor invades submucosa	**N3a**	Metastasis in 7-15 regional lymph nodes
T2	Tumor invades muscularispropria	**N3b**	Metastasis in 16 or more regional lymph nodes
T3	Tumor penetrates subserosal connective tissue without invasion of visceral peritoneum or adjacent structures		
T4	Tumor invades serosa (visceral peritoneum) or adjacent structures	**Distant metastasis (M)**	
T4a	Tumor invades serosa (visceral peritoneum)	**M0**	No distant metastasis
T4b	Tumor invades adjacent structures	**M1**	Distant metastasis

Table 1. TNM Classification for Gastric Cancer

Stage	T	N	M	Stage	T	N	M
0	Tis	N0	M0	**IIIA**	T4a	N1	M0
IA	T1	N0	M0		T3	N2	M0
IB	T2	N0	M0		T2	N3	M0
	T1	N1	M0	**IIIB**	T4b	N0	M0
IIA	T3	N0	M0		T4b	N1	M0
	T2	N1	M0		T4a	N2	M0
	T1	N2	M0		T3	N3	M0
IIB	T4a	N0	M0	**IIIC**	T4b	N2	M0
	T3	N1	M0		T4b	N3	M0
	T2	N2	M0		T4a	N3	M0
	T1	N3	M0	**IV**	Any T	Any N	M1

A tumor may penetrate the muscularispropria with extension into the gastrocolic or gastrohepatic ligaments, or into the greater or lesser omentum, without perforation of the visceral peritoneum covering these structures. In this case, the tumor is classified T3. If there is perforation of the visceral peritoneum covering the gastric ligaments or the omentum, the tumor should be classified T4.• The adjacent structures of the stomach include the spleen, transverse colon, liver, diaphragm, pancreas, abdominal wall, adrenal gland, kidney, small intestine, and retroperitoneum.

Δ Intramural extension to the duodenum or esophagus is classified by the depth of the greatest invasion in any of these sites, including the stomach.

◊ A designation of pN0 should be used if all examined lymph nodes are negative, regardless of the total number removed and examined.

Tables 1 & 2 Source: The original source for this material is the AJCC Cancer Staging Manual, Seventh Edition [2010] published by Springer New York, Inc.*

Table 2. Anatomic stage/prognostic groups

Criteria
1. High probability of en bloc resection
2. Tumor histology: a. Intestinal type adenocarcinoma b. Tumor confined to the mucosa c. Absence of venous or lymphatic invasion
3. Tumor size and morphology: a. Less than 20 mm in diameter, without ulceration b. Less than 10 mm in diameter if Paris classification IIb or IIc
(Extended criteria)
4. Mucosal tumors of any size without ulceration
5. Mucosal tumors less than 30 mm with ulceration
6. Submucosal tumors less than 30 mm confined to the upper 0.5 mm of the submucosa without lymphovascular invasion

Table 3. The criteria for EMR/ESD

http://dx.doi.org/10.5772/45896

2.15. Spread

GC initially infiltrates the submucosa and invades through the muscle wall into the fat of the omentum. Transcoelomic spread of the tumor cells is possible through peritoneal fluid when serosa is involved. Such metastases may involve to rectovesical pouch or ovary (Krukenberg tumor). Microscopic satellite nodules may be formed some distance away from the main mass by involvement through submucosal lymphatics. Lymphatic spread is responsible for the involvement of the nodes around the stomach. Also, when tumor spreads to involve left supraclavicular nodes, it is known as Virchow's nodes.

2.16. Clinical features

Most patients, who are diagnosed with GC in the US are in advanced stage III or IV disease at the time of diagnosis. GCs, when surgically curable and superficial, usually produce no symptoms. The clinical manifestations also depend on the anatomical location of the tumor. Large tumors which are present in the fundus and body may simply manifest with occult blood loss. In contrast, tumors of the antrum will delay gastric emptying and lead to anorexia, early satiety, and eventually the features of gastric outlet obstruction. Tumors of the proximal stomach can also involve the distal esophagus and present with dysphagia. As the cancer becomes more extensive, patients might complain of slight upper abdominal distress varying in intensity from a vague, postprandial fullness to a severe, sturdy pain. Symptoms are generally nonspecific and most frequently include abdominal pain, weight loss, nausea, decreased food intake due to anorexia and early satiety. Weight loss consequences from inadequate calorie intake rather than increased catabolism and may be attributable to nausea, anorexia, abdominal pain, early satiety, and dysphagia.

Abdominal pain tends to be epigastric in nature. Dysphagia is a common symptom in cancers involving proximal stomach or at the esophago-gastric junction. Other symptoms include nausea, early satiety, symptoms of gastric outlet obstruction. Occult gastrointestinal bleeding with or without iron deficiency anemia is not uncommon. Postprandial vomiting suggests pyloric obstruction. Nearly 25% of patients have a history of gastric ulcer, stressing the importance of eradication of *H. pylori* infection.

Patients may also present with signs or symptoms of distant metastatic disease. Since GC can spread through lymphatics, the physical examination may reveal a left supraclavicular adenopathy (a Virchow's node) which is the most common physical examination finding of metastatic disease, a periumbilical nodule (Sister Mary Joseph's node), or a left axillary node (Irish node). Peritoneal spread can present with an enlarged ovary (Krukenberg's tumor) or a mass in the cul-de-sac on rectal examination (Blumer's shelf). Ascites can also be the initial indication of peritoneal carcinomatosis. A liver mass that can be palpable may indicate metastases. Paraneoplastic manifestations may include skin findings such as rapid appearance of diffuse seborrheic keratoses (sign of Leser-Trelat) or acanthosis nigricans, which is characterized by velvety and darkly pigmented patches on skin folds. Other signs are: microangiopathic hemolytic anemia, membranous nephropathy, hypercoagulable states (Trousseau's syndrome) and polyarteritis nodosa.

2.17. Tumor markers and screening

There is no single marker that has been identified as the marker of GC. A study conducted in Japan reported that screening program for GC has limited value. For the same reason, there are no recommendations for screening the cancer. Some of the high risk factors have been identified though. These include elderly patients with atrophic gastritis, pernicious anemia, patients with partial gastrectomy, patients with FAP/HNPCC (familial adenomatous polyposis / hereditary nonpolyposis colorectal cancer), patients with sporadic gastric adenoma. Periodic upper GI endoscopy can be of little benefit to those who are considered to be at risk. Recently, KAI1/CD82 has been researched as a possible marker for the cancer, but results are inconclusive [15]. Annexin II [16] and S100A6 proteins have shown promising results in predicting prognosis as these two proteins are associated with tumor invasion, metastasis, TNM stage and poor prognosis. Similarly PIWI protein and ADAM17 glycoprotein correlate with cancer occurrence, development and metastasis [17, 18]

2.18. Serologic markers

Serum levels of carcinoembryonic antigen (CEA), the glycoprotein CA 125 antigen (CA 125], CA 199, and CA 724 may be elevated in patients with GC [19, 20]. Nevertheless, low rates of sensitivity and specificity stop the use of any of these serologic markers as diagnostic tests for GC. Some GCs may mark elevated serum levels of α-fetoprotein (AFP); which are referred to as α-fetoprotein producing GCs [21-22]. A subset, hepatoid adenocarcinomas of the stomach, has a histologic appearance that is analogous to that of HCC. Regardless of morphology, AFP-producing GCs are aggressive and associated with a poor prognosis.

2.19. Investigations and preoperative evaluation

- Patients >45 years of age who have new-onset dyspepsia, as well as all patients with heart burn and alarm symptoms (dysphagia, weight loss, recurrent vomiting, evidence of bleeding, or anemia) or with a family history of GC should have timely upper endoscopy and biopsy if a mucosal lesion is noted by endoscope.
- All patients in whom GC is one of the differential diagnoses should undergo endoscopic and biopsic procedures. If the biopsy is negative and suspicion for cancer is high, the patient should be re-endoscoped and more aggressively biopsied.
- In some patients with gastric tumors, upper GI series can be useful in planning treatment. Although a good double-contrast barium upper GI examination is sensitive for gastric tumors (up to 75% sensitive), endoscopy has become the gold standard for the diagnosis of gastric malignancy.

2.20. Endoscopy

Tissue identification and anatomic localization of the primary tumor are best accomplished by upper gastrointestinal endoscopy. The early usage of upper endoscopy in patients presenting with gastrointestinal complaints may be related with a higher rate of finding of early GCs. Endoscopy allows a close inspection of the mucosa, which is generally the only way to detect early GC. The presence of dysplasia, however, should always be regarded as significant because it could be a sign of malignant transformation, or presence of adjacent malignancy.

The diagnosis of a particularly aggressive form of diffuse-type GC, called "linitis plastica", can be cumbersome with endoscopy owing to the nature of these tumors to infiltrate into the submucosa and muscularis propria, and hence, biopsies of superficial mucosal may be false negative. For this reason, a combination of strip and bite biopsy technique should be used when there is a suspicion of diffuse type GC.

2.21. Ultrasonography

Ultrasonography of the abdomen may be helpful for assessing the spread of GC. It may detect evidence of lymphadenopathy but can be particularly precious in detecting metastases within the liver. A number of studies advocate that endoscopic ultrasound has an accuracy of 90% in defining the depth of invasion within the stomach itself. It is also sensitive to wall thickening and will detect diffuse carcinomas, and carcinomas associated with peripheral lymph nodes.

2.22. Barium studies

Barium studies can make out both malignant gastric ulcers and infiltrating lesions. However, false-negative barium studies can occur in as many as 50% of cases. Thus, in most settings, upper endoscopy is the chosen initial diagnostic test for patients in whom GC is suspected.

The only scenario where barium study may be superior to upper endoscopy is in patients with linitis plastica. The decreased distensibility of the stiff, "leather-flask" appearing stomach is more obvious on radiography, while the endoscopic image may appear relatively normal.

2.23. Positron emission tomography scanning

Whole-body PET scanning uses a principle whereby tumor cells preferentially amass positron-emitting ^{18}F fluorodeoxyglucose. This modality is most helpful in the evaluation of distant metastasis in GC but can also useful in loco-regional staging. PET scan is most useful when combined with spiral CT (PET-CT) and should be considered before major surgery in patients with predominantly high-risk tumors or multiple medical co morbidities.

2.24. Abdominopelvic CT scan

Dynamic computerized tomography (CT) imaging is generally performed early during preoperative assessment after a diagnosis of GC is made. CT is widely available and noninvasive. It is best suited in evaluating widely metastasized disease, especially hepatic or adnexal metastases, ascites, or distant nodal spread. Patients who have CT-defined visceral metastatic disease can evade unnecessary surgery, although biopsy confirmation is recommended because of the risk of false-positive findings. Peritoneal metastases and hematogenous metastases smaller than 5 mm are often missed by CT, even using modern CT techniques [23].

2.25. Endoscopic ultrasonography [24-27]

Endoscopic ultrasonography (EUS) is considered to be the most reliable nonsurgical method available for evaluating the depth of invasion of primary gastric cancers, particularly for early (T1) lesions. The precision of EUS for differentiation of individual tumor stages (T1 to T4) ranges from 77 to 93%, with the experience of the operator markedly influencing these rates.

2.26. PET scan

The role of positron emission tomography (PET) using 18-fluorodeoxyglucose (FDG) in preoperative staging of GC is rapidly developing. From the stand point of loco-regional staging, integrated PET/CT imaging may assist in the confirmation of CT-detected malignant lymphadenopathy [28]. The main advantage of PET is that it is more sensitive than CT for the detection of distant metastases [29, 30]. An important caution is that the sensitivity of PET scanning for peritoneal carcinomatosis is only approximately 50% [31]. Thus, PET is not a satisfactory replacement for staging laparoscopy.

2.27. Chest imaging

A preoperative chest x-ray is recommended in patients with GC [32]. However, the sensitivity for metastases is limited, and a chest CT scan is preferred (particularly for patients with a proximal GC) if the detection of intrathoracic disease would modify the treatment plan.

2.28. Staging laparoscopy

Laparoscopy, while more invasive than CT or EUS, has the advantage of directly visualizing the liver surface, the peritoneum, and local lymph nodes. Between 20 and 30 percent of patients who have disease that is beyond T1 stage on EUS will be found to have peritoneal metastases in spite of having a negative CT scan [34]. Particularly among patients with advanced (T3 or 4) primary tumors, performance of a diagnostic laparoscopy may alter management (typically by avoiding an unnecessary laparotomy) in up to one-half [35]. As noted previously, the sensitivity of PET scans for the detection of peritoneal carcinomatosis is only about 50%. Another advantage to laparoscopy is the chance to perform peritoneal cytology in patients who have no visible evidence of peritoneal spread. In most (but not all) series this is a poor prognostic sign, even in the absence of overt peritoneal dissemination, and predicts for early peritoneal relapse. Diagnostic laparoscopy should also be performed in patients who are being considered for neoadjuvant therapy.

2.29. Preoperative evaluation

The rationale of the preoperative evaluation is to primarily stratify patients into two clinical groups: those with loco-regional, potentially resectable (stage I to III) disease and those with systemic (stage IV) involvement.

2.30. Treatment (EGC)

Treatment options available for early GC (EGC) are endoscopic resection, gastrectomy, antibiotic therapy to eradicate *H. pylori* and adjuvant therapies. Endoscopic resection is achieved either by endoscopic mucosal resection (EMR) or endoscopic submucosal dissection (ESD). The criteria for EMR or ESD are outlined in the table: 2 [36, 37]:

Even though *en bloc* resection of the tumor mass has the ideal outcome following mucosal resection, when it fails gastrectomy is the option. Gastrectomy is the most widely practiced treatment modality for GC with a very high five-year survival rates [39-44]. Recently laparoscopic gastrectomy is gaining popularity with high success rates observed in several centers [40, 41, 45-50].

Anti-H.pylori therapy: As noted above, *H. pylori* is declared as a definite carcinogen. Its occurrence is associated with cancer recurrence necessitating its eradication [51]. According to a randomized trial and a case series, eradication of *H. pylori* following endoscopic resection of EGC is found to be associated with reduced risk of metachronous cancers [52].

Adjuvant therapy: The adjuvant therapy with either systemic chemotherapy, radiotherapy, or intraperitoneal chemotherapy following treatment for EGC is not completely established especially for patients with node-negative cancer. On the other hand, for all patients with positive nodes, adjuvant therapy is recommended irrespective of T stage.

2.31. Treatment of invasive GC

The only curative treatment for GC is surgical excision of tumorous mass [53, 54]. Usually abdominal exploration is considered with the curative intent unless there is doubt regarding dissemination, vascular invasion, patient has a medical contraindication for surgery, or a neoadjuvant therapy is considered.

Linitis plastica: In ~5 percent of GC, most of the stomach wall or sometimes the entire stomach wall is infiltrated by malignancy resulting in a rigid thickened wall called linitis plastica. It is more prevalent in younger population [55]. Sometimes this form of cancer represents spread from lobular breast cancer, and is associated with poor prognosis [56, 57]. As there will be nodal involvement frequently, complete excision is the goal even though surgeons consider it to be a contraindication to curative resection.

Total versus subtotal gastrectomy: Total gastrectomy is in vogue for the treatment of invasive GC, even though endoscopic resection is performed for superficial cancers. To note, total gastrectomy is indicated for lesions in the proximal (i.e. upper third) of the stomach, and distal lesions (lower two-thirds) require subtotal gastrectomy with resection of adjacent lymph nodes. Importantly, the patients presenting with large mid gastric or infiltrative lesions like linitis plastica require total gastrectomy.

Proximal and esophagogastric junction tumors: The precise guidelines for surgical excision of proximal tumors are complex. Those tumors that do not invade the esophagogastric junction (EGJ) are managed by either a total or a proximal subtotal gastrectomy. Most surgeons prefer total gastrectomy for the following reasons: 1. The incidence of reflux esophagitis is extremely low following Roux-en-Y reconstruction performed during total gastrectomy compared to those who have undergone proximal subtotal gastrectomy in whom roughly one third patients had reflux esophagitis. 2. It is highly unlikely to remove the lymph nodes along the lesser curvature following proximal subtotal gastrectomy. This may make the metastases escape from surgery.

Degree of lymph node dissection: Again this is the controversial area in the surgical management of GC. Japanese surgeons routinely perform extended lymphadenectomy, which may partially account for the better survival rates among Asian series as compared to Western series [58]. 'Extended lymphadenectomy' refers to either a D2 or D3 nodal dissection.

D1, D2, and D3 terminologies: Japanese surgeons have divided the draining lymph nodes of stomach into 16 stations: stations 1-6 are perigastric, remaining 10 are located side by the major vessels, posterior to pancreas and along the aorta. D1 lymphadenectomy involves limited dissection of only the perigastric lymph nodes. D2 lymphadenectomy involves extended lymph node dissection encompassing removal of nodes along the hepatic, left gastric, celiac and splenic arteries and splenic hilum (stations 1 to 11). D3 lymphadenectomy involves super extended lymph node dissection. In short it is the D2 lymphadenectomy along with resection of nodes within portahepatis and periaortic regions (referred to as stations 1 to 16). Others use the term to denote a D2 dissection plus periaortic nodal dissection (PAND) [59].

Factors in favor of extended lymphadenectomy are, removing more number of nodes accurately stages the disease extent and failure to remove these nodes leaves behind the disease in nearly one third of patients [60]. This would explain the better stage specific survival rates in Asian patients.

Factors against the extended lymphadenectomy are, higher incidence of associated morbidity and mortality especially if splenectomy if done so as to achieve extended lymphadenectomy. Also, most of the randomized trials have shown low survival benefits which discourage surgeons to go for extended lymphadenectomy.

In summary, considering the impact of D2 lymphadenectomy on disease specific survival, most of the cancer hospitals perform D2 as compared to D1 dissection. National Comprehensive Cancer Network has published its treatment guidelines, according to which D2 node dissection is better than D1 dissection. Considering the higher rates of operative mortality in randomized trials, the choice of surgery is at the discretion of the surgeon. D2 lymphadenectomy that preserves pancreas and spleen provides superior staging benefit at the same time avoiding excess morbidity. If splenectomy performed during resection of gastric tumors not adjacent to or invading the spleen or the pancreatic tail will increase the morbidity and mortality without improving the survival [61]. Hence splenectomy is not recommendable unless the tumor has extended directly.

2.32. Adjuvant chemoradiotherapy

It is apt to consider adjuvant radiation therapy as nearly 80 percent of patients who succumb to GC would have experienced local recurrence. Also, three randomized trials (Inter-group 0116, CALGB 80101 and ARTIST trials) have shown significant survival benefit for postoperative combined chemoradiation therapy compared to surgery alone following resection of GC [63].

Neoadjuvant/Perioperative chemotherapy: prior to operating for a locally advanced malignancy, neoadjuvant therapy if used will help to 'downstage' the disease process. Two of the three large trials (MAGIC, French FNLCC/FFCD, EORTC trial 40954) compared surgery alone and surgery with neoadjuvant chemotherapy showed a significant survival benefit for this approach [62, 64, 65].

2.33. Adjuvant chemotherapy

There are more than 30 trials which compared adjuvant systemic chemotherapy to surgery alone. The overall results were negative. Few of the trials to name are Japanese S-1 trial, CLASSIC trial.

2.34. Prognosis

Unless treatment is instituted, the doubling time for EGC is of the order of several years indicating a very stable biologic state compared to a doubling time of less than a year for advanced cancer [66]. A very interesting Nomogram has been developed based on various clinical and pathological statuses by Kim's group for predicting the disease-free survival probability [67]. With the treatment on, the overall five year survival rate is more than 90 percent [68]. According to a Korean study, long term survival rate was 95 percent in patients without nodal involvement; 88% with one to three nodes involved; 77% with more than 3 nodes involvement.

3. Conclusion

Adenocarcinoma is the commonest type of GC. It is one of the top 10 causes of death in USA, twice more common in blacks. Infection with H.pylori, consumption of salt-preserved and smoked foods, achlorhydric stomach are few of the important insults for the development of GC. E-cadherin, a key protein on the cell surface responsible for intercellular connections, is absent in diffuse type of carcinoma enabling tumor cells to invade and metastasize. TNM staging is the most widely used system for staging the disease. As there are no screening tests available for diagnosis of GC, patients usually present in the stage 3 or 4 cancer. Early Gastric Cancer is treated with Endoscopic resection, gastrectomy, antibiotic therapy to eradicate H.pylori and adjuvant therapies. Surgery is the mainstay of treatment for invasive GC. Adjuvant chemoradiotherapy is essential as 80% treated cases develop local recurrence. With the treatment being initiated the prognosis is better as the overall five year survival rate becomes more than 90 percent.

Author details

Rokkappanavar K. Kumar[1], Sajjan S. Raj[2], Esaki M. Shankar[3], E. Ganapathy[4], Abdul S. Ebrahim[5*] and Shukkur M. Farooq[6*]

*Address all correspondence to: eabdulsh@med.wayne.edu, mabdulsh@med.wayne.edu

1 Biochemistry and Molecular Biology,Wayne State University, Detroit, USA

2 Physiology & NeuroScience, St. George's University, Grenada, West Indies

3 Dept. of Medical Microbiology, University of Malaya, Kuala Lumpur, Malaysia

4 Dept. of Obstetrics and Gynecology, University of California Los Angeles, Los Angeles, USA

5 Internal Medicine, Wayne State University, Detroit, USA

6 Pharmacy Practice, Wayne State University, Detroit, USA

[1,2] These authors contributed equally to this review article.

References

[1] Ferlay J, Shin HR, Bray F, et al. Estimates of worldwide burden of cancer in 2008: GLOBOCAN 2008. Int J Cancer 2010; 127:2893. PMID: 21351269.

[2] Jemal A, Siegel R, Xu J, et al. Cancer statistics, 2010. CA Cancer J Clin 2010; 60:277. PMID: 20610543.

[3] Anderson WF, Camargo MC, Fraumeni JF Jr, et al. Age-specific trends in incidence of noncardia gastric cancer in US adults. JAMA 2010; 303:1723. PMID:20442388.PMID: 20442388.

[4] Kang HJ, Kim DH, Jeon TY, et al. Lymph node metastasis from intestinal-type early gastric cancer: experience in a single institution and reassessment of the extended criteria for endoscopic submucosal dissection. GastrointestEndosc 2010; 72:508.PMID: 20554277.

[5] SEER. SEER Stats Facts Sheet. Available from: http://www.seer.cancer.gov/statfacts/html/ stomach.html. [Cited 2009 December 27, 2009].

[6] Edgren G, Hjalgrim H, Rostgaard K, et al. Risk of gastric cancer and peptic ulcers in relation to ABO blood type: a cohort study. Am J Epidemiol 2010; 172:1280. PMID: 20937632.

[7] Fox JG, Wang TC: Inflammation, atrophy, and gastric cancer. J Clin Invest 117:60, 2007. PMID:17200707.

[8] Correa P, Houghton J: Carcinogenesis of Helicobacter pylori. Gastroenterology, 2007, 133:659. PMID: 17681184.

[9] Yang P, Zhou Y, Chen B, et al. Overweight, obesity and gastric cancer risk: results from a meta-analysis of cohort studies. Eur J Cancer 2009; 45:2867. PMID: 19427197.

[10] Freedman ND, Abnet CC, Leitzmann MF, et al. A prospective study of tobacco, alcohol, and the risk of esophageal and gastric cancer subtypes. Am J Epidemiol 2007; 165:1424. PMID:17420181.

[11] Wu CY, Wu MS, Kuo KN, et al. Effective reduction of gastric cancer risk with regular use of nonsteroidal anti-inflammatory drugs in Helicobacter pylori-infected patients. J ClinOncol 2010; 28:2952. PMID:20479409.

[12] Epplein M, Nomura AM, Wilkens LR, et al. Nonsteroidalantiinflammatory drugs and risk of gastric adenocarcinoma: the multiethnic cohort study. Am J Epidemiol 2009; 170:507. PMID:19584132.

[13] Yasui W, Sentani K, Motoshita J, et al. Molecular pathobiology of gastric cancer. Scand J Surg 2006; 95:225.PMID:17249269.

[14] Ushiku T, Chong JM, Uozaki H, et al. p73 gene promoter methylation in Epstein-Barr virus-associated gastric carcinoma. Int J Cancer 2007; 120:60. PMID: 17058198.

[15] Knoener M, Krech T, Puls F, et al. Limited value of KAI1/CD82 protein expression as a prognostic marker in human gastric cancer. Disease markers. 2012; 32(6):337-42. PMID:22684230.

[16] Zhang Q, Ye Z, Yang Q, et al. World J SurgOncol. Upregulated expression of Annexin II is a prognostic marker for patients with gastric cancer.2012; 10(1):103. PMID: 22681645.

[17] Wang Y, Liu Y, Shen X, et al. The PIWI protein acts as a predictive marker for human gastric cancer. Int J ClinExpPathol. Epub 2012;5(4):315-25. PMID:22670175.

[18] Shou ZX, Jin X, Zhao ZS. Upregulated Expression of ADAM17 Is a Prognostic Marker for Patients With Gastric Cancer. Ann Surg. 2012 Jun 29. PMID:22668812.

[19] Carpelan-Holmström M, Louhimo J, Stenman UH, et al. CEA, CA 19-9 and CA 72-4 improve the diagnostic accuracy in gastrointestinal cancers. Anticancer Res 2002; 22:2311.PMID:12174919.

[20] Lai IR, Lee WJ, Huang MT, et al. Comparison of serum CA72-4, CEA, TPA, CA19-9 and CA125 levels in gastric cancer patients and correlation with recurrence. Hepatogastroenterology 2002; 49:1157.PMID:12143226.

[21] Liu X, Cheng Y, Sheng W, et al. Clinicopathologic features and prognostic factors in alpha-fetoprotein-producing gastric cancers: analysis of 104 cases. J SurgOncol 2010; 102:249.PMID:20740583.

[22] Ushiku T, Uozaki H, Shinozaki A, et al. Glypican 3-expressing gastric carcinoma: distinct subgroup unifying hepatoid, clear-cell, and alpha-fetoprotein-producing gastric carcinomas. Cancer Sci 2009; 100:626.PMID:19243386.

[23] Kim SJ, Kim HH, Kim YH, et al. Peritoneal metastasis: detection with 16- or 64-detector row CT in patients undergoing surgery for gastric cancer. Radiology 2009; 253:407. PMID:19789243.

[24] Yoshida S, Tanaka S, Kunihiro K, et al. Diagnostic ability of high-frequency ultrasound probe sonography in staging early gastric cancer, especially for submucosal invasion. Abdom Imaging 2005; 30:518.PMID:15688103.

[25] Kelly S, Harris KM, Berry E, et al. A systematic review of the staging performance of endoscopic ultrasound in gastro-oesophageal carcinoma. Gut 2001; 49:534.PMID: 11559651.

[26] Byrne MF, Jowell PS. Gastrointestinal imaging: endoscopic ultrasound. Gastroenterology 2002; 122:1631.PMID:12016428.

[27] Ganpathi IS, So JB, Ho KY. Endoscopic ultrasonography for gastric cancer: does it influence treatment? SurgEndosc 2006; 20:559.PMID:16446988.

[28] Yun M, Lim JS, Noh SH, et al. Lymph node staging of gastric cancer using (18)F-FDG PET: a comparison study with CT. J Nucl Med 2005; 46:1582.PMID:16204706.

[29] Chen J, Cheong JH, Yun MJ, et al. Improvement in preoperative staging of gastric adenocarcinoma with positron emission tomography. Cancer 2005; 103:2383.PMID: 15856477.

[30] Kinkel K, Lu Y, Both M, et al. Detection of hepatic metastases from cancers of the gastrointestinal tract by using noninvasive imaging methods (US, CT, MR imaging, PET): a meta-analysis. Radiology 2002; 224:748.PMID:12202709.

[31] Yoshioka T, Yamaguchi K, Kubota K, et al. Evaluation of 18F-FDG PET in patients with advanced, metastatic, or recurrent gastric cancer. J Nucl Med 2003; 44:690.PMID:12732669.

[32] National Comprehensive Cancer Network (NCCN) guidelines. Available at: www.nccn.org (Accessed on May 15, 2012).

[33] Power DG, Schattner MA, Gerdes H, et al. Endoscopic ultrasound can improve the selection for laparoscopy in patients with localized gastric cancer. J Am CollSurg 2009; 208:173.PMID:19228527.

[34] Sarela AI, Lefkowitz R, Brennan MF, et al. Selection of patients with gastric adenocarcinoma for laparoscopic staging. Am J Surg 2006; 191:134.PMID:16399124.

[35] Leake PA, Cardoso R, Seevaratnam R, et al. A systematic review of the accuracy and indications for diagnostic laparoscopy prior to curative-intent resection of gastric cancer. Gastric Cancer 2011.PMID:21667136.

[36] Gotoda T. Endoscopic resection of early gastric cancer: the Japanese perspective. CurrOpinGastroenterol 2006; 22:561. PMID:16891890.

[37] Soetikno R, Kaltenbach T, Yeh R, et al. Endoscopic mucosal resection for early cancers of the upper gastrointestinal tract. J Clin Oncol 2005; 23:4490. PMID:16002839.

[38] Gotoda T, Yanagisawa A, Sasako M, et al. Incidence of lymph node metastasis from early gastric cancer: estimation with a large number of cases at two large centers. Gastric Cancer 2000; 3:219. PMID:11984739.

[39] Morita S, Katai H, Saka M, et al. Outcome of pylorus-preserving gastrectomy for early gastric cancer. Br J Surg 2008; 95:1131. PMID:18690631.

[40] Mochiki E, Kamiyama Y, Aihara R, et al. Laparoscopic assisted distal gastrectomy for early gastric cancer: Five years' experience. Surgery 2005; 137:317. PMID:15746786.

[41] Lee JH, Yom CK, Han HS. Comparison of long-term outcomes of laparoscopy-assisted and open distal gastrectomy for early gastric cancer. SurgEndosc 2009; 23:1759. PMID: 19057958.

[42] Hiki N, Sano T, Fukunaga T, et al. Survival benefit of pylorus-preserving gastrectomy in early gastric cancer. J Am CollSurg 2009; 209:297. PMID: 159717032.

[43] Katai H, Morita S, Saka M, et al. Long-term outcome after proximal gastrectomy with jejunal interposition for suspected early cancer in the upper third of the stomach. Br J Surg 2010; 97:558. PMID: 20169569.

[44] Ikeguchi M, Hatada T, Yamamoto M, et al. Evaluation of a pylorus-preserving gastrectomy for patients preoperatively diagnosed with early gastric cancer located in the middle third of the stomach. Surg Today 2010; 40:228. PMID: 20180075.

[45] Watson DI, Devitt PG, Game PA. Laparoscopic Billroth II gastrectomy for early gastric cancer. Br J Surg 1995; 82:661. PMID: 7613945.

[46] Kim MC, Kim KH, Kim HH, et al. Comparison of laparoscopy-assisted by conventional open distal gastrectomy and extraperigastric lymph node dissection in early gastric cancer. J SurgOncol 2005; 91:90. PMID: 15999352.

[47] Hayashi H, Ochiai T, Shimada H, et al. Prospective randomized study of open versus laparoscopy-assisted distal gastrectomy with extraperigastric lymph node dissection for early gastric cancer. SurgEndosc 2005; 19:1172. PMID: 16132323.

[48] Kitano S, Shiraishi N, Uyama I, et al. A multicenter study on oncologic outcome of laparoscopic gastrectomy for early cancer in Japan. Ann Surg 2007; 245:68. PMID: 17197967.

[49] Kim YW, Baik YH, Yun YH, et al. Improved quality of life outcomes after laparoscopy-assisted distal gastrectomy for early gastric cancer: results of a prospective randomized clinical trial. Ann Surg 2008; 248:721. PMID: 18948798.

[50] Fujiwara M, Kodera Y, Misawa K, et al. Longterm outcomes of early-stage gastric carcinoma patients treated with laparoscopy-assisted surgery. J Am CollSurg 2008; 206:138. PMID: 18155579.

[51] Fuccio L, Zagari RM, Eusebi LH, et al. Meta-analysis: can Helicobacter pylori eradication treatment reduce the risk for gastric cancer? Ann Intern Med 2009; 151:121.

[52] Fukase K, Kato M, Kikuchi S, et al. Effect of eradication of Helicobacter pylori on incidence of metachronous gastric carcinoma after endoscopic resection of early gastric cancer: an open-label,randomised controlled trial. Lancet 2008; 372:392. PMID: 18675689

[53] Dicken BJ, Bigam DL, Cass C, et al: Gastric adenocarcinoma: Review and considerations for future directions. Ann Surg 241:27, 2005. PMID: 15621988.

[54] Cho CS, Brennan MF: Gastric adenocarcinoma, in Cameron JL (ed): Current Surgical Therapy, 9th ed. Philadelphia: Mosby, 2008.

[55] Windham TC, Termuhlen PM, Ajani JA, et al. Adenocarcinoma of the stomach in patients age 35 years and younger: no impact of early diagnosis on survival outcome. J SurgOncol 2002; 81:118. PMID: 12407722.

[56] Henning GT, Schild SE, Stafford SL, et al. Results of irradiation or chemoirradiation following resection of gastric adenocarcinoma. Int J RadiatOncolBiolPhys 2000; 46:589.

[57] Najam AA, Yao JC, Lenzi R, et al. Linitis plastica is common in women and in poorly differentiated and signet ring cell histologies: an analysis of 217 patients (abstract). Proc Am Soc Clin Oncol 2002; 21:166a.

[58] Noguchi Y, Yoshikawa T, Tsuburaya A, et al. Is gastric carcinoma different between Japan and the United States? Cancer 2000; 89:2237. PMID: 11147594.

[59] Sasako M, Sano T, Yamamoto S, et al. D2 lymphadenectomy alone or with para-aortic nodal dissection for gastric cancer. N Engl J Med 2008; 359:453. PMID: 18669424.

[60] Roukos DH, Kappas AM. Targeting the optimal extent of lymph node dissection for gastric cancer. J SurgOncol 2002; 81:59. PMID : 12355403.

[61] Csendes A, Burdiles P, Rojas J, et al. A prospective randomized study comparing D2 total gastrectomy versus D2 total gastrectomy plus splenectomy in 187 patients with gastric carcinoma. Surgery 2002; 131:401. PMID: 11935130.

[62] Cunningham D, Allum WH, Stenning SP, et al. Perioperative chemotherapy versus surgery alone for resectablegastroesophageal cancer. N Engl J Med 2006; 355:11. PMID: 16822992.

[63] Macdonald JS, Smalley SR, Benedetti J, et al. Chemoradiotherapy after surgery compared with surgery alone for adenocarcinoma of the stomach or gastroesophageal junction. N Engl J Med 2001; 345:725. PMID: 11547741.

[64] Boige V, Pignon J, Saint-Aubert B, et al. Final results of a randomized trial comparing preoperative 5-fluorouracil/cisplatin to surgery alone in adenocarcinoma of stomach and lower esophagus (ASLE): FNLCC ACCORD07-FFCD 9703 trial (abstract). J CliNOncol 2007; 25:200s.

[65] Schuhmacher C, Gretschel S, Lordick F, et al. Neoadjuvant chemotherapy compared with surgery alone for locally advanced cancer of the stomach and cardia: European Organisation for Research and Treatment of Cancer randomized trial 40954. J Clin Oncol 2010; 28:5210. PMID : 21060024.

[66] Tsukuma H, Oshima A, Narahara et al. Natural history of early gastric cancer: a non-concurrent, long term, follow up study. Gut 2000; 47:618. PMID: 11034575.

[67] Kim JH, Kim HS, Seo WY, et al. External validation of nomogram for the prediction of recurrence after curative resection in early gastric cancer. Ann Oncol 2012; 23:361. PMID: 21566150.

[68] Okada K, Fujisaki J, Yoshida T, et al. Long-term outcomes of endoscopic submucosal dissection for undifferentiated-type early gastric cancer. Endoscopy 2012; 44:122. PMID: 22271022.